Extraordinary Science and Psychiatry

Philosophical Psychopathology

Jennifer Radden and Jeffrey Poland, editors

Extraordinary Science and Psychiatry: Responses to the Crisis in Mental Health Research, Jeffrey Poland and Şerife Tekin, editors (2017)

Disturbed Consciousness: New Essays on Psychopathology and Theories of Consciousness, Rocco J. Gennaro, editor (2015)

Being Amoral: Psychopathy and Moral Incapacity, Thomas Schramme, editor (2014)

A Metaphysics of Psychopathology, Peter Zachar (2014)

Classifying Psychopathology: Mental Kinds and Natural Kinds, Harold Kincaid and Jacqueline Sullivan, editors (2014)

The Ethical Treatment of Depression: Autonomy through Psychotherapy, Paul Biegler (2011)

Addiction and Responsibility, Jeffrey Poland and George Graham, editors (2011)

Brain Fiction: Self-Deception and the Riddle of Confabulation, William Hirstein (2004)

Imagination and Its Pathologies, James Phillips and James Morley, editors (2003)

Imagination and the Meaningful Brain, Arnold H. Modell (2003)

Divided Minds and Successive Selves, Jennifer Radden (1996)

Extraordinary Science and Psychiatry

Responses to the Crisis in Mental Health Research

edited by Jeffrey Poland and Şerife Tekin

The MIT Press
Cambridge, Massachusetts
London, England

This book was set in ITC Stone Serif Std by Toppan Best-set Premedia Limited. Printed and bound in the United States of America.

Library of Congress Cataloging-in-Publication Data

Names: Poland, Jeffrey Stephen, editor. | Tekin, Şerife, editor.
Title: Extraordinary science and psychiatry : responses to the crisis in mental health research / edited by Jeffrey Poland and Şerife Tekin.
Other titles: Philosophical psychopathology. \
Description: Cambridge, MA : The MIT Press, [2017] | Series: Philosophical psychopathology | Includes bibliographical references and index.
Identifiers: LCCN 2016018927 | ISBN 9780262035484 (hardcover : alk. paper)
Subjects: | MESH: Mental Health | Empirical Research | Evidence-Based Medicine
Classification: LCC RC454 | NLM WM 20 | DDC 616.89—dc23 LC record available at https://lccn.loc.gov/2016018927

10 9 8 7 6 5 4 3 2 1

JP: For Barbara, Alisa, and David
ŞT: For Tekin women, Bahriye, Eylem, Süda; and for my father, Hasan

Contents

Acknowledgments

Extraordinary Science and Psychiatry: Responses to the Crisis in Mental Health Research brings together a number of perspectives on the current crisis in psychiatric research. The idea for the volume emerged following the Psychiatric Taxonomy and Mental Disorder Symposium, at the Philosophy of Science Association Meeting, in 2012, in San Diego. We wish to thank the participants, Kenneth Schaffner, Peter Zachar, Dominic Murphy, Brian Keeley, and the audience for the stimulating discussion at the symposium. We also express our deepest gratitude to George Graham, Jennifer Radden, and Owen Flanagan for their help in numerous forms since the project's inception. And many thanks to Phil Laughlin, Senior Editor at the MIT Press, for helpful guidance and support. ŞT thanks Jacob Robert Smith, Kristin Andrews, Jacqueline Sullivan, the fellows of University of Pittsburgh's Center for Philosophy of Science, Shawn Kelley, and Daemen College for their support during the development of this project. JP thanks the Rhode Island School of Design for a sabbatical leave that facilitated work on this project and thanks Michael Frank and Barbara Von Eckardt for numerous invaluable conversations.

1 Introduction: Psychiatric Research and Extraordinary Science

Jeffrey Poland and Şerife Tekin

A climate of crisis and controversy exists in contemporary mental health research and practice, stemming partially from tensions within psychiatry. On the one hand, as a branch of medicine, psychiatry aims at clinically addressing the complaints of individuals with mental disorders, including unwanted behavior and the subjective, mental, and first-person aspects of psychopathology (such as feelings of unwarranted guilt and hallucinations); yet there are serious concerns regarding overdiagnosis and overtreatment, and there is no consensus on which treatment methods are most effective in addressing mental health problems. On the other hand, as a branch of science, psychiatry targets the objective, embodied, and third-person causes and correlates of behavioral problems and mental distress (such as atypical brain mechanisms and genetic anomalies); however, there is no agreement on what kinds of scientific constructs will best help probe these phenomena, and there has been a notable lack of scientific progress. At the center of these controversies is *The Diagnostic and Statistical Manual of Mental Disorders* (DSM), the psychiatric taxonomy used in the United States and widely around the world, which has been developed to identify both the scientific and clinical targets of psychiatry, as well as to be used in the service of sociological, pedagogical, and forensic projects (American Psychiatric Association 2013, xli; American Psychiatric Association 1994, xv). It is widely agreed, however, that the DSM is seriously flawed. Common and widely acknowledged problems include problems concerning the validity and reliability of the psychiatric diagnoses, poorly understood comorbidities, heterogeneity of diagnostic groupings, and overinclusiveness of diagnostic criteria. As a consequence, the DSM is seen by many as a major source of the current crisis in mental health research and practice.

The goal of the present volume is to focus directly on research-related issues in this crisis and to explore both the nature and sources of the crisis as well as whether and, if so, how, it can be responded to, or at best, overcome. There has been an increased focus on the scientific research of mental disorders, not only by scientists, but also by philosophers. However, both in areas where this research exemplifies the problems characteristic of the crisis (e.g., problems of scientific validity of DSM categories) and in areas where it constitutes a source of responses to those problems (e.g., the conviction that the more we understand the brain, the better we will address mental disorders), a thorough philosophical investigation of the current crisis is missing. Moreover, given the existing crisis, whether and, if so how, research in psychiatry can make progress is not adequately addressed in the relevant literature.

Several recent philosophical and scientific discussions and developments set the stage. First, underlying the conviction that the DSM is seriously flawed as a guide for research is the concern that the mental disorder constructs found in the DSM are not appropriate for scientific research (Frances 2013; Hacking 2013; Horwitz and Wakefield 2007; Schwartz and Wiggins 1987; Poland, Von Eckardt, and Spaulding 1994; Poland 2001; Sadler 2005; Tekin 2014). Critics argue that the DSM categories, being based on atheoretical, polythetic, and symptom-based criteria, are too general and that they do not include specific details that square with the features of mental disorder. Because of this, a wide range of phenomena—sometimes problems in ordinary living, such as grief—are included as mental disorders. Further, this nonspecificity of DSM categories leads to problems of their validity as scientific constructs, heterogeneity of diagnostic groupings, overinclusiveness of diagnostic criteria, and problems of false positives. In addition, because diagnostic groupings are heterogeneous, diagnostic criteria for different categories sometimes overlap, and boundaries of the constructs are fuzzy and loose, it becomes challenging to detect and investigate comorbidities (i.e., simultaneous occurrence of multiple mental disorders). These various problems make DSM categories ill-suited for scientific research.

Second, there are various explanations tracking the source of the crisis in psychiatric research. Some point to the lack of an adequate scientific foundation of the DSM-III (American Psychiatric Association 1980) classification scheme—which marked the transition from a psychoanalytically oriented etiological taxonomy to a symptom and sign oriented descriptive taxonomy—and its successors (DSM-III-R, DSM-IV, DSM-IV-TR, DSM-5). Others, more specifically, focus on the lack of an adequate scientific foundation due to the immaturity of neuroscience and genetics (Schwartz and Wiggins 1987; Sadler 2005; Zisook, Shear, and Kendler 2007; Frances 2013; Kleinman 2012; Kendler et al. 2008; Tekin 2011; Radden 1994). An alternative view sees the crisis as resulting partially from a failure of the DSM to effectively map the domain of mental illness, which exhibits multidimensional, hierarchical, dynamical, and interactive causal complexity as well as personal perspectives and considerable individual variation (Poland and Von Eckardt 2013; Tekin and Mosko 2015). Correspondingly, there are multiple proposals on what would constitute an adequate response to this crisis. For example, some phenomenologically oriented critics prioritize psychiatry's medical target and argue that the way to overcome the crisis in psychiatry is focusing on the needs of the clinic (Parnas 2005; Parnas and Zahavi 2002; Tekin 2015). Some of those who see psychiatry as a branch of science, on the other hand, believe that psychiatry should work harder to resemble the basic sciences such as genetics and neuroscience (Andreasen 2001; Insel and Lieberman 2013). Scientific explanations, framed in terms of the genetic and neurological underpinnings of mental disorders, are viewed by them as the best way to develop effective psychiatric interventions. Others, however, emphasize the importance of integrating resources from a broader range of relevant sciences (Murphy 2006; Poland 2014). Further, with respect to such proposed remedies, there is no consensus on whether an adequate response to current problems in psychiatric research and practice needs to provide a single unified solution applicable to all contexts in which psychiatric classifications are deemed necessary or whether a pluralistic approach is required where the multifaceted complexity of mental health related issues are addressed in a piecemeal manner.

Third, the existing crisis recently became explosive following the publication of the just revised DSM, namely, the DSM-5. Some critics have proposed that the DSM needs more revising and tinkering to be made fit for research (and clinical) purposes. For instance, Allen Frances, the chair of the DSM-IV Task Force, argued vehemently against some of the changes in the DSM-5, insisting, for example, that grief should remain conceptualized as a normal response to loss, as opposed to being categorized as depression (Frances, 2013). Others, on the other hand, push toward a rejection of the DSM project altogether, declaring the DSM-5 to be unfit for scientific research. For example, the National Institute of Mental Health (NIMH), the division of the US government that funds most research in psychiatry, has declared the DSM unsuitable for research purposes (Insel 2013; Insel and Lieberman 2013). The arguments put forward are that the DSM categories are no longer appropriate for research purposes because they lack validity, and that a diagnostic system that aims to scrutinize mental illness should more directly reflect modern brain science, as "mental illness will be best understood as disorders of brain structure and function that implicate specific domains of cognition, emotion, and behavior" (Insel and Lieberman 2013). As an alternative to the DSM for research purposes, the NIMH announced the Research Domain Criteria (RDoC) project (Insel et al. 2010), which attempts to create a new conceptual framework for psychiatric research that identifies domains of functioning that can be analyzed at several levels of analysis, thereby integrating resources provided by various basic sciences, especially genetics, neuroscience, and cognitive science. Critics of the NIMH's approach have suggested that emphasizing the primacy of neuroscientific and genetic research in psychopathology continues an unfortunate trend that ignores the crucial role of the phenomenology of mental illness (Graham and Flanagan 2013). Others are concerned that in the RDoC there may be a lack of suitable attention to relational problems, social processes, and cultural context (Poland 2014). Whether to choose the revise-and-tinker approach to the DSM project or go with a more radical approach that completely abandons the DSM is a philosophy of science question that needs attention.

Finally, the current landscape of responses to the crisis in psychiatric research also includes abundant work of numerous individuals and research groups concerned with probing the problems exhibited by DSM categories (e.g., the development of methods and models for understanding the heterogeneity and unexplained comorbidities of DSM categories; Poland and Von Eckardt 2013 provide some examples) and with targeting various aspects of mental illness in novel ways (e.g., creating meta-clusters of DSM categories, focusing on specific symptoms or cognitive impairments, introducing novel measures of biological, psychological, and behavioral functioning, and building on genetic, biochemical, neurostructural, and neurofunctional findings). Special attention has been given to a focus on "endophenotypes" and the use of novel sampling methods, measurement technologies, multidimensional functional profiles, and modeling techniques (Wiecki, Poland, and Frank 2015 provide some examples).

Current research is in a state of flux and increasingly directed at responding to the problems of conventional diagnostic categories and developing novel ways of studying and understanding mental illness. Although such approaches are promising, it is our view that more needs to be done at a deeper level in response to the current crisis. General philosophy of science, in particular, gives us some conceptual resources to engage in such analysis.

The probing of the problems of the dominant research framework of psychiatry (viz., the DSM by critics and institutions such as the NIMH), as well as the emergence of alternative scientific initiatives (e.g., the RDoC project and the work of various research groups) is suggestive of Thomas Kuhn's characterization of periods of crisis that can arise in scientific research during "normal science" and of the "extraordinary science" that ensues in response to such periods of crisis (Kuhn 1962/1996, 77–91). Extraordinary science takes several forms in Kuhn's view, which, we believe, are mimicked in contemporary psychiatry. Consider a few of these here: (1) attempts to shore up and defend a reigning paradigm (exemplified by the American Psychiatric Association's insistence that the DSM-5 is a potentially useful research framework given its new organizational structure; American Psychiatric Association 2013, 10), (2) attempts to isolate and probe anomalous research results encountered during the normal science[1] period (exemplified by research aimed at explaining the heterogeneity of diagnostic categories), (3) the loosening of standard forms of research practice (exemplified by the NIMH's RDoC initiative which eliminates the necessity of using DSM diagnoses), and (4) the exploration of alternative research frameworks (again exemplified by the NIMH's RDoC initiative as well as the work of various research groups). Kuhn also emphasizes another feature of this stage of research: namely, the turning to philosophical analysis for an identification and evaluation of the constitutive frameworks of research programs and the exploration of their foundational assumptions (e.g., identification of questions and problems deemed important by the scientific community, analysis and evaluation of constitutive concepts and assumptions concerning the domain of research, and analysis and evaluation of various substantive and methodological assumptions that structure research practices).

Following Kuhn, we suggest that the current crisis in mental health research provides an important opportunity for a critical examination of the foundations of research in this area and that such philosophical analysis is a crucial component in efforts to effectively respond to, and perhaps overcome, the current crisis. It is especially called for because of the nature of the domain of scientific investigation (viz., mental illness) insofar as this domain is (1) causally complex (e.g., processes involve multiple dimensions, hierarchical organizations, dynamic interactivity spanning numerous levels of analysis, context sensitivity, etc.) and (2) concerned with physically embodied human agents with a personal perspective who are embedded in sociocultural contexts. Such factors complicate both the research agenda and the application of research findings in practical (e.g., clinical, educational, social) contexts. This is especially the case for (2) since, although the sciences are well equipped for tackling problems of causal analysis, they are not as advanced and well equipped for dealing with either the personal or the sociocultural dimensions of mental illness. Arguably, given (2) and the social and personal significance of mental illness, a special premium should be placed on pursuing scientific research agendas that are compatible with maintaining an important focus on personal perspective, agency, and sociocultural context.

Philosophical analysis concerning this domain and the research agendas focused upon it can contribute to a deeper understanding of the features of mental illness and to the pursuit of responsive and robust research programs that will contribute to understanding and managing the current crisis. This volume brings together a collection of original chapters that share this goal. The authors develop and apply various analytical ideas and strategies from the philosophy of science, and from other relevant areas of philosophy and science, with the aim of clarifying some aspect of the current crisis and the associated extraordinary science. The various purposes of these chapters include understanding the research domain of mental illness, clarifying the nature of the problems that constitute the current crisis in mental health research, identifying key substantive and methodological assumptions concerning classification and research focused on the domain, identifying ideas bearing on how best to respond to the current crisis with respect to the scientific research agenda (e.g., identification of promising pathways forward for scientific research), and constructively addressing the tension between pursuing a progressive scientific research program concerning mental illness and maintaining a place of prominence for individual persons and their contexts. Such philosophical analyses can help in the process of engaging and resolving the current crisis. They can also contribute to reconciling the claims that a study of psychopathology needs to be scientific and that it needs to put the person/self/individual suffering from psychopathology at the center. Further, such work may provide new insights for the philosophy of science based on the special features of this sort of case study.

Overview of the Chapters

The volume starts with two chapters by Edouard Machery and Robyn Bluhm that trace the source of the current crisis to fundamental epistemological problems about the ontological status of mental disorders, and the nature of evidence that guides psychiatric research. Machery ("Kinds or Tails?") focuses on a pivotal epistemological problem at the heart of determining whether psychiatric conditions are best conceived as distinct kinds or whether they are the tail of a distribution of some trait in the general population (e.g., are individuals suffering from depression a distinct kind or are they at the tail of a distribution of, say, neuroticism?). The epistemological problem is how to know whether psychiatric syndromes are taxons or the tails of a distribution defined over the general population. Machery addresses this question by contrasting informal (e.g., clinical judgment) and formal (e.g., cluster analysis) methods and argues for the superiority of the latter. However, he shows that specific procedures can have built-in assumptions about the nature of taxons (e.g., that they are classes characterized by causal essences or that symptoms are uncorrelated among patients), and he notes that such commitments can be at odds with certain features of psychiatric syndromes (e.g., they can be more or less severe or they can have a heterogeneous etiology). Thus, an aspect of extraordinary science is the pursuit of research programs that require vigilance for inherent assumptions that may or may not fit well with features of the domain under investigation.

Robyn Bluhm ("Evidence-Based Medicine, Biological Psychiatry, and the Role of Science in Medicine") focuses on the current crisis in psychiatry by evaluating how current psychiatric research practices frame the nature of evidence in psychiatry. She identifies a tension between evidence-based medicine (EBM), an instance of medical empiricism that focuses on the efficacy of treatments without regard to mediating causal mechanisms, and biological psychiatry, an instance of medical rationalism which aims to improve clinical efficacy by focusing on the causes that give rise to clinical outcomes. Using the examples of research concerning post-traumatic stress disorder and attachment, Bluhm argues that EBM is shortsighted and proposes that EBM be integrated with rationalist concerns with pathophysiology. She then applies this framework to compare NIMH's RDoC initiative with the pre-DSM-III Feighner criteria, cautioning against the possibility of reifying RDoC criteria and constructs before the assumptions of RDoC are fully examined and the clinical relevance of such constructs and criteria is established.

The next two chapters focus on the NIMH's RDoC project and evaluate whether the project is indeed an effective response to the crisis in psychiatric research. Ginger A. Hoffman and Peter Zachar ("RDoC's Metaphysical Assumptions: Problems and Promises") identify two key features of the current crisis: a lack of validity of DSM categories (with associated problems of "therapeutic impact") and toxic "reflective impact" of DSM diagnoses on patients' reasoning about their illness. They proceed to present the RDoC initiative of the NIMH as an important research program aimed at meeting problems of validity and (ultimately) therapeutic impact. With respect to RDoC's promise for promoting "etiopathological validity" they discuss several obstacles that must be negotiated (e.g., problems of multiple mappings across levels of analysis), but (somewhat ironically) they note that the complexities of the RDoC approach may undermine toxic reflective impact by inhibiting the incorporation of pathology concepts into an individual's self-narrative and identity.

Claire Pouncey ("Psychopathology without Nosology: The Research Domain Criteria Project as Normal Science") identifies the RDoC as a response to the stagnation of DSM-based research but argues that the shift of focus to the RDoC framework is not a paradigm shift as many maintain since the core theoretical and methodological assumptions of biological psychiatry are maintained across this shift in research focus. Rather, RDoC is a version of the normal science tradition of which DSM-based research is a part. In both instances, the aim is to translate basic and clinical neuroscience research relating brain structure, brain function, and behavior into a classification of psychiatric disorders based on etiology and pathophysiology. The standards of research (e.g., a focus on construct validity and the development of nomological networks) are also maintained across this shift.

The next four chapters each focus on a particular research practice in psychiatry, namely, computational psychiatry, personalized psychiatry, mechanistic approaches, and user-led research initiatives, assessing their ability to effectively respond to the crisis in research. In their chapter ("The Promise of Computational Psychiatry"), Jeffrey Poland and Michael Frank focus on computational psychiatry. They offer an explanation of why the crisis in psychiatric research exists that helps to identify four sorts of challenge that researchers must face during the current period of extraordinary science: ideological, methodological, clinical, and transitional. They then proceed to identify the foundational substantive and methodological assumptions and resources of the research program of computational psychiatry, and they demonstrate the promise of this research program for meeting various of the challenges using case studies focused on Parkinson's disease and schizophrenia.

Aaron Kostko and John Bickle ("Personalized Psychiatry and Scientific Causal Explanations: Two Accounts") focus on personalized psychiatry. They explore the tension in psychiatry between striving to be individualized and patient centered on the one hand and scientific on the other. To do this, they pursue a strategy of applying two accounts of causal explanation (viz., Woodward's 2003, 2008 interventionist account and Silva, Landreth, and Bickle's 2013 metascientific account) to research bearing on psychopathology in social neuroscience and environmental epigenetics. While each account has strengths and weaknesses, two main lessons are gleaned from the analysis: (1) properly understood, basic scientific research is not inconsistent with the aims of personalized psychiatry, and (2) non-epistemic considerations (e.g., clinical utility and therapeutic applicability) partly determine which account of scientific causal explanation best fits with personalized psychiatry (e.g., with respect to questions about the most appropriate level at which to explain psychiatric disorders). Of special importance in their discussion is the epistemic value placed on pursuing fundamental research into mechanisms that mediate high-level causal relations (e.g., identification of such mechanisms helps secure confidence in causal claims).

Kelso Cratsley ("The Shift to Mechanistic Explanation and Classification") focuses on mechanistic approaches to psychiatric research. He takes on the question of how mechanistic explanation fits into the effort to build a scientifically sound etiological and nosological framework for psychiatry. After sketching what mechanistic explanation should look like in the context of psychiatric research, Cratsley identifies several challenges posed by features of the domain under investigation (e.g., the role of social and environmental factors, the relatively transient nature of symptoms, the complexity of underlying systems, and the significance of nonstandard developmental course for many psychiatric conditions). Cratsley argues that such challenges can be met with a broad notion of mechanism that allows for something less than flawless execution of internal operations, that attends to organizational relations both within the mechanism itself and across the wider cognitive system, and that appeals to the influence of contextual factors. His discussion exemplifies the general theme that, among the challenges to researchers in this period of extraordinary science, the features of the target domain call for conceptual and methodological resources that are up to the task of representing and managing them.

Next, Rachel Cooper ("Classification, Rating Scales, and Promoting User-Led Research") focuses on user-led research initiatives in psychiatry. She notes that a critical dimension of the current crisis in psychiatric research concerns a crisis of trust and confidence in reported research findings. For a variety of reasons, such confidence has been eroded, and a part of navigating this period of extraordinary science is to identify research practices and processes that will help restore confidence in research. Cooper observes that one widely believed cause of the loss of confidence is the perception that much research serves the interests of industry rather than the interests of patients. And she suggests that one way to ameliorate such concerns is by the development of more "amateur/citizen/user-led" research, something which would constitute a dramatic shift from current research practices.

Cooper argues that promoting user-led research conducted outside traditional academic settings promises a range of benefits, and she engages certain objections to such research (e.g., amateur/user researchers are not competent and have nothing to contribute). After arguing that user-led research is worth pursuing, she goes on to discuss how research by users is impacted by the informational infrastructure of science (e.g., different styles of classification and rating scale can facilitate or interfere with the work of amateur/user-led research communities). Thus, changes to such informational infrastructure might be required for effectively engaging the challenges of extraordinary science.

The next three chapters focus on specific psychiatric categories, namely, schizophrenia, major depressive disorder, and bipolar disorder, and address some problems that underlie the research on these. Richard P. Bentall ("Six Myths about Schizophrenia: A Paradigm Well Beyond Its Use-By Date?") provides a brief history of the schizophrenia concept and identifies six "myths" concerning the diagnostic category bearing on reliability, boundaries with normality and other diagnostic categories, genetics, environmental factors, and brain disease. In all cases, he argues that, although widely endorsed within conventional psychiatry, these assumptions about the nature of schizophrenia lack scientific support and in some cases are refuted by the research record. Bentall concludes by drawing some important lessons for extraordinary science. First, the endurance of the schizophrenia concept and the associated myths, despite the increasingly countervailing research record, is testament to the power that paradigms can hold over the minds of researchers. Further, the impact of such powerful paradigms can lead to a failure of normal processes of empirical refutation. For example, deeply entrenched assumptions about schizophrenia can lead to a relaxation of standards in order to accommodate recalcitrant data and thereby protect paradigms, and they can lead to a stifling of research that challenges the paradigm, as well as to blindness to the significance of research findings.

With a focus on DSM-led research on schizophrenia, Şerife Tekin ("Looking for the Self in Psychiatry: Perils and Promises of Phenomenology–Neuroscience Partnership in Schizophrenia Research"), like Bentall, reviews some criticisms of the schizophrenia concept and the research based upon it. Her special target is a research initiative she calls the "phenomenology–neuroscience partnership (PNP)," which takes the phenomenology approach as a starting point to investigate schizophrenia. Although largely supportive of the initiative, Tekin identifies a weakness in much extant research. Specifically, she identifies a critical conceptual distinction concerning two senses of "self-experience" (viz., a subjective sense and an objective sense), and she argues that PNP researchers have typically failed to honor the distinction, focusing exclusively on the objective sense when it is the subjective sense that is putatively disturbed in schizophrenia. She dubs this the problem of "wandering terminology." The upshot is that, while PNP has promise for engaging subjective dimensions of severe mental illness, there is a need to be vigilant regarding the problem of wandering terminology so as to maintain contact with the person who is the subject of mental illness. She concludes by pointing out some of the strengths of PNP and offers suggestions for improvement.

Harold Kincaid ("DSM Applications to Young Children: Are There Really Bipolar and Depressed Two-Year-Olds?") responds to critics who reject the DSM wholesale and suggests that the DSM exhibits "heterogeneous validity," that is, while many DSM categories lack established validity and research utility, some categories do not. He reviews a range of research findings supportive of the idea that both adult major depressive disorder (MDD) and adult bipolar disorder (BPD) have established validity and research utility. However, Kincaid contends that the application of categories of adult psychopathology (specifically MDD and BPD) to young children, for either research or clinical purposes, is entirely unwarranted by the research record. He argues that, given that this is true for "best case scenarios" (i.e., categories that have been validated for adults), great caution should be exercised when applying any DSM categories to children, especially in clinical contexts where drugs are routinely prescribed. Kincaid points to possible social explanations for the persistent use of psychiatric diagnostic categories, and especially the increase in diagnoses of BPD in children.

The volume concludes with a provocative chapter by Owen Flanagan and George Graham ("Truth and Sanity: Positive Illusions, Spiritual Delusions, and Metaphysical Hallucinations") that targets the psychiatric enterprise as a whole. They strongly criticize what they take to be the worrisome trend in contemporary psychiatry that pathologizes normalcy on dubious epistemic grounds. They specifically target the dual ideas that mental health has a clear, precise, and firm link to true belief and that mental disease/disorder has some clear, precise, and firm link to false or misbegotten belief. Using a broad range of examples of experiences, they argue that illusions, delusions, and hallucinations are not categorically or even typically unhealthy or abnormal. As a consequence, the assumptions that link truth/falsity with mental health/illness are suspect and should raise doubts about our understanding of what might make illusions and so forth unhealthy or abnormal. Such concerns reach to the normative underpinnings of contemporary mental health research and practice and, more importantly, to the challenges for effectively engaging such norms during this period of extraordinary science.

Concluding Comment

This is an exciting time for the philosophy of psychiatry. Within the current climate of crisis and controversy and given recent developments in the landscape of psychiatric research, this is a moment in time when philosophy is substantially relevant to mental health research and practice and philosophers have opportunities to address fundamental questions in ways that might contribute to scientific change.

Using the analytical resources offered by history and philosophy of science, philosophy of mind, and ethics, philosophers are actively engaging questions about the causes of the current crisis; the nature of mental illness; the validity and reliability of psychiatric diagnoses; the substantive, methodological, and normative assumptions in psychiatric research; the criteria for good constructs; the pathways for progress in psychiatric research; the tensions among scientist, practitioner, and patient perspectives; and the morality of various clinical practices. With *Extraordinary Science and Psychiatry: Responses to the Crisis in Mental Health Research* we aim to further the impact of philosophy of psychiatry by providing a sampling of work that examines and responds to some of these questions.

Note

1. Of course, it is doubtful that psychiatric research ever entered a period of "normal science" as Kuhn understood that term; nonetheless, we think the Kuhnian apparatus is useful for understanding the current situation in psychiatric research.

References

American Psychiatric Association. 1980. *Diagnostic and Statistical Manual of Mental Disorders*. 3rd ed. Washington, DC: American Psychiatric Association.

American Psychiatric Association. 1994. *Diagnostic and Statistical Manual of Mental Disorders*. 4th ed. Washington, DC: American Psychiatric Association.

American Psychiatric Association. 2013. *Diagnostic and Statistical Manual of Mental Disorders*. 5th ed. Arlington, VA: American Psychiatric Association.

Andreasen, N. 2001. *Brave New Brain: Conquering Mental Illness in the Era of the Genome*. New York: Oxford University Press.

Frances, A. 2013. Last plea to DSM-5: Save grief from the drug companies. Huffington Post. January 7. http://www.huffingtonpost.com/allen-frances/saving-grief-from-dsm-5-a_b_2325108.html.

Graham, G., and O. Flanagan. 2013. Psychiatry and the brain. Oxford University Press Blog; August 1. https://blog.oup.com/2013/08/psychiatry-brain-dsm-5-rdoc/.

Hacking, I. 2013. Lost in the forest. *London Review of Books* 35 (15) (August 8).

Horwitz, A. V., and J. C. Wakefield. 2007. *The Loss of Sadness: How Psychiatry Transformed Normal Sadness into Depressive Disorder*. New York: Oxford University Press.

Insel, T. 2013. Director's blog: Transforming diagnosis. http://www.nimh.nih.gov/about/director/2013/transforming-diagnosis.shtml.

Insel, T., B. Cuthbert, M. Garvey, R. Heinssen, D. S. Pine, K. Quinn, C. Sanislow, and P. Wang. 2010. Research Domain Criteria (RDoC): Toward a new classification framework for research on mental disorders. *American Journal of Psychiatry* 167 (7): 748–751.

Insel, T. R., and J. A. Lieberman. 2013. DSM-5 and RDoC: Shared interests. Press Release, May 13. http://www.nimh.nih.gov/news/science-news/2013/dsm-5-and-rdoc-shared-interests.shtml.

Kendler, K. S., S. H. Aggen, N. Czajkowski, E. Roysamb, K. Tambs, S. Torgersen, M. C. Neale, and T. Reichborn-Kjennerud. 2008. The structure of genetic and environmental risk factors for *DSM-IV* personality disorders. *Archives of General Psychiatry* 65 (12): 1438–1446.

Kleinman, A. 2012. The art of medicine: Culture, bereavement, psychiatry. *Lancet* 379 (9816): 608–609.

Kuhn, T. S. 1962/1996. *The Structure of Scientific Revolutions*. 3rd ed. Chicago: University of Chicago Press.

Murphy, D. 2006. *Psychiatry in the Scientific Image*. Cambridge, MA: MIT Press.

Parnas, J. 2005. Clinical detection of schizophrenia-prone individuals: Critical appraisal. *British Journal of Psychiatry* 187 (Suppl. 48): s111–s112.

Parnas, J., and D. Zahavi. 2002. The role of phenomenology in psychiatric classification and diagnosis. In *Psychiatric Diagnosis and Classification*, ed. M. Maj, W. Gaebel, and J. J. Lopez-Ibor, 137–162. World Psychiatric Association Series in Evidence and Experience in Psychiatry. Chichester, UK: Wiley.

Poland, J. 2001. Review of *DSM-IV Sourcebook*, Vol. 1, *Metapsychology Online Reviews* 5 (14). http://metapsychology.mentalhelp.net/poc/view_doc.php?type=book&id=557&cn=392.

Poland, J. 2014. Deeply rooted sources of error and bias in psychiatric classification. In *Psychiatric Classification and Natural Kinds*, ed. H. Kincaid and J. Sullivan, 29–63. Cambridge, MA: MIT Press.

Poland, J., and B. Von Eckardt. 2013. Mapping the domain of mental illness. In *The Oxford Handbook of Philosophy and Psychiatry*, ed. K. W. M. Fulford, M. Davies, R. G. T. Gipps, G. Graham, J. Z. Sadler, G. Stanghellini, and T. Thornton, 735–752. Oxford: Oxford University Press.

Poland, J., B. Von Eckardt, and W. Spaulding. 1994. Problems with the DSM approach to classification of psychopathology. In *Philosophical Psychopathology*, ed. G. Graham and L. Stevens, 235–260. Cambridge, MA: MIT Press.

Radden, J. 1994. Recent criticism of psychiatric nosology: A review. *Philosophy, Psychiatry, & Psychology* 1 (3): 193–200.

Sadler, J. 2005. *Values and Psychiatric Diagnosis*. Oxford: Oxford University Press.

Schwartz, M. A., and O. P. Wiggins. 1987. Diagnosis and ideal type: A contribution to psychiatric classification. *Comprehensive Psychiatry* 28 (4): 227–291.

Silva, A. J., A. Landreth, and J. Bickle. 2013. *Engineering the Next Revolution in Neuroscience: The New Science of Experiment Planning*. Oxford: Oxford University Press.

Tekin, Ş. 2011. Self-concept through the diagnostic looking glass: Narratives and mental disorder. *Philosophical Psychology* 24 (3): 357–380.

Tekin, Ş. 2014. Self-insight in the time of mood disorders: After the diagnosis, beyond the treatment. *Philosophy, Psychiatry, & Psychology* 21 (2): 139–155.

Tekin, Ş. 2015. Against hyponarrating grief: Incompatible research and treatment interests in the DSM-5. In *The DSM-5 in Perspective: Philosophical Reflections on the Psychiatric Babel,* ed. P. Singy and S. Demazeux, 179–195, History, Philosophy and Theory of the Life Sciences Series. Dordrecht, the Netherlands: Springer.

Tekin, Ş., and M. Mosko. 2015. Hyponarrativity and context-specific limitations of the DSM-5. *Public Affairs Quarterly* 29 (1): 111–136.

Wiecki, T., J. Poland, and M. Frank. 2015. Model-based neuroscience approaches to computational psychiatry: Clustering and classification. *Clinical Psychological Science* 3 (3): 378–399.

Woodward, J. 2003. *Making Things Happen: A Theory of Causal Explanation*. Oxford: Oxford University Press.

Woodward, J. 2008. Cause and explanation in psychiatry. In *Philosophical Issues in Psychiatry: Explanation, Phenomenology, and Nosology*, ed. K. S. Kendler and J. Parnas, 132–184. Baltimore: Johns Hopkins University Press.

Zisook, S., K. Shear, and K. S. Kendler. 2007. Validity of the bereavement exclusion criterion for the diagnosis of major depressive episode. *World Psychiatry: Official Journal of the World Psychiatric Association (WPA)* 6 (2): 102–107.

2 Kinds or Tails?

Edouard Machery

Psychiatric nosology, the branch of psychiatry dealing with the classification of psychiatric syndromes, has attracted much attention from philosophers of psychiatry (e.g., Kendler and Parnas 2012), but much of the philosophical debate has focused on a narrow set of topics: whether psychiatric syndromes (e.g., psychopathy) can be defined objectively, whether psychiatric syndrome labels (e.g., "depression" or "schizophrenia") refer to natural kinds (whatever a natural kind is), and whether the current nosology will be radically transformed by focusing on the endophenotypes emerging from neuroscience (on the former issue, see, e.g., Zachar 2000; Murphy 2006; Cooper 2014; Kincaid and Sullivan 2014; on the latter issue, see, e.g., Schaffner 2012). There has been comparatively little attention among philosophers to the following vexed question (*the taxon issue*): Are psychiatric syndromes the tails of distributions of particular traits in the general population, or do they form distinct kinds or taxa? For instance, do individuals suffering from depression form a distinct kind, or are they rather the tail of the distribution of neuroticism in the general population? Do people suffering from delusions form a distinct kind, or rather are they individuals with an extreme openness to experience? While the taxon issue may have little practical implications when it comes to alleviating distressing symptoms—it may not really matter whether depression is an extreme form of neuroticism or a distinct taxon when the goal is to reduce suicidal thoughts in a patient—it may have important implications for research on the etiology of psychiatric syndromes: although this issue calls for further reflection (Meehl 1999), it is plausible that tails of distributions and taxa result from different causal structures.

I will not address the taxon issue head on in this chapter; rather, my aim is to address a preliminary epistemological question: How can we determine whether psychiatric syndromes should be treated as kinds or taxa rather than as the tails of distributions defined over the general population?

I will argue that formal methods are required to address this epistemological question, but that their assumptions should be carefully scrutinized.

In the first section, I elaborate on the taxon issue. In the second section, I argue for the superiority of formal methods over informal ones for addressing the taxon issue. In the third section, I show that cluster analysis is not an adequate approach to resolve the taxon issue. In the fourth section, I discuss Meehl's taxometric methods.

The Taxon Issue

Taxa and Distributions

People differ from one another and resemble one another in all kinds of ways. We do not have the same height, tall women are similar in being tall and female, small men in being small and male. French people are like each other in that they speak French and differ from Germans in this respect. Nouns are more or less concrete; "chair" and "dog" are similar in that both are concrete, "love" and "democracy" in that both are abstract. "Chair" and "dog" are also similar in that they are common nouns, and they differ from "Napoleon" in this respect.

Similarities and differences defined over a population of items (words, people, cities, planets, etc.) can be explained in various ways. It is convenient to distinguish two competing accounts. On the one hand, two items can resemble one another or differ from one another because they belong, respectively, to the same taxon or to different taxa (*the taxon account*). What makes two members of a taxon similar qua members of this taxon and what makes them different from the member of another taxon qua members of different taxa is that they possess, respectively, the same property or different properties instead of having more or less of an underlying dimension. For instance, it is not the case that "Napoleon" and "the Eiffel Tower," two proper names, are similar to one another with respect to their semantic properties (e.g., both refer to an individual) and syntactic properties and differ from "dog," a common noun, with respect to those same properties (e.g., "dog" is satisfied by a class of particulars) because "Napoleon," "the Eiffel Tower," and "dog" have more or less of an underlying dimension: proper names do not differ from common nouns in having more (or less) of something. What makes "Napoleon" and "the Eiffel Tower" similar and different from "dog" qua proper names is that both have the same property, *being a proper name*, which "dog" does not have. On the other hand, two items can resemble one another or differ from one another because they have similar or different values with respect to one or several underlying dimensions (*the dimensional account*). For example, people high on neuroticism are similar to one another in having fewer social connections and in being more prone to anxiety because they have more of a given underlying personality dimension—neuroticism—and they differ from people low on neuroticism because the latter have less of this dimension.

More generally, let's distinguish *indicators*—roughly observable properties—from *latent variables*, underlying properties that explain why some items have the indicators. Indicators can, but need not be, graded; they can, but need not be, continuous. Body temperature, muscle pain intensity, or pain location could be indicators. Items differ from one another and are similar to one another with respect to these indicators. People who have the flu differ from healthy people in having a higher body temperature and more muscle pain. The taxon account is correct for a collection of items if and only if the relevant latent variable is categorical. For instance, whether or not one has the flu is a categorical variable (whether one has the flu depends on whether one has been contaminated by some influenza virus); it explains the similarities and differences between healthy people and patients with flu: healthy people have a lower body temperature (i.e., no fever) and less muscle pain than sick people because they do not have the flu. The dimensional account is correct if and only if the relevant latent variable is graded. What explains the differences and similarities of items with respect to the indicators is that they have more or less of this graded underlying latent variable.

A few further clarifications of the taxon and distribution accounts are in order. First, the dimensional account is compatible with the definition of distinct classes or groupings by setting cutoff points over the relevant latent variable (e.g., Haslam 2002; Gärdenfors 2004). We could distinguish people high on neuroticism or on openness to experience (another fundamental personality dimension) from the remainder of the population by setting some cutoff point. The distinctions obtained by setting cutoff points over the underlying latent variables need not be arbitrary, and they can be drawn on various grounds (including on practical grounds in the case of psychiatric syndromes; see Zachar 2000). Second, the notion of taxon is not characterized by appealing to a bimodal distribution of the indicators. Even if the latent variable is not categorical (i.e., if the dimensional account of the similarities and differences in the relevant domain is correct), it is possible to have bimodal indicators (for discussion, see Meehl 1999). Third, that two particulars belong to two distinct taxa does not entail that the indicators or cues that are used to assign them to these taxa cannot be values of a variable distributed over the general population. Flu is a pretty good taxon, but the symptoms of flu (body aches, fever, weariness, and cough) are all distributed over the general population (Meehl 1999). As Meehl (1999, 167) writes, it is not the case "that if the latent structure is categorical, then quantitative indicators of the conjectured latent taxon should be bimodally distributed."

In some parts of the world (in some "domains") such as organic diseases or social roles, items are organized in taxa; in other parts they form distributions defined over some noncategorical variables. Since some of these domains are areas of scientific inquiry, some sciences focus on taxa, and others on distributions. It is sometimes assumed that sciences are in the business of identifying the kinds in their domains (e.g., Machery 2009, chapter 7), but if by "kinds" we mean taxa, this generalization is mistaken. Science can instead focus on identifying the underlying dimensions and how the items in their domain are distributed with respect to these dimensions. It is often a matter of serious scientific controversy whether or not the items in the domain of a given science form taxa. In addition, in some areas of psychology, whether or not one believes in dimensional or taxon accounts almost defines the professional identity of scientists. Meehl reports the following anecdote (1999, 165):

> A highly capable postdoctoral student, someone who had thought deeply about trait theory and psychometric factors (...) was being considered for a job at a prestigious psychology department. After giving a first-rate talk on the well-corroborated eye-tracking anomaly in schizophrenics and their first-degree relatives, he thought he had a pretty good chance at the job. No offer was made, however; and a friendly faculty member consoled him, saying, "Oh, there's no doubt about your excellent qualifications, but, you see, we are dimension people, and you are a category person."

Taxa, Tails, and the Mind

Psychologists often disagree about whether psychological constructs are best understood as taxa or as regions within complex multidimensional spaces. Emotions provide a good example of such disagreement. Some leading psychologists of emotions view them as taxa (although they do not use this terminology). Ekman (1992) identifies a subset of emotions—the "basic emotions": fear, happiness, surprise, disgust, anger, sadness—with discrete complex patterns of facial expressions, body changes, feelings, and behavioral dispositions. Ekman often refers to "discrete emotions" (e.g., Ekman and Friesen 1971, 124). Cognitivists about emotions such as Lazarus disagree with Ekman about pretty much everything, but they too treat emotions as taxa. For Lazarus, for instance, emotions are to be identified with complex patterns of appraisals (roughly, patterns of evaluative judgments about what one's relation with the environment means for one's well-being). On this view, to feel happy just is to assess that one is "making reasonable progress toward the realization of a goal" (Lazarus 1991, 122). The different types of appraisal differ from one another in a discrete manner. On the other hand, an influential tradition in the psychology of emotions views them as regions of a space. Russell's (1980) classic circumplex model of emotions distinguishes two dimensions, arousal (roughly, how energized one feels when one has an emotion) and valence. For instance, surprise is an aroused state of a person whose valence is neutral. Similar debates can take place, and have taken place, about many other issues in psychology, such as sexual orientation.

Disagreements about whether psychological constructs are taxa or regions of multidimensional spaces are naturally not limited to the psychology of neurotypical individuals, but they are found throughout psychiatry and clinical psychology. One can, for instance, wonder whether depression is a taxon or whether it is the tail of a latent variable distributed in the general population (perhaps anxiety or neuroticism). From a sociological point of view, clinical psychologists seem to prefer dimensional models of psychiatric syndromes, perhaps because of the influence of nonclinical psychology, psychiatrists categorical models, perhaps because of the influence of medicine and the need to make yes/no diagnostic judgments (Haslam 2002).

The taxon question in psychiatry has, of course, a long history, which can't be reviewed in detail here. Suffice it to highlight the fact that since the 1950s, Eysenck has done extensive work on the statistical methods that could be brought to bear on the taxon issue (e.g., Eysenck 1950, 1952, 1955). Kendell (1968) also raised it forcefully in his influential *The Classification of Depressive Illnesses*, arguing for a dimensional approach to depressions.

Clearing Up Misconceptions

The claim that a psychiatric syndrome is a distinct taxon instead of the tail of the distribution of one or several traits in the general population is often misunderstood (Meehl 1995, 1999). First and foremost, the fact that a syndrome forms a taxon does not entail that its etiology is biological (a fortiori genetic) in contrast to social (however this contrast is drawn). Taxa can result from social causes or, perhaps more commonly, from the complex interplay of social and biological causes. There is little doubt that the existence of "mad travelers" (Hacking 1998) is at least partly due to social causes, but this nineteenth-century syndrome may have been a distinct taxon. (Naturally, whether it was is an empirical question, which will probably never be settled.) As we have seen above, cognitivists in the psychology of emotions treat emotions as taxa although cognitivism leaves room for emotions to be socially constructed (e.g., Averill 1980). Conversely, that a syndrome has biological causes does not entail that it forms a taxon. Degrees of neuroticism in the general population are partly determined by genetic factors, but they do not form taxa.

Second, whether a syndrome forms a taxon or is the tail of a distribution over the general population says nothing about its reality or its severity. Tails of distributions are as real (whatever that means) as taxa; they can be as distressing for patients as taxa, or even more so. As Haslam (2002, 206) puts it, "The case of neuroticism serves to show how the study of mental disorders can encompass differences between people that are not differences in kind. People who fall relatively high on the dimension are at increased risk of various forms of psychiatric disturbance, and extreme emotional lability is clearly of psychiatric interest."

Third, taxa need not have sharp boundaries (Meehl 1999). Membership in a syndrome that happens to be a taxon tolerates vagueness, and vagueness does not entail that a syndrome should be viewed as the tail of a distribution defined over the general population.

Finally, it is important not to confuse the properties of the syndromes with the properties of their representations. Taxa can be represented dimensionally. As noted above (see the flu example above), taxa members and nonmembers differ with respect to the taxon's diagnostic properties (i.e., its indicators) and can thus be located in a multidimensional space. So, even if emotions (or a subset thereof) are distinct taxa, they can still be represented dimensionally—for instance, in Russell's two-dimensional space. Conversely, dimensional syndromes can be represented categorically. One can always define a cutoff point on an underlying dimension. We can distinguish neurotic from nonneurotic individuals by defining a cutoff point on the dimension of neuroticism.

The Failure of Informal Approaches to the Taxon Issue

Judgment

Let's suppose that some psychiatrists have access to the symptoms of a psychiatric syndrome and want to decide whether it is a genuine kind—a taxon—or rather the tail of a distribution. How should they proceed? An *informal* approach is available: they can rely on clinical experience and judgment. According to this strategy, experience with, on the one hand, genuine psychiatric taxa and, on the other hand, tails of distributions has endowed psychiatrists with a capacity to determine whether a syndrome is a taxon. Psychiatrists may not be able to justify their judgments, a characteristic often found in clinical judgments, but this limitation does not speak against psychiatrists' genuine capacity to identify taxa.

This approach is unlikely to be successful. First, it assumes that psychiatrists have already identified a substantial number of genuine taxa among psychiatric syndromes. By training their judgment against known taxa and known tails and by receiving feedback in case of mistaken classification, psychiatrists would be able to hone their judgment, exactly as one can improve one's judgment that something is an *F* by learning to classify *F*'s as *F*'s and getting feedback when one is mistaken. It is however quite dubious that psychiatric nosology has had much success in resolving the taxon issue. Since acquiring an expertise in distinguishing *x*'s from *y*'s typically requires training on genuine *x*'s and *y*'s as well as feedback in the event of erroneous classification, psychiatrists cannot have acquired by training and experience a capacity to decide whether some syndrome is a genuine taxon if existing psychiatric classifications do not reliably distinguish between taxa and tails of distributions.

Second, psychiatrists have only access to the distribution of symptoms in the population of patients and nonpatients. For instance, they may have access to the distributions of anxiety, sex drive, frequency of suicidal thoughts, and so on. Symptoms and indicators are not limited to the first-person reports made by patients in psychiatric interviews or on checklists; they also include the measurable results of psychometric or neuroscientific tests. The problem is that, as noted in the first section of this chapter, the indicators of taxa and of tails of distributions may be very similar. Bimodal indicators can be produced by noncategorical latent variables, and taxa need not produce bimodal distributions of symptoms. Because categorical and continuous latent variables can produce symptoms similarly distributed, it is extremely difficult, if not utterly impossible, to examine these distributions in order to decide whether the syndromes form taxa.

More generally, inducing from psychiatry's scientific record, we should be skeptical of the prospects of clinical judgment based on experience. Scientists have plausibly appealed to judgment to resolve the taxon issue, but little progress has been made, suggesting that clinical judgment does not have the resources for distinguishing taxa from tails of distributions.

A Pragmatic Argument

It has sometimes been argued that one should choose between dimensional and taxonic representations of psychiatric syndromes on pragmatic grounds. In an influential article discussed at greater length below, Paykel

(1971, 286) contends that, while dimensional models may be correct, in practice "it seems likely that psychiatric classification will continue to be based not on dimensions but on the familiar model of diagnostic categories to which individual patients are assigned (…)." On his view, dimensional models would only be useful if we could measure the relevant dimensions with sufficient precision, which he doubts is possible; furthermore, the relations between patients on high-dimensional models are often opaque.

Pragmatic arguments are not to be dismissed as a matter of principle, but embracing pragmatic arguments similar to Paykel's is tantamount to accepting that the taxon issue cannot be properly resolved. We should thus only appeal to this type of pragmatic argument as a last resort.

The Need for Formal Methods

Psychiatrists have not merely relied on judgment or on pragmatic considerations to resolve the taxon issue. For at least fifty years they have appealed to contemporary developments in statistics—for example, factor analysis, drawn from IQ research and personality psychology, or cluster analysis, drawn from biological taxonomy and phenetics—to resolve this issue (e.g., Eysenck 1950). Meehl (1995, 266) captures this effort when he writes,

> Classification in psychopathology is a problem in applied mathematics; it answers the empirical question "Is the latent structure of these phenotypic indicator correlations taxonic (categories) or nontaxonic (dimensions, factors)?" It is not a matter of convention or preference.

There are naturally many possible formal methods—cluster analysis, latent class analysis (e.g., Magidson and Vermunt 2004), the taxometric methods developed by Meehl, and so forth—and space prevents examining all these methods here (for discussion of the prospects of factor analysis for taxometric purposes, see, e.g., Meehl 1999). In what follows, I will focus on cluster analysis and on Meehl's methods.

Examining the potential contribution of these statistical methods raises at least two types of questions, which for sake of a better terminology we can call "statistical" and "interpretative":

1. *Statistical questions*: What are the statistical assumptions made by the formal methods, and are they justified for the problem at hand? What are their statistical limitations (e.g., extreme sensitivity to outliers) or their boundary conditions? Are their error probabilities known (or at least estimated by simulations), and are these acceptable?
2. *Interpretative questions*: What assumptions about kinds or taxa are made for these formal methods to be reliable in determining whether

a psychiatric syndrome is a taxon instead of the tail of a distribution? When a method allows us to infer that a syndrome is a taxon, what commitments does the formalism impose on us?

Philosophers of psychiatry interested in the epistemological issues underlying the taxon issue should pay attention to both types of questions. In what follows, I will address both, although I will focus more on interpretative questions.

Cluster Analysis

What Is Cluster Analysis?

"Cluster analysis" refers to a family of algorithms that divide items (participants in an experiment, organisms, cities, words on the Web, etc.) into groups (e.g., Everitt et al. 2011). It is commonly used in psychology, biology (including genetics), and sociology. It has been extensively used to classify organisms into taxa (Sneath and Sokal 1973). In general, cluster analysis algorithms divide items into groups so as to maximize the similarity of items within a group and minimize it across groups. Clustering algorithms differ from one another, among other things, because they involve different strategies to maximize the similarity of items within a group and minimize it across groups. Clustering can take many forms; in particular, it can be hierarchical (clusters are subclusters of larger clusters) or partitional (i.e., nonhierarchical).

As noted, there are several clustering algorithms. The K-means algorithm is one of the oldest, most commonly used, and simplest clustering algorithms. It produces partitional clusters, where each cluster member is more similar to the prototype of its cluster (also called "centroid") than to the prototypes of the other clusters. K items are selected (according to one of several selection procedures). The first step of the algorithm assigns the remaining items to K clusters depending on their similarity (or proximity) with these selected K prototypes. Similarity is a function of (typically the square of) the distance between each item and the prototypes according to some metric (e.g., Euclidean distance). Different metrics (more generally, different proximity measures) can be used depending on the items to be clustered. The second step determines the prototypes of these newly formed K clusters. The algorithm then goes back to step 1, assigning all the items to K clusters depending on their similarity with the newly computed K prototypes. Iteration stops when the computation of the prototypes at stage 2 does not change the prototypes on the basis of which clusters were created at stage 1 (or changes less than *x*%—e.g., 1%—of these prototypes).

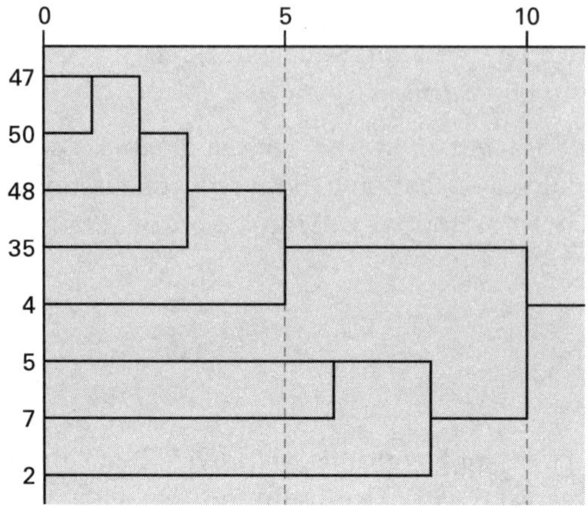

Figure 2.1
Fragment of a dendogram of numbered items (on the y-axis) grouped hierarchically.

Hierarchical cluster analysis outputs can be represented by dendograms, which group together items in a hierarchical manner (see figure 2.1). Visually, a dendogram seems to describe a hierarchy of increasingly inclusive kinds, reminiscent of biological taxonomies.

Cluster Analysis in Psychiatry

Cluster analysis has been extensively used in psychiatry to identify subgroups of various syndromes (e.g., Paykel 1971; Everitt, Gourlay, and Kendell 1971; Achenbach and Edelbrock 1978; for more recent discussion, see Kendell and Jablensky 2003). In an influential paper, Paykel (1971) applied a clustering algorithm to 165 depressed patients and reported that they clustered into four "readily interpretable" groups (1971, 275): psychotic, anxious, hostile, depressive patients with personality disorders. Thirty-five variables (mostly clinical symptoms ratings and biographical variables) characterized the 165 patients. These 35 variables were reduced to 6 dimensions by factor analysis, and these 6 dimensions were used to characterize the items (i.e., the patients) for clustering purposes (resulting in a 6-dimensional space over which a proximity measure was defined). Several partitional analyses were conducted, with two to five groups specified a priori. The analysis with four groups was judged to be the best of these four analyses. Paykel (1971, 286) concluded, "[T]he cluster analysis technique employed here is specifically intended to isolate groups of individuals and is capable of working in multidimensional hyperspace to do so. It is a very powerful technique."

Cluster analysis may seem a good candidate to resolve the taxon issue. It classifies items into clusters. Items within a cluster are more similar to one another than to members of other groups, according to some similarity measure, a property expected of kinds (Quine 1977). It can produce outputs that are similar to biological taxonomies. And it has been used to identify variants of psychiatric syndromes.

A word of caution is however needed. It is not clear that when psychiatrists used cluster analysis, they meant to resolve the taxon issue for the relevant syndromes (e.g., depression or schizophrenia). Indeed, it is noteworthy that most studies based on cluster analysis do not involve samples of patients and nonpatients, as they should if their point was to resolve the taxon issue. Rather, these studies examine only samples of patients (e.g., the 165 depressed patients in Paykel 1971). These studies may in fact be *assuming* that the psychiatric syndromes are taxa; they may be using cluster analysis to identify the relevant taxa instead of trying to decide whether the syndromes are taxa.

The Limitations of Cluster Analysis

Whether or not the actual use of cluster analysis in psychiatric studies was intended to resolve the taxon issue, cluster analysis is in any case badly tailored for this purpose. First, like other data compression techniques such as factor analysis (McCaffrey and Machery 2016), which, incidentally, has also been used to bear on taxonomic issues in psychiatry (e.g., Fahy, Brandon, and Garside 1969; for discussion, see Meehl 1999), cluster analysis suffers from an underdetermination problem. As mentioned above, "cluster analysis" refers to a family of clustering algorithms, and these can produce very different partitions (Blashfield 1976; Everitt et al. 1971; Golden and Meehl 1980). Furthermore, when the number of clusters must be specified a priori, as is the case in the K-means algorithm described above, cluster analysis can produce inconsistent partitions for different numbers of clusters. The fact that there are many distinct clustering algorithms is not necessarily problematic for cluster analysis since data analysis can be robust across clustering procedures (Everitt et al. 1971). In fact, examining the robustness of clustering is common advice in textbooks on cluster analysis. However, when clustering is *not* robust (as in Golden and Meehl 1980), it can be underdetermined which partition to embrace. For instance, in Paykel (1971), clustering the 165 patients into three clusters split one of the clusters obtained when the patients were clustered into two clusters, and the clustering of these patients into four clusters split one of the clusters obtained when the patients were clustered into three clusters. These three partitions were thus consistent with one another, but when patients were clustered into five clusters, "in the change from four to five groups the hierarchical structure was lost" (1971, 278).

Second, and more important, in contrast to factor analysis, cluster analysis partitions the set of items to be divided into a number of (sometimes hierarchically organized) clusters, and this capacity explains why in the late 1960s and early 1970s psychiatrists proposed to replace factor analysis with cluster analysis for nosological purposes. However, the capacity of cluster analysis of forming kinds does not show that the kinds so formed are taxa. As noted in the first section of this chapter, even when items belong to a single distribution, as tall and small people do, it is possible to define kinds. We can, for instance, set up a threshold above which people are defined as being tall, and below which people are defined as being small. (We seem to do precisely this when we distinguish tall and small people intuitively: LeBron James is tall, Nicolas Sarkozy small.) Thus, the fact that cluster analysis produces similarity-based kinds does not by itself show that the outputted kinds are taxa.

The point just made is connected to the fundamental limitation of cluster analysis with respect to the taxon issue. This statistical method is merely a way of representing the similarity of a set of items according to some similarity measure. Items are classified in clusters depending on their respective similarity. However, whether patients suffer from a psychiatric syndrome that is a taxon or the tail of a distribution defined over the general population, patients and nonpatients belong to a similarity space defined by the relevant symptoms (or indicators), exactly as patients with flu and healthy people can be represented in a similarity space defined by body temperature, muscle pain intensity, and so forth. Cluster analysis merely divides the items in such a space into clusters, and it is thus insensitive to the distinction between taxa and tails of distributions.

The upshot is that cluster analysis is badly suited to resolve the taxon issue. Other tools are therefore needed (see also Meehl 1979).

Meehl's Contribution to Taxometry

MAXCOV

Among Paul Meehl's many noteworthy contributions to philosophy and the behavioral sciences, one of the most important is the development of new formal methods for deciding whether a psychiatric syndrome is a taxon, including MAMBAC and MAXCOV (e.g., Grove and Meehl 1993; Meehl and Yonce 1994, 1996; Meehl 1973, 1992, 1995, 1999, 2004; Waller and Meehl 1998; Ruscio and Ruscio 2004; Beauchaine 2007; Ruscio, Haslam, and Ruscio 2013). I will focus exclusively on MAXCOV, which stands for "maximum of covariance," in this chapter.

MAXCOV (Meehl and Yonce 1996) relies on three indicators or symptoms that discriminate between patients and nonpatients (e.g., patients suffering from major depressive disorder and nonpatients). Examples include various cognitive measures such as reaction times in a cognitive task, how much one sleeps per day, frequency of anxiety attacks, sex drive, and so on. The indicators discriminate between the two populations in that they are not identically distributed over the two populations. (Meehl recommends indicators whose means are at least 1.25 SD apart.) For instance, patients with major depressive disorder can have lower sex drive on some scale than nonpatients. One of the three indicators (called "the input") is then divided into intervals (see figure 2.2). The covariance of the two other intervals is then computed for each of the intervals of the input. So, for instance, if the frequency of anxiety attacks is the input, and the two other indicators

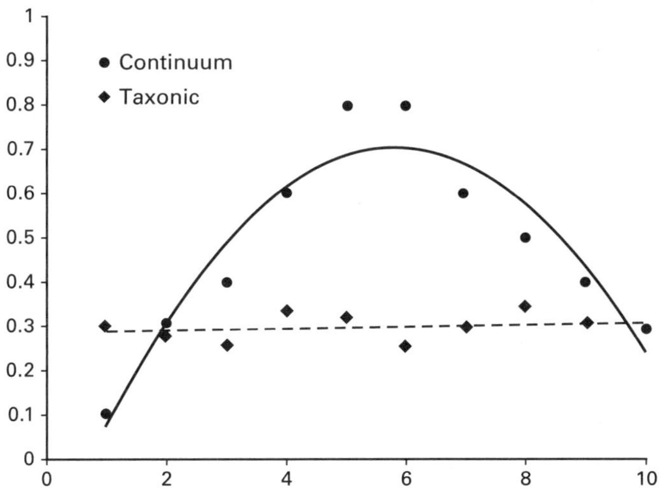

Figure 2.2
Ten intervals of an input indicator are plotted on the x-axis; the covariance of the two other indicators is plotted on the y-axis. If the covariance line is flat (diamonds), the psychiatric syndrome is not a taxon; if the covariance peaks (round dots), the syndrome is a taxon.

are sex drive and amount of sleep per day, the covariance of sex drive and amount of sleep per day is computed for those participants in the sample (with and without major depressive disorder) who have few anxiety attacks (who are in the bottom third, say), some anxiety attacks, and many anxiety attacks (the top third).

Meehl and Yonce (1996) then propose an informal decision rule to decide whether the psychiatric syndrome (e.g., major depressive disorder) is a taxon. If the covariance line is flat (see the dotted line in figure 2.2), then the psychiatric syndrome is the tail of a distribution defined over the general population: in this case, depressed people would be very anxious people. If it is concave (see the solid line in figure 2.2), then it is a taxon: in this case, either one is depressed or one is not depressed, exactly as either one has the flu or one does not have it. (The lower the proportion of patients in the sample, the more the peak is shifted toward the right.) Furthermore, from the apex of the concave line one can estimate the parameters of the populations (base rate of the psychiatric syndrome, means with respect to the indicators, hit and false positive rates).

This decision rule is underwritten by the following reasoning. If the population of patients forms a taxon, then the two indicators are plausibly not correlated within the syndrome and its complement because considering the correlation of the two indicators within the syndrome and its complement amounts to conditionalizing on their common cause (see figure 2.3A). The two indicators will then only be correlated in mixed samples, that is, when a sample contains patients and nonpatients (figure 2.3A). The covariance between the two indicators will then vary across the samples defined by the intervals of the input indicator as a function of the proportion of patients and nonpatients in each of these samples, and it will reach its maximum value for a sample composed of the same number of patients and nonpatients. This predicts a concave covariance curve. Thus, if a concave covariance curve is observed, psychiatrists can then infer that the syndrome is a taxon. By contrast, if the population of patients is not a taxon, then the two indicators remain correlated within the populations of patients and nonpatients, and the covariance line must be roughly flat (see figure 2.3B).

Meehl recognizes that the MAXCOV decision rule is fallible and emphasizes the virtue of robustness. If different taxometric procedures, based on different assumptions, such as MAXCOV and MAMBAC, converge on the same conclusion, one has good grounds for inferring that a psychiatric syndrome is a taxon. As he puts it (1999, 169):

> My method involves several distinct, minimally redundant procedures which, if the taxon exists and the inferred latent values are fairly accurate, must agree with

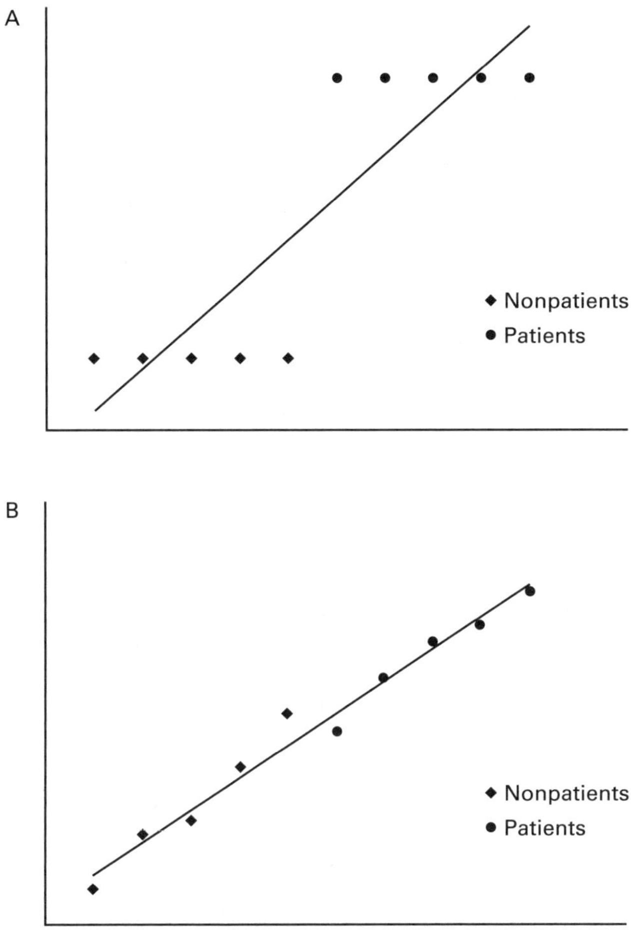

Figure 2.3
The x-axis shows the value of indicator 1; the y-axis shows the value of indicator 2; dots represent patients and diamonds nonpatients. (A) No correlation within the syndrome and its complement, correlation in mixed samples. (B) Correlation within the syndrome and its complement as well as in mixed samples.

> one another within tolerance. Agreement of these distinct procedures already constitutes a kind of consistency or coherency test.

Moving away from the details of the MAXCOV procedure, what is assumed about taxons? What commitments does one take on when one infers that a syndrome is a taxon based on this procedure? Let's call "the MAXCOV condition" the situation where two indicators are correlated in mixed samples composed of patients and nonpatients, but not within the syndrome and its complement. The MAXCOV condition (as in figure 2.3A) allows psychiatrists to infer that a syndrome is a taxon; the absence of this condition (as in figure 2.3B) that a syndrome is the tail of a distribution. In effect, the MAXCOV condition is treated by Meehl as a quasi-necessary and sufficient condition for a syndrome to be a taxon. The MAXCOV condition holds of a syndrome when syndrome membership is a proxy for the common cause of its symptoms (i.e., the indicators that distinguish patients from nonpatients). It plausibly also holds only when syndrome membership is such a proxy. If this is right, then, according to the MAXCOV procedure, a taxon is a class of entities that have distinctive properties (properties that distinguish this taxon from its complement), each of which has a common cause. This cause can be intrinsic (as is the flu virus) or extrinsic (as is the case for social roles). So, here is the commitment one undertakes by using the MAXCOV procedure to identify genuine taxa in psychiatry: syndromes are classes with a causal essence, that is, a common cause of its symptoms.

Critical Discussion

The MAXCOV procedure has been examined critically on various grounds. The discussion has often focused on its boundary conditions, that is, on the situations where this procedure would result in a false conclusion (e.g., Maraun, Slaney, and Goddyn 2003; Maraun and Slaney 2005; Ruscio and Kaczetow 2009). In particular, Maraun and Slaney (2005) have proven that for continuous indicators it is not the case that the covariance function is peaked if and only if the latent variable is categorical. Engaging with this technical literature is however better left for another paper.

In the remainder of this chapter, I want to focus on the philosophical assumption that taxa are characterized by the presence of a causal essence and that conditionalizing on syndrome membership—a proxy for the presence of this causal essence—makes the symptoms probabilistically independent. I will start with the second commitment. At least without emendation, this account of taxa cannot easily accommodate the fact that psychiatric syndromes can be more or less severe. Some people suffer from major depressive disorder more than others, exactly as one can have the flu to a greater or smaller extent. People who suffer from more severe forms of major depressive disorder have more extreme symptoms than people who suffer from less severe forms of this syndrome. Similarly, people who have a more severe flu have a higher fever, more muscle pain, and so forth. That is, when syndromes can be more or less severe, which is plausibly the case for most, if not all, syndromes, symptoms remain correlated even after conditionalizing on syndrome membership. That is the case because syndrome membership is then a poor proxy for the common cause of the symptoms: the common cause is graded; syndrome membership is not. Think about the following analogy. Smoking causes yellow teeth and yellow fingers and, plausibly, yellow teeth and yellow fingers distinguish smokers from nonsmokers. Yellow teeth and yellow fingers are not correlated among nonsmokers, but they are among smokers. So, conditionalizing on smoking does not make the correlation between yellow teeth and yellow fingers disappear. That is the case because, while smoking versus nonsmoking is a categorical variable, there is a dose–response relationship between how much one smokes and the yellowness of one's teeth and fingers.

Turning now to the first commitment, syndromes that are taxa have a causal essence (which, keep in mind, need not be biological or even intrinsic). The problem here is that some syndromes may result from several different causal pathways, in which case they are not associated with a single causal essence. Furthermore, some causal pathways may result in more extreme symptoms than other pathways. If this situation occurs, the symptoms will be correlated after conditionalizing on syndrome membership. The MAXCOV procedure is badly suited to identify this kind of taxon.

Conclusion

The main goal of this chapter was to bring to the attention of philosophers of psychiatry a hitherto ignored epistemological question: how can we justifiably decide whether a syndrome is a taxon or the tail of a distribution defined over the general population? Resolving the taxon issue cannot rest on expert judgment or on pragmatic considerations. There is however a rich literature on this issue in statistics and in machine learning (e.g., latent class analysis), and this article has merely touched upon two approaches, cluster analysis and Meehl's taxometric methods. Examining these methods calls for attention to statistical and to interpretative questions. With respect to the latter, formal methods for resolving the taxon issue may embody a particular, and possibly problematic, conception of taxa or kinds. To illustrate, I have shown how Meehl's MAXCOV procedure involves a commitment to a particular understanding of a taxon—taxa are classes characterized by causal essences and symptoms are uncorrelated among patients—and that these commitments may be at odds with the fact that psychiatric syndromes can be more or less severe and with the fact that they may have a heterogeneous etiology.

Acknowledgments

Many thanks to Şerife Tekin and Jeff Poland for comments.

References

Achenbach, T. M., and C. S. Edelbrock. 1978. The classification of child psychopathology: A review and analysis of empirical efforts. *Psychological Bulletin* 85:1275–1301.

Averill, J. R. 1980. A constructivist view of emotion. *Emotion: Theory, Research, and Experience* 1:305–339.

Beauchaine, T. P. 2007. Methodological article: A brief taxometrics primer. *Journal of Clinical Child and Adolescent Psychology* 36:654–676.

Blashfield, R. K. 1976. Mixture model tests of cluster analysis: Accuracy of four agglomerative hierarchical methods. *Psychological Bulletin* 83:377–388.

Cooper, R. 2014. *Psychiatry and Philosophy of Science*. New York: Routledge.

Ekman, P. 1992. An argument for basic emotions. *Cognition and Emotion* 6:169–200.

Ekman, P., and W. V. Friesen. 1971. Constants across cultures in the face and emotion. *Journal of Personality and Social Psychology* 17:124–129.

Everitt, B. S., A. J. Gourlay, and R. E. Kendell. 1971. An attempt at validation of traditional psychiatric syndromes by cluster analysis. *British Journal of Psychiatry* 119:399–412.

Everitt, B., S. Landau, M. Leese, and D. Stahl. 2011. *Cluster Analysis*. Chichester, UK: Wiley.

Eysenck, H. J. 1950. Criterion analysis: An application of the hypothetico-deductive method to factor analysis. *Psychological Review* 57:38–53.

Eysenck, H. J. 1952. *The Scientific Study of Personality*. Oxford: Macmillan.

Eysenck, H. J. 1955. Cortical inhibition, figural aftereffect, and theory of personality. *Journal of Abnormal and Social Psychology* 51:94–106.

Fahy, T. J., S. Brandon, and R. F. Garside. 1969. Clinical syndromes in a sample of depressed patients: A general practice material. *Proceedings of the Royal Society of Medicine* 62:331–335.

Gärdenfors, P. 2004. *Conceptual Spaces: The Geometry of Thought*. Cambridge, MA: MIT Press.

Golden, R., and P. E. Meehl. 1980. Detection of biological sex: An empirical test of cluster methods. *Multivariate Behavioral Research* 15:475–496.

Grove, W. M., and P. E. Meehl. 1993. Simple regression-based procedures for taxometric investigations. *Psychological Reports* 73:707–737.

Hacking, I. 1998. *Mad Travelers: Reflections on the Reality of Transient Mental Illnesses*. Charlottesville: University of Virginia Press.

Haslam, N. 2002. Kinds of kinds: A conceptual taxonomy of psychiatric categories. *Philosophy, Psychiatry, & Psychology* 9:203–217.

Kendell, R. E. 1968. *The Classification of Depressive Illnesses*. Oxford: Oxford University Press.

Kendell, R., and A. Jablensky. 2003. Distinguishing between the validity and utility of psychiatric diagnoses. *American Journal of Psychiatry* 160:4–12.

Kendler, K. S., and J. Parnas. 2012. *Philosophical Issues in Psychiatry II: Nosology*. Oxford: Oxford University Press.

Kincaid, H., and J. Sullivan, eds. 2014. *Classifying Psychopathology: Mental Kinds and Natural Kinds*. Cambridge, MA: MIT Press.

Lazarus, R. S. 1991. Progress on a cognitive-motivational-relational theory of emotion. *American Psychologist* 46:819–834.

Machery, E. 2009. *Doing without Concepts*. New York: Oxford University Press.

Magidson, J., and J. Vermunt. 2004. Latent class models. In *Handbook for Quantitative Methodology*, ed. D. Kaplan, 175–198. Thousand Oaks, CA: Sage.

Maraun, M. D., and K. Slaney. 2005. An analysis of Meehl's MAXCOV-HITMAX procedure for the case of continuous indicators. *Multivariate Behavioral Research* 40:489–518.

Maraun, M. D., K. Slaney, and L. Goddyn. 2003. An analysis of Meehl's MAXCOV-HITMAX procedure for the case of dichotomous indicators. *Multivariate Behavioral Research* 38:81–112.

McCaffrey, J., and E. Machery. 2016. The reification objection to bottom-up cognitive ontology revision. *Behavioral and Brain Sciences* 39:e125.

Meehl, P. E. 1973. MAXCOV-HITMAX: A taxonomic search method for loose genetic syndromes. *Psychodiagnosis: Selected Papers*, 200–224. Minneapolis: University of Minnesota Press.

Meehl, P. E. 1979. A funny thing happened to us on the way to the latent entities. *Journal of Personality Assessment* 43:564–581.

Meehl, P. E. 1992. Factors and taxa, traits and types, differences of degree and differences in kind. *Journal of Personality* 60:117–174.

Meehl, P. E. 1995. Bootstraps taxometrics: Solving the classification problem in psychopathology. *American Psychologist* 50:266–275.

Meehl, P. E. 1999. Clarifications about taxometric method. *Applied & Preventive Psychology* 8:165–174.

Meehl, P. E. 2004. What's in a taxon? *Journal of Abnormal Psychology* 113:39–43.

Meehl, P. E., and L. J. Yonce. 1994. Taxometric analysis: I. Detecting taxonicity with two quantitative indicators using means above and below a sliding cut (MAMBAC procedure). *Psychological Reports* 74:1059–1274.

Meehl, P. E., and L. J. Yonce. 1996. Taxometric analysis: II. Detecting taxonicity using covariance of two quantitative indicators in successive intervals of a third indicator (MAXCOV procedure). *Psychological Reports* 78:1091–1227.

Murphy, D. 2006. *Psychiatry in the Scientific Image*. Cambridge, MA: MIT Press.

Paykel, E. S. 1971. Classification of depressed patients: A cluster analysis derived grouping. *British Journal of Psychiatry* 118:275–288.

Quine, W. V. O. 1977. Natural kinds. In *Naming, Necessity, and Natural Kinds*, ed. S. P. Schwartz, 155–175. Ithaca, NY: Cornell University Press.

Ruscio, J., N. Haslam, and A. M. Ruscio. 2013. *Introduction to the Taxometric Method: A Practical Guide*. New York: Routledge.

Ruscio, J., and W. Kaczetow. 2009. Differentiating categories and dimensions: Evaluating the robustness of taxometric analyses. *Multivariate Behavioral Research* 44:259–280.

Ruscio, J., and A. M. Ruscio. 2004. A nontechnical introduction to the taxometric method. *Understanding Statistics* 3:151–194.

Russell, J. A. 1980. A circumplex model of affect. *Journal of Personality and Social Psychology* 39:1161–1178.

Schaffner, K. F. 2012. A philosophical overview of the problems of validity for psychiatric disorders. In *Philosophical Issues in Psychiatry II: Nosology*, ed. K. S. Kendler and J. Parnas, 169–189. Oxford: Oxford University Press.

Sneath, P. H., and R. R. Sokal. 1973. *Numerical Taxonomy. The Principles and Practice of Numerical Classification*. San Francisco: Freeman.

Waller, N. G., and P. E. Meehl. 1998. *Multivariate Taxometric Procedures: Distinguishing Types from Continua*. Thousand Oaks, CA: Sage.

Zachar, P. 2000. Psychiatric disorders are not natural kinds. *Philosophy, Psychiatry, & Psychology* 7:167–182.

3 Evidence-Based Medicine, Biological Psychiatry, and the Role of Science in Medicine

Robyn Bluhm

At first glance, evidence-based medicine (EBM) and biological psychiatry may seem to be natural allies. Both were motivated by concerns about the way that medicine/psychiatry were being practiced, and both aim explicitly to make clinical practice more scientific by encouraging a stronger link between research and practice. Both also believe that doing so will result in improved patient care. Yet a closer look at each of these influential movements reveals that there is a deep tension between them. Moreover, I suggest, this tension may mean that neither approach can make the contribution to improved patient care that it desires to make. In this chapter, I trace the development of EBM and of biological psychiatry in order to begin to make this tension and its causes clear. I then introduce the distinction between empiricist and rationalist approaches to medicine; EBM is an empiricist approach while biological psychiatry is, or at least aspires to be, a form of rationalism. I then show that EBM's empiricism is shortsighted and could be a better approach to patient care if it incorporated some aspects of the rationalist approach. By contrast, biological psychiatry should incorporate some aspects of EBM's empiricism. In particular, the Research Domain Criteria (RDoC), which is the most recent incarnation of biological psychiatry, needs to ensure that it ties physiological research back to clinically important outcomes. I close by examining a case of research in psychiatry that shows why a combined rationalist/empiricist approach is promising.

Evidence-Based Medicine

Throughout the chapter, I assume that "evidence-based psychiatry" (EBP) is nothing but the basic tenets of EBM, as applied to psychiatry. That is, there is nothing about the methods of EBP that differs from EBM in other areas of medicine. This assumption seems to reflect the general discussion about EBP. For example, Joel Paris argues that psychiatry has become more "evidence-based" and cites the developers of EBM in order to show what he means by the term (Paris 2000, 34). (See also Geddes and Carney 2001.) Because the explicit rationale of an evidence-based approach has been described in greatest detail by the developers of EBM, I will use this literature to describe the background, as well as the merits and shortcomings, of EBP.

Evidence-based medicine was developed primarily at McMaster University in Hamilton, Ontario, Canada, though it was influenced by earlier work such as Alvin Feinstein's "clinical epidemiology" (Feinstein 1985) that aimed to use the methods of epidemiology in a clinical setting. The developers of EBM consolidated these ideas and presented them in ways that were readily appreciable by busy practicing clinicians and medical educators.

The term "evidence-based medicine" first appeared in print in a 1991 article in the journal *ACP Journal Club*, but it was introduced to the larger medical community the following year in a manifesto published in *JAMA* by the Evidence-Based Medicine Working Group (1992). This article describes "the way of the past" in medicine, in which medicine was practiced primarily on the basis of information obtained from authority figures. The article illustrates this outdated approach with a case of a resident consulting her senior resident, who in turn checks with the attending physician, for advice about what to tell a patient about his likely prognosis (specifically the probability that he will have another seizure). By contrast, "the way of the future" shows the resident developing a search strategy on the basis of her patient's question, finding research papers that address the issue, and critically appraising the papers in order to determine what to tell her patient. This approach leaves both the resident and the patient with a clearer sense of the patient's prognosis, showing clearly that an evidence-based approach was intended—and expected—to improve clinical practice.

In addition to their concerns about the dependence of medical practice on authority, the developers of EBM also noted that prescribing practice varied considerably (perhaps in part because of the influence of authority figures with differing views) (Wennberg 1984) and that when evidence supporting the superiority of a treatment over alternatives existed, it did not readily affect clinical practice (Laupacis 2001). Moreover, in many situations, there was simply no reliable evidence in support of commonly used therapies. A common theme in expositions of EBM is to point to cases in which a well-designed randomized controlled trial (RCT) showed definitively that a common therapy was useless or, worse, harmful.[1] All in all, the proponents of EBM felt that there should be a much clearer framework in place to ensure that treatment was based on solid evidence.

It became the central aim of EBM to provide such a framework. Although the term "evidence" in "evidence-based medicine" does not provide any guidance regarding what *sort* of evidence is the best basis for medicine, the core idea of EBM, the "hierarchy of evidence," does provide just that.[2] The hierarchy of evidence ranks different study methods according to the quality of evidence that they provide in support of a therapy's effectiveness.[3]

Although there are a number of different versions of the hierarchy, they have in common a basic structure on which RCTs are at the top because they are held to provide the best evidence. Below these are nonrandomized studies. These two levels of epidemiological research are, in turn, superior to studies that examine physiological mechanisms (rather than outcome differences in populations of patients) and to the unsystematic experience of individual clinicians, as reported, for example, in case reports or case series (see, e.g., Guyatt and Rennie 2001, 7).

EBM also offers guidance for critically appraising the quality of a study; these guidelines focus mainly on whether the method of randomization was adequate, whether patients and clinicians involved in the study were (throughout the study) unaware of whether patients were allocated to the treatment or to the control group, and whether outcome data were collected on enough patients in each group to provide an adequate basis for determining whether patients in the treatment group had better outcomes than those in the control group. If the study does all of these things well, its results can be considered valid, and clinicians can be assured that they are drawing on the best available research evidence in making decisions about patient care (Guyatt and Rennie 2001, chapter 1B1).

Even though much of the published work explicating the principles of EBM has focused on the technical aspects of appraising research, it has always been expected that following an evidence-based approach will improve clinical practice. For example, the most commonly cited definition of EBM focuses on patient care, saying that EBM is "the conscientious, explicit and judicious use of current best evidence in making decisions about the care of the individual patient" (Sackett et al. 1996, 71). I show below that EBM has some serious epistemological shortcomings that prevent it from attaining this goal. Before doing so, however, I will describe and trace the history of biological psychiatry, drawing out some of the similarities and differences between it and EBM.

Biological Psychiatry

Unlike EBM, biological psychiatry is not a unified, self-conscious movement with a number of papers that explicitly outline its position. (I will show, however, that it does stem from such a movement.) I will therefore begin by clarifying what I mean by "biological psychiatry." A good starting point for this is in the work of the philosopher Dominic Murphy (2011, 425). Murphy links biological psychiatry to the "medical model" of psychiatry, saying that psychiatry "has become more biological and more closely affiliated with medicine and the life sciences." He then distinguishes between two senses in which people tend to use the term "medical model" in psychiatry. On the "minimal interpretation," the medical model in psychiatry "thinks of diseases as collections of symptoms that occur together and unfold in characteristic ways, but it makes no commitments about the underlying causes of mental illness" (Murphy 2011, 425). In other words, it *describes* different mental disorders, but does not *explain* how they arise. By contrast, "[t]he strong interpretation argues that mental illnesses are caused by distinctive pathophysiological processes in the brain" (Murphy 2011, 425). Murphy then argues that psychiatry needs to adopt the strong interpretation of the medical model; a focus on causal explanation is necessary for psychiatry to make progress in characterizing mental disorders and, ultimately, for improvements in patient care.

I agree with Murphy that the strong interpretation is more likely to lead to long-term progress in psychiatry, particularly in terms of the development of more fine-grained diagnostic categories and of treatments targeted to these new categories. I disagree, however, that the minimal interpretation is best viewed as a (somewhat fainthearted) *alternative* to the strong interpretation. Rather, the distinction reflects the tension between the need to work with the best available knowledge (in particular, in this case, the best available characterization of mental disorders) in order to be able to help current patients, and the need to *improve* knowledge of mental disorders and, on the basis of this knowledge, to provide better care for patients in the future. Below, I will show how this tension has played out in psychiatry; I will later argue that it also has implications for EBM.

The minimalist interpretation of the medical model is exemplified by, and perhaps originates with, the development of the Feighner criteria in the late 1960s and early 1970s. But, I will show, the developers of these criteria intended that the criteria should be understood as a starting point for research that would ultimately lead to the emergence of a (strong interpretation) medical model in psychiatry.

The Feighner criteria were developed by a group of psychiatrists working at Washington University in St. Louis. The work was motivated in large part by the lack of consistency in psychiatric diagnoses, as shown, for example, in studies by Ash (1949) and Beck (1962) (see Kendler, Muñoz, and Murphy 2010). They viewed this problem as arising from the vagueness of descriptions of psychiatric illnesses—for example, in the second edition of the *Diagnostic and Statistical Manual of Mental Disorders* (DSM-II)—and therefore aimed to develop standardized diagnostic categories that would enable different clinicians to reach the same diagnosis for a patient.[4] In his own description of the development of the criteria, Feigner says that the process began with his providing a literature review and a draft set of criteria for a condition. The six coauthors of the eventual publication then debated and revised the criteria. The result of this process was published in 1972 and provided a set of diagnostic criteria for fifteen different categories of mental illness.

There are several points that need to be made with regard to the Feighner criteria. First, they were intended to be used for research rather than for treatment. The authors explain that their work "is meant to provide common ground for different research groups so that diagnostic definitions can be emended constructively as further studies are completed" (Feighner et al. 1972, 57). Second, the criteria were deliberately "atheoretical" in that they did not make any attempt to identify the *causes* of the mental disorders they described. This decision was in part a reflection of the state of psychiatry at the time; the majority of psychiatrists still took a psychodynamic approach while others were influenced by behaviorism or by the medical model. Despite the disagreement that was inevitable among these different orientations, there was an expectation that all could agree on "whether patients described by different groups are comparable" (Feighner et al. 1972, 57). Yet it was also in part a recognition of the state of science at the time; little was known about the biology of mental illness. Further, it was felt that diagnosis—understood by Feighner et al. to consist in the careful observation of current symptoms, and a knowledge of the course and outcome of illness—was *prior to* a deeper understanding of the nature of the disorders they described. Grouping people with similar symptoms together would help researchers to determine when and whether this similarity was due to shared underlying pathophysiology. To put the point somewhat differently, the Feighner criteria were concerned with the *reliability* of diagnosis, which was relatively easy to achieve. Further research needed to be conducted before the *validity* of the diagnostic categories could be determined and, where necessary, improved.[5]

Yet the authors of the Feighner paper clearly felt that this next stage would—and should—follow from the use of their diagnostic criteria as a result of the kind of "constructive emendation" they recommend. Moreover, the group at Washington University were themselves engaged in biological research. Beginning well before the development of the Feighner criteria, Eli Robins published papers on neurochemistry and histology, while George Winokur and Samuel Guze both investigated the role of heredity in mental illness (Decker 2007). This suggests that despite the atheoretical nature of the Feighner criteria themselves, the authors viewed biological psychiatry as the theoretical approach most likely to lead to progress in psychiatry.

Perhaps the most sustained discussion of the medical model in psychiatry, and its relation to a specifically biological approach to psychiatry, is in Guze's 1992 book, *Why Psychiatry Is a Branch of Medicine*. In this work, Guze describes the medical model in detail and links it explicitly with neurobiological research. Although he says that the idea of applying the medical model to psychiatry "means simply that the concepts, strategies, and jargon of general medicine are applied to psychiatric disorders" (Guze 1992, 4), he further explains that this also involves taking a biological approach to psychiatry:

> There is another fundamental assumption underlying modern medical thinking that has its counterpart in the application of the medical model to psychiatry. All physicians believe that improvements in diagnosis and treatment will depend to a large degree on advances in basic biomedical knowledge. The more we learn about the body's development, structure, and function, at all levels, from the integrative activity of the whole body to cellular and molecular processes, the more likely we are to become effective in understanding, healing, and preventing disease. For psychiatry, of course, this assumption includes special emphasis on advances in understanding the brain. (Guze 1992, 11)

This quotation captures the idea that the Feighner criteria, as an example of the "minimal" medical model, were intended to guide further research in psychiatry that was ultimately expected to lead to a better understanding of the underlying neurobiology. This means that they were intended not as an alternative, but as a pathway, to the development of a strong medical model approach to psychiatry. To quote Guze again, biological psychiatry "is not so much based on current knowledge of anatomy and physiology in psychiatric conditions as a strategic way of thinking and the expectation that this will lead us to the relevant knowledge" (Guze 1992, 56).

Despite the intention that the Feighner criteria should serve as a starting point in the development of better diagnostic categories, the symptom-based approach they exemplify has merely become more entrenched over time. The Feighner criteria influenced the development of the Research Diagnostic Criteria (RDC; Spitzer, Endicott, and Robins 1978), which in turn informed the DSM-III and subsequent editions. Although there has been a great deal of research examining the biology of mental illness, this has not resulted in significant changes in psychiatric diagnosis.

This lack of progress has recently led the National Institute of Mental Health (NIMH) to propose a new approach to research in biological psychiatry, the Research Domain Criteria. The categories proposed by RDoC do not map neatly onto current diagnostic categories. Instead, they comprise a two-dimensional matrix that encourages researchers to examine various domains of functioning (e.g., cognitive processes involved with attention, attachment formation and maintenance, or sleep and wakefulness) at different "levels" of analysis (e.g., genes, brain circuits, behavior). The categories identified on the basis of this dimensional approach may include individuals with different DSM diagnoses or may make distinctions among individuals with the same diagnosis. The aim is to better understand mental disorders by identifying *specific* pathological markers, which can then be used as the basis for a new set of diagnostic categories.

Although RDoC does include behavioral measures, they aim explicitly to improve our understanding of the biology of mental disorders, placing them firmly in the tradition of biological psychiatry. Moreover, like the earlier Feighner criteria, RDoC is based on the idea that the existing situation in psychiatry is problematic. Both also claim explicitly to be only a starting place that needs to be tested and refined through further research. With regard to this latter point, for the Feighner criteria, this revision did not occur to the extent that the developers had hoped. There may be reason to be more optimistic about the prospects for the RDoC criteria, though, since several decades of research in neuroscience and psychiatry have at least identified candidate biological and psychological entities that appear to be affected in different mental illnesses. At the same time, however, the developers of RDoC realize that what will be most important is to determine whether this research is useful for clinical practice: "[T]he critical test is how well the new molecular and neurobiological parameters predict prognosis and treatment" (Insel et al. 2010).

Conducting this critical test, however, requires bringing together biological psychiatry's pathophysiological research with the kind of clinical research that is the focus of EBM. In the next section, I show that bringing these kinds of research together is not straightforward. They exemplify very different approaches to medicine. Moreover, EBM, in particular, is very skeptical of integrating the two approaches.

Rationalism and Empiricism in Medicine

Philosophers of medicine distinguish between rationalist and empiricist approaches to medicine (see, e.g., Newton 2001; Wulff et al. 1990). (The meanings of the terms "rationalism" and "empiricism" in this context are not the same as their standard use in philosophy.) Medical empiricism emphasizes careful observation and description of *how* things are but does not examine the causes of the phenomena described. Warren Newton (2001, 299) describes empiricism as emphasizing "the outcomes of individual patients and groups of patients" while Henrik Wulff and colleagues say that it emphasizes the importance of clinical observations, including the description of disease entities "on the basis of their clinical manifestations" (Wulff et al. 1990, 33). By contrast, medical rationalism focuses on causes, on explaining *why* things are the way they are. For Newton, this involves "the search for and emphasis on basic mechanisms of disease" (Newton 2001, 299). Wulff et al., who use the term "realism" to characterize rationalist approaches, add that diseases may be defined in terms of "a mixture of anatomical, physiological, microbiological and other criteria" (Wulff et al. 1990, 33).

Based on these descriptions, EBM is an empiricist approach to medicine. First, as described above, it views the highest form of evidence in medicine as large RCTs, which show *that* a treatment leads, or fails to lead, to better outcomes than a control intervention. It does not, however, concern itself with the rationalist question of *why* the treatment works. In fact (and this is a second reason that it is strongly empiricist, which I will elaborate on later), it has explicitly downplayed pathophysiological explanations for the accuracy of a diagnostic test, the different prognoses of demographic groups, or (most importantly, given its emphasis and impact on treatment decisions) the effectiveness, or ineffectiveness, of therapy. The hierarchies of evidence for both treatment and prognosis clearly place epidemiological studies at a higher level than physiological studies, on the grounds that the results of physiological research cannot directly inform clinical practice while the results of epidemiological studies are taken to be directly applicable to practice. For example, one of the founders of EBM, David Sackett, describes research on vitamin E therapy for the prevention of heart disease. A large body of laboratory research suggested that this treatment would work, but an RCT testing vitamin E showed that this was not the case (Sackett 1999). His conclusion, translated into my terminology, is that rationalist (physiological) explanations cannot be trusted to predict accurately the effects of a treatment in clinical practice.

Yet a closer look at Sackett's example suggests that things are more complicated than he acknowledges. The study he cites did show that there was no significant difference between the group receiving vitamin E and the control group, but when the *causes* of death within each group were examined, people who took vitamin E were significantly less likely to suffer a cardiac death (defined as cardiac death, coronary death, or sudden death) (Gruppo Italiano per lo Studio della Sopravvivenza nell'Infarto miocardico 1999). The authors of this study also point out that different doses of vitamin E, or a longer course of therapy than was measured in this study, might show greater benefit than was observed in their trial. Moreover, the participants in the study had already suffered a myocardial infarction; vitamin E may have a stronger protective effect in people who do not already have heart problems. I raise these points here not to argue for the benefits of vitamin E, but to show that the idea that a single RCT can provide a definitive result that outweighs all others is a strongly empiricist view that does not take seriously enough the many factors that may affect treatment outcomes.

By contrast with EBM, biological psychiatry is rationalist; it views progress in psychiatry as dependent upon a better understanding of the pathophysiology of mental illness. Biological research is taken to be the best way to develop better diagnostic categories since it will group patients according to similarities in the pathophysiology underlying their symptoms rather than just the symptoms themselves. Guze and, more recently, the developers of RDoC predict that these physiologically informed categories will allow clinicians to make better predictions about prognosis and to develop more targeted treatment strategies. In short, EBM and biological psychiatry have opposing views on the best way to use science to improve clinical practice.

Historically, rationalist and empiricist approaches to medicine have been contrasted, and there is, in fact, some tension between them. Newton (2001, 300) considers this tension to be "fundamental" though he acknowledges that the two approaches can complement each other. Wulff et al. (1990, 38), by contrast, believe that both approaches should work together; they describe the optimal approach as "realism under empirical control." Historically, they acknowledge, rationalist approaches to medicine tended to be "speculative," in that they drew on an overarching theory of medicine, such as humoral theory, to make diagnoses and treatment recommendations, rather than on observation, and "believed that it was possible by armchair reasoning alone to ascertain the nature of [a] disease mechanism" (Wulff et al. 1990, 31). Yet this is not the case with contemporary rationalist approaches, on which the aim of medical research is to develop theories about the nature of disease that are well supported by empirical data drawn from sciences such as physiology or molecular biology. Despite their defense of rationalism, Wulff et al. further (echoing the developers of EBM) emphasize that, when it comes to clinical practice, we should be empiricists, testing *whether* treatments actually work even when they are well supported by theory.

This characterization suggests that rationalism is concerned with the causes of disease whereas empiricism focuses on treatment outcomes. However, the relationship between the two approaches is not that simple. As Wulff et al. point out, rationalist theories about disease must be supported by empirical evidence. Similarly, I would add that the staunchly empiricist EBM would be better able to achieve its goals if it incorporated the rationalist concern with causes and with distinguishing among patients based on physiological differences.[6] Next, I will show why EBM's version of empiricism leads to problems and suggest an alternative approach.

EBM as Shortsighted Empiricism

I have characterized EBM as an empiricist approach to medicine. To a certain extent, its empiricism is warranted. What matters to patients and to their physicians is that a treatment *does* work, in the sense that it achieves desired clinical outcomes, even if we don't know exactly why. Moreover, a treatment that appears likely to work on the basis of laboratory research does need to be tested in a clinical trial before it is adopted in practice. Yet EBM's empiricism is ultimately shortsighted: it focuses on statistical relationships between treatments and clinical outcomes but ignores or downplays other important factors that influence this observed relationship. Understanding these factors requires using a rationalist perspective that is focused on causal claims; this will allow a better understanding of variability of treatment results due to demographic, physiological, or other differences among patients.

EBM, however, is skeptical of explanations of the results of clinical research in terms of physiological or other (e.g., demographic) characteristics. This is reflected in its hierarchy of evidence, which places physiological research near the bottom. Granted, physiological research on its own does not provide good evidence for the effectiveness of a treatment. But EBM is also skeptical of the use of physiological considerations in interpreting the results of clinical trials. In discussing the use of subgroup analyses in clinical trials, the *Users' Guides* warns: "The human mind is sufficiently fertile that there is no shortage of biologically plausible explanations, or indirect evidence, in support of almost any observation" (Guyatt and Rennie 2001, 562). Moreover, EBM tends to view the use of physiological "surrogate outcomes" for clinical outcomes with skepticism, noting that "[m]any biologically plausible surrogates are associated only weakly with clinically important outcomes" (Guyatt and Rennie 2001, 397).[7]

Yet this attitude ignores the fact that not all "biologically plausible" claims are *equally* plausible. Some are speculative, but others are both grounded in a solid understanding of the physiological mechanisms and well supported by empirical observations. For example, in oncology, it is well recognized that it may be important to identify the genetic properties of tumors for effective treatment. Biology makes a big difference to outcomes; it can be used to identify subgroups of patients that will respond to the same treatment very differently than the other groups. This example shows that an empiricist approach to medicine can take into account both knowledge of pathophysiological mechanisms and clinical tests of treatment outcomes; EBM should also embrace a "deeper" form of empiricism that addresses rationalist concerns with pathophysiology.

One possible objection to my characterization is that I am missing the point of EBM. Because it aims to use current evidence to treat patients *now*, its empiricist approach is warranted. The results of subgroup analyses provide hypotheses to be tested in the future, but it would be premature to change practice now. This objection, however, misses *my* point. I noted above, in describing the strong and weak medical models in psychiatry, that they are best understood as reflecting the tension between treating current patients and making scientific progress in psychiatry. The same tension applies to EBM. Although EBM does focus on treating current patients, it also makes very strong claims about what counts as good research. Specifically, it says that the highest form of evidence is provided by RCTs that focus on clinically important outcomes (rather than physiological measures) and that results from subgroups of trial participants are not to be trusted. It does acknowledge that subgroup analyses and research on physiological processes can provide hypotheses to be tested in later RCTs, but its overall message of skepticism is influential, even when there is good reason to distinguish among subgroups, as the following example shows.

Mona Gupta discusses a case that provides an example of the influence of EBM's shortsighted empiricism on research on major depression (Gupta

2007). She notes that both atypical depression and melancholic depression are subsumed under the category of major depression and that because of this, patients participating in clinical research will be included in the same category despite real differences in their symptoms. While all of the patients will share some features of major depression, those with atypical depression experience "symptom reversal" compared with those with the melancholic subtype. For example, they gain weight instead of losing it and experience hypersomnia instead of insomnia. Gupta also points out that there is evidence that patients with the two subtypes respond better to different therapies (Kennedy et al. 2001; cited in Gupta 2007). As a result, combining the two subtypes in one group in a clinical trial, and considering only the overall average outcomes, may confound the results of the study, so that "the result may not be helpful in guiding practice for either group" (Gupta 2007, 111).

In the case of the distinction between melancholic and atypical depression, there is solid empirical evidence that the groups *are* different; this is why they are recognized as different subtypes and why these subgroups should be distinguished in clinical research. Yet, as Gupta also points out, not all variability in patients' clinical presentation clusters as neatly as the distinction between the atypical and the melancholic subtypes of major depression. In addition, patients may well describe their symptoms differently, and in ways that do not reflect current diagnostic criteria. Here, Gupta gives the example of a patient who, when asked to describe her mood, replies that she feels "dead" rather than using more common adjectives such as "sad," "despairing," or "hopeless." In order to make a diagnosis, her psychiatrist must decide whether her state is equivalent to those described by these alternative terms.

Gupta's argument also shows that the value of a clinical trial for informing practice depends on how similar the patients participating in a clinical trial are to each other (e.g., do they have the same subtype of depression?) and to patients whose treatment will be informed by the results of the study. This problem is perhaps most pressing in psychiatry, given the criticisms raised regarding psychiatric diagnosis, but I would also argue that it is a problem for all areas of medicine. Instead of EBM's empiricist approach, clinical research in psychiatry should search for factors that cause a difference in treatment outcomes (or, more broadly, in prognosis). In some cases, these factors will be symptoms or combinations of symptoms; in others, they may be demographic factors. And particularly in psychiatry, a better understanding of pathophysiology might be the best way to group patients who can be expected to have a similar prognosis and/or response to treatment. This is precisely the bet made by those who espouse some form of biological psychiatry.

More generally, progress in medicine is best served by taking an approach that combines rationalism and empiricism, thereby looking for relationships among clinical signs and symptoms, demographic characteristics, and biological markers and then linking these with treatment outcomes. Such an approach also makes it clear that questions about diagnosis (the main concern of biological psychiatry) are best not separated from questions about treatment (the focus of EBM). The goal underlying research in both areas is to improve patient outcomes, and an important prerequisite for doing so is to group patients based on characteristics that are clinically relevant, in that they affect prognosis and/or response to treatment.

The problem with EBM, I have argued, is that it does not pay sufficient attention to those patient characteristics that may help to predict outcomes. The entire project of biological psychiatry can be understood as a search for those characteristics, or at least the physiological ones. In the next section, I return to the analysis of biological psychiatry, in order to show how the framework I have sketched in this section can inform research based on RDoC.

What Can RDoC Learn from EBM's Shortcomings?

As I noted above, compared with other areas of medicine, relatively little is known about the biology of mental disorders. This was true in the 1960s and 1970s when the Feighner criteria and the DSM-III were being developed, and it is scarcely less true now. Despite several decades of research on genetics, neuroanatomy, and neurophysiology, the pathophysiology of mental illnesses remains unclear.

This last claim, however, requires some qualification. Researchers *have* identified a number of genes and many anatomical or physiological characteristics that appear to be associated with a particular mental illness. In fact, these are nicely captured by the RDoC matrix. Recall that RDoC is a two-dimensional framework; the columns of the framework are different levels of analysis (e.g., genes, neural circuits, behaviors) while the rows consist of various domains of functioning, divided into "constructs." These constructs are "the fundamental units of analysis" in the RDoC system (NIMH 2014). Constructs include a wide variety of things, including attachment formation and maintenance, declarative memory, reward learning, and self-knowledge. The cells of the RDoC matrix are filled with the *specific* genes, neural circuits, hormone systems, and so forth that have been previously identified as relevant to the particular construct in that row.

RDoC thus builds on previous research, summarizing what is currently known about the biology and psychology of each construct. Future research drawing on RDoC will essentially involve developing a deeper understanding of each construct; the NIMH says that "it is anticipated that most studies would focus on one construct (or perhaps compare two constructs on relevant measures)" (NIMH 2014). Again, as noted above, focusing on constructs might involve making distinctions within a current diagnostic category since individuals with the same diagnosis may differ in the specific functional impairments they experience, and/or it might group together people with the same impairment but different diagnoses. Thus, although it builds on what is known now, RDoC replaces current diagnostic categories with a set of constructs that reflect functional impairments.

According to the RDoC project, the lack of progress to date in understanding the biological bases of mental illness is due to the fact that the neuroscientific findings do not map neatly onto current diagnostic categories for mental illness. The constructs are held to be a more promising way to link behavior with pathophysiology, and the hope is that, ultimately, they will form the basis for a new set of diagnostic categories. The developers of RDoC (Insel et al. 2010, 750) acknowledge that "the critical test is how well the new molecular and neurobiological parameters predict prognosis and treatment." They further acknowledge that this outcome is not guaranteed: "[W]e recognize that there are many 'ifs' at this stage. We are still a long way from knowing if this approach will succeed." So far, this sounds promising. But it should be noted that the developers of RDoC sound very much like the developers of the Feighner criteria. Both groups propose a radical new way of understanding and categorizing psychiatric disorders (but a way that is, all the same, rooted in current science). Both also see their taxonomy as a starting point, to be refined by future research. Yet this refinement of diagnostic criteria did not happen with the Feighner criteria. Instead, the symptom-based approach took on a life of its own, and relatively little change in the original criteria has occurred through the development of the DSM-III and its subsequent editions. The NIMH has now chosen to base further research on RDoC because, like the earlier biological psychiatrists, they believe that a better understanding of pathophysiology will lead to the development of psychiatric diagnoses that are more clinically useful, that is, ones that are more informative about patients' prognosis and response to treatment.

The current danger, however, is that RDoC will result in a wealth of knowledge about the neurobiology of the proposed constructs but will supply little information of clinical relevance. According to the NIMH (2014), RDoC is "agnostic about current disorder categories" and "begins with current understandings of behavior-brain relationships and links them to clinical phenomena." It is not clear, though, what these clinical phenomena are, only that they are *not* psychiatric disorders identified on the basis of current criteria.

One possibility is that the clinical phenomena referred to are the constructs themselves, as all of the constructs are dimensions of psychological functioning that are affected in various psychiatric disorders. If this is the case, however, RDoC risks becoming just as shortsighted as I have argued that EBM has become. To see this, consider one way that research using RDoC may be conducted, one that is suggested by the quotation above that says that most research will focus on one construct. A research group interested in attachment formation and maintenance may operationalize this construct in a variety of ways (perhaps drawing on the measures listed under the "behavioral" and "paradigm" columns of the RDoC matrix) and may investigate the molecular, neural, or hormonal processes that appear to be altered in people who have functional problems associated with this construct. (I will ignore the fact that a significant amount of this research will actually be done in animal models, and that it will be difficult to extrapolate from these models to humans.)

Following this approach, we may come to learn quite a bit about the neurophysiology of attachment. The clinical value of this information, however, is not clear. Attachment disorders do occur in a number of psychiatric disorders, including schizophrenia, post-traumatic stress disorder (PTSD), and autism. But it does not seem plausible that such a diverse group of patients is best viewed as united by an underlying malfunction in attachment neurocircuitry. This is because, despite the problems with current diagnostic criteria, they do at least have the merit of incorporating clinical features that are important to patients and clinicians.

Instead, research based on RDoC should take to heart EBM's insistence on careful observation of clinically important outcomes. A better understanding of the pathophysiology of attachment is only clinically useful if it improves clinicians' ability to predict prognosis and treatment response. This means that RDoC will have to incorporate a healthy dose of medical empiricism into its rationalist concerns with pathophysiology. If it does not do so, then RDoC will result in a form of medical rationalism that, while not speculative, will be as useless as earlier forms of rationalism for patient care. Just as I argued above that EBM needs to look for clinically relevant pathophysiological differences among patients, RDoC needs to ensure that the pathophysiological differences it seeks to understand are indeed clinically relevant. The following example illustrates the approach I advocate.

The Dissociative Subtype of PTSD

A common research paradigm in investigating PTSD uses script-driven imagery. Patients describe their experiences of a traumatic event, and a script based on their description is read to them during the neuroimaging session. Patients use the script to help them to remember the event in detail, focusing in particular on sensory and emotional aspects of the experience. In a series of neuroimaging experiments, Ruth Lanius and her colleagues have shown that patients tend to respond to the script in one of two ways. The majority of patients have vivid recollections of the event and both emotional and physiological (as measured by increased heart rate) arousal. Others "dissociate" from the experience, report feeling emotionally numb, and do not tend to show an increase in heart rate. Moreover, different patterns of neural activity characterize the two responses (Lanius et al. 2001, 2002).

Further research suggests that these two responses may characterize two distinct subtypes of PTSD (Lanius et al. 2010, 2012). The "hyperarousal" response may be more common in patients who have experienced a single traumatic event as an adult. By contrast, patients with a long history of exposure to psychological trauma, particularly those who have a history of childhood abuse, seem to be more likely to dissociate in response to trauma reminders. Moreover, the types of therapy appropriate for each group seem to differ. The former group often responds well to treatments that involve exposure and desensitization to trauma reminders, but in the latter group, the tendency to dissociate may prevent patients from fully engaging with the trauma reminders and the treatment is therefore not as successful (Foa and Kozak 1986). Alternative approaches that help patients to learn to regulate their own emotions may be more promising (Cloitre et al. 2002). Lanius et al. (2010, 645) conclude that "[g]rouping all PTSD patients, regardless of their different symptom patterns, in the same diagnostic category will hinder our understanding of posttraumatic psychopathology. … Classification of different PTSD subtypes will enable a more careful analysis of differential responses to psychological trauma and eventually lead to a more sophisticated understanding of the neurobiology and treatment of PTSD."

This example shows that pathophysiological differences within a patient group can help to identify clinically important differences among patients. I do *not* mean here that knowing that the pathophysiology of dissociative and hyperarousal responses are distinct somehow makes the experiential and clinical differences among patients more real. Rather, I believe that this example shows that information about pathophysiology can be used *together with* patients' reports and clinical observations to develop better diagnostic categories. This is because it combines the rationalist concern with disease mechanisms with empiricism's focus on clinical outcomes.

Conclusion

In summary, both EBM and biological psychiatry aim to use scientific research to improve patient care, though they do this in very different ways. I have shown in this chapter that biological psychiatry's emphasis on causes need not be the sort of "speculative" approach of early modern medicine, despite EBM's mistrust of pathophysiological reasoning. At the same time, even well-grounded claims about pathophysiology must be shown to be clinically relevant; knowledge of pathophysiological mechanisms is not guaranteed to improve clinical care. Rather, combined with the empiricist emphasis on careful description and observation, the rationalism of biological psychiatry can lead to (and is already leading to) a better understanding of the relationship between clinical characteristics, pathophysiology, and therapeutic decision-making.

Acknowledgments

I would like to thank Mona Gupta, Jeffrey Poland, Şerife Tekin, and Sarah Wieten for comments on earlier versions of this chapter.

Notes

1. Probably the most frequently cited example is that of the Cardiac Arrhythmia Suppression Trial (Echt et al. 1991), which demonstrated that the frequently prescribed antiarrhythmic drugs encainide and flecainide significantly increased the risk of cardiac arrest and of death.

2. Montori and Guyatt (2008) identify the hierarchy of evidence as the first fundamental principle of EBM. While other sources (e.g., Sackett et al. 1996) describe EBM as involving (1) clinical research, ranked according to the hierarchy; (2) knowledge of patient values; and (3) the clinician's best judgment, in practice most discussions of EBM focus on how to appraise clinical research.

3. There are different evidence hierarchies for other aspects of medicine, such as studies of prognosis and studies examining a diagnostic test (Guyatt and Rennie 2001). Yet EBM focuses, as I shall discuss later in the chapter, primarily on the assessment of treatments.

4. For a discussion of the problems of reliability as they pertained to the development of the DSM-III, which was strongly influenced by the Feighner criteria, see Kirk and Kutchins (1992/2008). Although a detailed discussion of the development of the DSM-III is beyond the scope of this chapter, it should be noted that it, too, is an example of a minimalist medical model of psychiatry.

5. Although there is broad agreement that it is important that psychiatry develop valid diagnostic categories, there is disagreement on what, exactly, validity is. For a survey of different kinds and interpretations of validity, see Haslam (2013) and Zachar et al. (2015).

6. Demographic, socioeconomic, and lifestyle factors may also be relevant to patient outcomes and may in some cases be the best way to group patients. Rationalists, however, would emphasize that all of these differences must ultimately make a physiological difference in order to affect patient outcomes.

7. EBM advocates instead using "patient important" clinical outcomes, such as mortality, stroke, symptom abatement, and ability to function on a daily basis. Surrogate end points should only be used when they have been shown to accurately predict these clinical outcomes.

References

Ash, P. 1949. The reliability of psychiatric diagnoses. *Journal of Abnormal Psychology* 44:272–276.

Beck, A. T. 1962. Reliability of psychiatric diagnoses, 1: A critique of systematic studies. *American Journal of Psychiatry* 119:210–216.

Cloitre, M, K. C. Koenen, L. R. Cohen, and H. Hyemee. 2002. Skills training in affective and interpersonal regulation followed by exposure: A phase-based treatment for PTSD related to childhood abuse. *Journal of Consulting and Clinical Psychology* 70:214–222.

Decker, H. S. 2007. How Kraepelinian was Kraepelin? How Kraepelinian are the neo-Kraepelinians—from Emil Kraepelin to *DSM-III*. *History of Psychiatry* 18 (3): 337–360.

Echt, D. S., P. R. Liebson, L. B. Mitchell, R. W. Peters, D. Obias-Manno, A. H. Barker, D. Arensberg, A. Baker, L. Friedman, H. L. Greene, M. L. Huther, D. W. Richardson, and the CAST investigators. 1991. Mortality and morbidity in patients receiving encainide, flecainide, or placebo—The Cardiac Arrhythmia Suppression Trial. *New England Journal of Medicine* 324:781–788.

The Evidence-Based Medicine Working Group. 1992. Evidence-based medicine: A new approach to teaching the practice of medicine. *Journal of the American Medical Association* 268:2420–2425.

Feighner, J. P., E. Robins, S. B. Guze, R. A. Woodruff, G. Winokur, and R. Munoz. 1972. Diagnostic criteria for use in psychiatric research. *Archives of General Psychiatry* 26:57–63.

Feinstein, A. R. 1985. *Clinical Epidemiology: The Architecture of Clinical Research.* Philadelphia: W.B. Saunders.

Foa, E. B, and M. J. Kozak. 1986. Emotional processing of fear: Exposure to corrective information. *Psychological Bulletin* 99 (1): 20–35.

Geddes, J., and S. Carney. 2001. Recent advances in evidence-based psychiatry. *Canadian Journal of Psychiatry* 42:403–406.

Gruppo Italiano per lo Studio della Sopravvivenza nell'Infarto miocardico. 1999. Dietary supplementation with n-3 polyunsaturated fatty acids and vitamin E after myocardial infarction: Results of the GISSI-Prevenzione trial. *Lancet* 354 (9177): 447–455.

Gupta, M. 2007. Does evidence-based medicine apply to psychiatry? *Theoretical Medicine and Bioethics* 28 (2): 103–120.

Guyatt, G., and D. Rennie, eds. 2001. *Users' Guides to the Medical Literature.* Chicago: AMA Press.

Guze, S. 1992. *Why Psychiatry Is a Branch of Medicine.* New York: Oxford University Press.

Haslam, N. 2013. Reliability, validity, and the mixed blessings of operationalism. In *The Oxford Handbook of Philosophy and Psychiatry*, ed. K. W. M. Fulford, M. Davies, R. G. T. Gipps, G. Graham, J. Z. Sadler, G. Stanghellini, and T. Thornton. Oxford: Oxford University Press. doi:10.1093/oxfordhb/9780199579563.013.0058

Insel, T., B. Cuthbert, M. Garvey, R. Heinssen, D. S. Pine, K. Quinn, C. Sanislow, and P. Wang. 2010. Research Domain Criteria (RDoC): Toward a new classification framework for research on mental disorders. *American Journal of Psychiatry* 167 (7): 748–751.

Kendler, K. S., R. A. Muñoz, and G. Murphy. 2010. The development of the Feighner criteria: A historical perspective. *American Journal of Psychiatry* 167:134–142.

Kennedy, S. H., R. W. Lam, N. L. Cohen, A. V. Ravindran, and the CANMAT Depression Work Group. 2001. Clinical guidelines for the treatment of depressive disorders. IV. Medications and other biological treatment. *Canadian Journal of Psychiatry* 46 (Suppl. 1): 38S–58S.

Kirk, S. A., and H. Kutchins. 1992/2008. *The Selling of DSM: The Rhetoric of Science in Psychiatry*. Hawthorne, NY: Aldine de Gruyter.

Lanius, R. A., B. Brand, E. Vermetten, P. A. Frewen, and D. Spiegel. 2012. The dissociative subtype of posttraumatic stress disorder: Rationale, clinical and neurobiological evidence, and implications. *Depression and Anxiety* 28 (8): 701–708.

Lanius, R. A., E. Vermetten, R. J. Loewenstein, B. Brand, C. Schmahl, J. D. Bremner, and D. Spiegel. 2010. Emotion modulation in PTSD: Clinical and neurobiological evidence for a dissociative subtype. *American Journal of Psychiatry* 167 (6): 640–647.

Lanius, R. A., P. C. Williamson, K. Boksman, M. Densmore, M. Gupta, R. W. J. Neufeld, J. S. Gati, and R. S. Menon. 2002. Brain activation during script-driven imagery induced dissociative responses in PTSD: A functional magnetic resonance imaging investigation. *Biological Psychiatry* 52 (4): 305–311.

Lanius, R. A., P. C. Williamson, M. Densmore, K. Boksman, M. A. Gupta, R. W. J. Neufeld, J. S. Gati, and R. S. Menon. 2001. Neural correlates of traumatic memories in posttraumatic stress disorder: A functional MRI investigation. *American Journal of Psychiatry* 158 (11): 1920–1922.

Laupacis, A. 2001. The future of evidence-based medicine. *Canadian Journal of Clinical Pharmacology* (Suppl. A): 6A–9A.

Montori, V., and G. Guyatt. 2008. Progress in evidence-based medicine. *Journal of the American Medical Association* 300 (15): 1814–1816.

Murphy, D. 2011. Conceptual foundations of biological psychiatry. In *Philosophy of Medicine*, ed. F. Gifford, 425–451. Amsterdam: Elsevier/North Holland.

National Institute of Mental Health. 2014. NIMH Research Domain Criteria (RDoC). Accessed November 30, 2014. http://www.nimh.nih.gov/research-priorities/rdoc/nimh-research-domain-criteria-rdoc.shtml.

Newton, W. 2001. Rationalism and empiricism in modern medicine. *Law and Contemporary Problems: Causation in Law and Science* 64:299–316.

Paris, J. 2000. Canadian psychiatry across 5 decades: From clinical inference to evidence-based practice. *Canadian Journal of Psychiatry* 45 (1): 34–39.

Sackett, D. L. 1999. Time to put the Canadian Institutes of Health Research on trial. *Canadian Medical Association Journal* 161:1414–1415.

Sackett, D. L., W. M. C. Rosenberg, J. A. Muir Gray, R. B. Haynes, and W. S. Richardson. 1996. Evidence-based medicine: What it is and what it isn't. *British Medical Journal* 312:71–72.

Spitzer, R. L., J. Endicott, and E. Robins. 1978. Research Diagnostic Criteria: Rationale and reliability. *Archives of General Psychiatry* 35 (6): 773–782.

Wennberg, J. E. 1984. Dealing with medical practice variations: A proposal for action. *Health Affairs* 3 (2) (summer): 6–32.

Wulff, H. R., S. A. Pederson, and R. Rosenberg. 1990. *Philosophy of Medicine: An Introduction*. 2nd ed. London: Blackwell Scientific.

Zachar, P., D. St. Stoyanov, M. Aragona, and A. Jablensky. 2015. *Alternative Perspectives on Psychiatric Validation*. Oxford: Oxford University Press.

4 RDoC's Metaphysical Assumptions: Problems and Promises

Ginger A. Hoffman and Peter Zachar

One of the clearest signs that psychiatry is undergoing a crisis of confidence in its classification system was Thomas Insel's (2013) surprising pronouncement, on the near-eve of its release, that the fifth edition of the *Diagnostic and Statistical Manual of Mental Disorders* (DSM-5), lacked *validity*:

> While DSM has been described as a "Bible" for the field, it is, at best, a dictionary, creating a set of labels and defining each. The strength of each of the editions of DSM has been "reliability"—each edition has ensured that clinicians use the same terms in the same ways. The weakness is its lack of validity. Unlike our definitions of ischemic heart disease, lymphoma, or AIDS, the DSM diagnoses are based on a consensus about clusters of clinical symptoms, not any objective laboratory measure. (Insel 2013)

Insel, a psychiatrist and director of the National Institute of Mental Health (NIMH), a long-time ally of the American Psychiatric Association (APA), shocked many by this opposition to a diagnostic manual in which the APA had invested so much time and effort. Insel (2013) cemented his opposition with his statement: "Patients with mental disorders deserve better."

But along with this denouncement, Insel offered a solution: a revamping of the psychiatric research framework. In this revamping, traditional DSM categories would be abolished in favor of the RDoC project, where *RDoC* stands for *Research Domain Criteria* (Insel et al. 2010; Sanislow et al. 2010). The implication was that this revamping would occur at the level of psychiatric research immediately and then would eventually result in a restructuring of psychiatric classification and clinical practice.

An initial, admittedly simplified, way to conceptualize RDoC is that, instead of organizing psychopathology[1] into familiar DSM categories such as schizophrenia, major depressive disorder, and obsessive–compulsive disorder (OCD), it seeks to understand psychopathology by studying basic psychological and behavioral functions (e.g., fear, attention, reward valuation (the assessment of the magnitude of benefit an action will produce)) and their biological mechanisms. More specifically, Insel proposes four fundamental tenets of RDoC:

- A diagnostic approach based on the biology as well as the symptoms must not be constrained by the current DSM categories,
- Mental disorders are biological disorders involving brain circuits that implicate specific domains of cognition, emotion, or behavior,
- Each level of analysis needs to be understood across a dimension of function,
- Mapping the cognitive, circuit, and genetic aspects of mental disorders will yield new and better targets for treatment. (Insel 2013)

The structure of RDoC is a matrix. The primary rows—the domains of RDoC—are five superordinate constructs. Within each domain is a set of other constructs representing basic psychological functions or processes like fear, attention, and reward valuation. These functions are to be studied with multiple levels of analysis (genes, molecules, etc.); these levels compose the columns of the RDoC matrix (see figure 4.1).

It is expected that these constructs will cut across current DSM categories like depression, schizophrenia, and substance use disorders. For instance, both depression and substance abuse presumably involve deviations in reward valuation.

Is RDoC the cure for what ails psychiatry? If patients "deserve better," can RDoC deliver? We will address these questions by exploring the following: (1) can RDoC offer an improvement in validity over current DSM categories? and (2) how might a classification system centered around RDoC affect patients' self-conceptions? These questions map onto two different possible effects of psychiatric research and its subsequent effects on psychiatric practice: its *therapeutic impact* and its *reflective impact* (Tekin 2014). Therapeutic impact refers to clinical treatments and therapies. We assume (but do not argue in detail) that a psychiatric research and classification system that improves validity will also heighten therapeutic impact since more accurate diagnosis would likely yield better knowledge about therapeutic options. Reflective impact, in contrast, refers to how psychiatry influences patients' reflections on their selves and lives beyond the clinical treatments they receive.

In the following two sections ("The Meaning of *Validity*" and "Can RDoC Improve Validity?"), we address the former question (question 1), and argue that even though RDoC can increase our understanding of lower

DOMAIN	Genes	Molecules	Cells	Circuits	Physiology	Behavior	Self-Report
Negative Valence Systems							
Positive Valence Systems							
Cognitive Systems							
Systems for Social Processes							
Arousal and Regulatory Systems							

Figure 4.1

The RDoC matrix, adapted from the NIMH website: https://www.nimh.nih.gov/research-priorities/rdoc/constructs/rdoc-matrix.shtml (accessed May 24, 2016). Note that the matrix depicted on this website contains an eighth column named "Paradigms" that follows "Self-Reports." However, the paradigms column is not included here because it refers to something completely different than do the initial seven columns.

level processes and thus advance the science of psychiatry in many ways, it faces hurdles in offering the "revolutionary" improvement in validity that it seeks. Afterwards, in the section titled "Can RDoC Improve Reflective Impact?," we address the latter question (question 2), outlining how RDoC may, nevertheless, introduce a valuable ethical goal for psychiatry at this stage, by highlighting a possible path to liberating patients from certain depersonalizing effects of diagnosis.

The Meaning of *Validity*

Validity as Representing Reality

In order to assess whether RDoC could offer an improvement in validity over DSM categories (question 1), we need some purchase on what *valid* means. This is not an easy task. *Validity* has a number of divergent meanings both in common usage and among different disciplines including logic, psychology, and medicine. Psychology, for example, traditionally differentiates between concurrent validity, predictive validity, and construct validity. And these three different concepts of validity—which were introduced to evaluate psychological tests—are different from medicine's concept of validity, which is based upon the notion of a disease entity (Zachar and Jablensky 2014).

Thus, a useful starting point for understanding psychiatric validity is to think of *validity* as a term for correctness, that is, a correct representation of reality. On this commonsense definition, a valid classification of disorders *correctly* demarcates disorders from nondisorders and *correctly* separates different disorders from one another. However, defining *valid* as *correctly representing reality* is not especially informative since the concept of *reality*, as the long history of metaphysics has shown, is often obscure. Although we seem to have some purchase on what might count as more or less real, claims such as *depression is valid because it is "real"* ultimately either beg the question or are simply obscure (see Zachar 2014; Cooper 2012).

Robins and Guze's Approach to Etiopathological Validity

A more informative way to construe *validity* in the context of psychiatric diagnosis is via the notion of *etiopathological validity*. A first pass at understanding this type of validity is expressed by psychiatrist Steven Hyman: "Validity: means that a diagnosis picks out a 'natural kind' based on etiology or pathophysiology" (Hyman 2010, 158). Thus, etiopathological validity is centered around the etiology—or cause—and the underlying pathology of disorders and is often considered by medicine to be a gold standard of validity. The best candidates in medicine for disorders that are etiopathologically valid (or, expressed another way, are validated by etiopathology) are infectious disease entities such as Ebola, strep throat, and tuberculosis. Take strep throat: all cases share a common cause—infection with a member of the genus of *Streptococcus* bacteria. Thus, if DSM categories were valid according to this notion of etiopathological validity, schizophrenia and depression would presumably be categorized according to their distinct underlying causal origins.[2] Thus, it seems clear that etiopathological validity is the type of validity toward which psychiatry aspires. Historically, however, there have been different ways of seeking this type of validity.

First, in an effort to work toward etiopathological validity in psychiatry, Eli Robins and Samuel Guze co-authored "Establishment of Diagnostic Validity in Psychiatric Illness: Its Application to Schizophrenia" (Robins and Guze 1970), the publication of which was one of the watershed events in late twentieth-century psychiatry. In this article, Robins and Guze claimed that valid classification is essential to the science of psychiatry, and they specifically linked the notion of validity to the ability to identify homogeneous categories of patients—categories of patients who have the same kind of disorder. The way to do this, they believed, was to establish the presence of "validators"—each providing a way to demarcate disorders or "clinical entities" from one another. Their five validators are as follows:

Clinical description: Clinical entities should have shared symptoms and onset conditions.
Laboratory studies: Clinical entities should have objectively measureable indicators—biological or psychological.
Delimitation from other disorders: Clinical entities should have unique, identifying features.
Follow-up study: People with the same disorder should have a similar prognosis.
Family study: Clinical entities should run in families (due to inheritance or learning).

Robins and Guze believed that psychiatrists would have a better chance of achieving etiopathological validity (which was, presumably, the ultimate goal) if they could start with diagnostic criteria composed of uniform and coherent presenting signs and symptoms. The idea here is that uniformity and coherence would pave the road toward shared causal processes.

This first step, identifying uniform disease entities or syndromes, was one of the main inspirations for the DSM-III. More specifically, the offspring of the Robins and Guze article—the Feigner criteria and the NIMH's *Research Diagnostic Criteria*—were the templates for the DSM-III (First 2012; Kendler, Muñoz, and Murphy 2010), which was published only a decade after Robins and Guze's article.

Problems with Robins and Guze's Approach to Etiopathological Validity

In retrospect, the Robins and Guze strategy for achieving diagnostic validity has not served psychiatry as hoped. Despite almost a half a century of research, psychiatry has not been able to develop diagnostic categories that have been clearly validated (i.e., able to fulfill the five criteria—validators—above) in the way Robins and Guze set forth (Bentall 1990; Chung, Fulford, and Graham 2007; Jablensky 2012). Take the current DSM-5 (APA 2013) category of schizophrenia, which arguably fulfills *none* of the five Robins and Guze validators:

Clinical description: The schizophrenia symptom pattern differs from patient to patient and within the same patient over time; the age of onset varies from the teen years to middle age (100, 102).

Laboratory studies: No diagnostically useful biomarkers have been discovered (101).

Delimitation from other disorders: Symptoms that were previously considered pathognomonic for schizophrenia, such as thought insertion, have been de-emphasized because they are not specific to schizophrenia (810).

Follow-up study: Outcome is variable—it is considered "deteriorating" in about 80% of cases and not "deteriorating" in about 20% of the cases (102).

Family study: What runs in families may be both a vulnerability to psychosis overall—including as a symptom of bipolar disorder—and a predisposition to odd and eccentric behavior that merges with normality; most people diagnosed with schizophrenia have no family history of psychosis (103).

In the 1970s and 1980s, psychiatrists believed that if any mental disorder was a valid disease syndrome, it was schizophrenia. Their expectation was that with the advances offered by DSM-III, in a decade or less, the biological basis of schizophrenia would be elucidated (Andreasen 1984). The failure to validate schizophrenia as expected is an exemplary reason for the current crisis of confidence in psychiatric research and classification.

Factorial Validity and the Role of Clinical Psychology

Given the historical centrality of Robins and Guze to the development of psychiatric classification, one might think that when advocates of RDoC trumpet the promise of increased validity, they are harkening back to Robins and Guze's vision. However, this does not seem to be the case: although RDoC shares Robins and Guze's ultimate goal of elucidating etiology and pathogenesis, fashioning a diagnostic system closely following RDoC will not help achieve validity in the same manner envisioned by Robins and Guze. This is because Robins and Guze's validity assumes the existence of *disorders* or *syndromes*, and one goal of the RDoC revolution is to move away from these kinds of clinical disease entities. Thus, for example, the Robins and Guze validator of "delimitation from other *disorders*" (emphasis ours) cannot be applied to the cells of the RDoC matrix in any literal way. This is because the matrix, technically speaking, does not contain disorders, but, rather, psychological constructs such as declarative memory and reward valuation that span the normal and the abnormal. This is reflected in RDoC's name: rather than NIMH Research *Diagnostic* Criteria (where "diagnostic" implies a diagnosis of disorders), RDoC is intentionally called NIMH Research *Domain* Criteria.

Thus, RDoC diverges from Robins and Guze in its strategy for achieving etiopathological validity. Much of this divergence may stem from the fact that RDoC is the result of a cross-disciplinary collaborative effort including both psychiatrists and psychologists who have different perspectives and training histories. In fact, RDoC's emphasis on dimensional (i.e., spanning normal and abnormal by matters of degree) constructs for basic psychological processes rather than categorical syndromes and disease entities (e.g., major depressive disorder, schizophrenia) is doubtlessly due to the important role played by clinical psychologists in RDoC's development (Cuthbert 2005; Cuthbert and Kozak 2013; Sanislow et al. 2010; Clark, Watson, and Reynolds 1995; Krueger, Watson, and Barlow 2005; Widiger and Samuel 2005).

To better understand the significance of the differences between the psychologists' and Robins and Guze's approaches, it is necessary to provide some stage setting. Both Robins and Guze and contemporary clinical psychologists believe that *homogeneity* is integral to validity. That is, a valid classification scheme should contain categories that pick out homogeneous groups. However, rather than trying to obtain homogeneity by looking to things like the natural history of disease, as proposed by Robins and Guze, psychologists rely on statistical approaches to achieve homogeneity (Krueger 1999; Smith and Combs 2010).

An important statistical technique used by psychologists for increasing the homogeneity of psychological constructs is called factor analysis. In the factor analytic paradigm, homogeneity is a property of factors (also called latent variables) that are *unidimensional*. A latent variable functions like a third variable that underlies a spurious correlation between other variables in the same way that population size (the third or latent variable) underlies a spurious positive correlation between the number of bars and churches in a town. That is, once population size is taken into account, the correlation between the number of bars and churches can be explained away. Likewise in clinical psychology, research has shown that the positive correlation between somatic symptoms such as headaches, stomach complaints, and fatigue can be explained away by statistically inferring a third variable—hypochondriasis—that is latent in the data (Tellegen et al. 2003; Morey 1991). In contrast, positive correlations between paranoia symptoms cannot be accounted for by a single latent variable; rather, one needs several latent variables including hypervigilance, resentment, persecutory ideas, and naïveté. Hence, hypochondriasis is a unidimensional factor whereas paranoia is not. In psychologists' terms, this statistical approach enhances what is known as *factorial validity* (and internal consistency).

Although it is not explicit in what the authors of RDoC say, we believe that factorial validity is a crucial ingredient in the path RDoC is mapping out for achieving etiopathological validity, and that this is one primary way in which it differs from Robins and Guze's approach. In fact, one of the "revolutionary" aspects of RDoC for psychiatry is not its emphasis on etiology and pathogenesis, which existed in psychiatry all along, but its emphasis on using validated psychological constructs that span the normal and the abnormal. Thus, it seems the hope of RDoC is that homogeneous constructs for basic processes will be better guides for discovering the kind of causes and underlying pathologies that are the best targets for treatment.

Consider Cuthbert and Kozak's quotation, which alludes to similar ideas:

> The RDoC initiative is intended to uncouple research questions from concepts that might be too heterogeneously large [e.g., DSM diagnostic categories like schizophrenia] for productive validation against biological phenomena of smaller "granularity." ... A working RDoC assumption is that granularity mismatch mitigates against successful multilevel analyses. (Cuthbert and Kozak 2013, 932)

According to this view, DSM syndromes such as schizophrenia (or subelements of them like psychosis) have not been validated because they have "too large a grain"—in other words, they are too coarse or heterogeneous, representing the confluences of too many different core psychological processes. Presumably, the unidimensional constructs of the factor analytic tradition will be of a "finer grain" and thus will be better able to "match" other "fine-grained" entities like neural circuits.

Given this understanding of the potential promise of RDoC in increasing factorial validity and, thereby, etiopathological validity, it is now time to examine its prospects of meeting that promise.

Can RDoC Improve Validity?

One way to chart RDoC's ultimate goal of increasing etiopathological validity is to look at whether its focus on homogeneous psychological constructs (a cornerstone of factorial validity) can help reveal causal mechanisms (a cornerstone of etiopathological validity). To this end, we will address two subquestions: (1) can the RDoC approach increase the homogeneity of constructs ("decrease the grain size") in a way that is needed to contribute to an accurate causal mechanistic analysis? And (2) can RDoC succeed in revealing causal connections by looking at "lower" levels like genes, molecules, and brain circuits? The first question addresses the nature of the *rows* of the RDoC matrix. The second addresses how the *columns* of the RDoC matrix relate to one another. We address the question of homogeneity first.

RDoC and Homogeneity

Psychological constructs such as reward valuation and fear are certainly more homogeneous (e.g., "smaller grained" and simpler) than DSM categories like bipolar disorder, but just because something is *more* homogeneous does not mean that it is homogeneous *enough* to be straightforwardly amenable to causal mechanistic analysis. In fact, many constructs within RDoC are much more heterogeneous than RDoC authors may be acknowledging. Take fear—one of the RDoC constructs. According to psychologist James Russell (2003, 2012), an emotion such as fear draws on many other basic process domains—including perception, cognition, and affect. For example, fear can be decomposed into cognitive processes (such as appraisal of dangerousness of certain stimuli), perceptual processes (including heightened auditory attention), and subjective moods (such as dread or discomfort). Since the underlying mechanisms of fear are likely distributed across each of these (and other) basic process domains, a comprehensive scientific theory of fear would need to incorporate a diverse array of mental processes (for more examples, see other work on the constructivist theory of emotions: e.g., Kiverstein and Miller 2015; Lindquist et al. 2012).

So a construct like fear may not be small-grained or homogeneous enough to adequately participate in causal mechanistic analyses. However, even if this is the case, RDoC could presumably overcome this obstacle by incorporating even more homogeneous latent variables that are the components of fear—like auditory attention, mentioned above. These, then, could serve as the proper building blocks of a causal mechanistic explanation. In fact, this is the solution that Cuthbert and Kozak propose for a similar worry raised by Berenbaum (2013) about the construct of belief. They suggest, "[P]erhaps a narrowly defined *kind* of belief or perception, such as "delusion" or "hallucination," could be limited enough to afford some likelihood of convergence with variables of the smaller granularity that characterize other levels of analysis" (Cuthbert and Kozak 2013, 933).

This solution seems promising, but the new concern is how we would know when we have hit upon a psychological construct that is homogeneous "enough" to participate in casual mechanistic explanations and still, in the end, be relevant to the original clinical phenomena that RDoC is meant to ameliorate. The worry is that in order to achieve the fineness of grain needed for elucidation of causal mechanisms, we risk losing connection to the "coarse" clinical phenomena of interest—given that the ultimate purpose of the NIMH (and, by extension, RDoC) is to reduce the burden of suffering from psychiatric disorders.

Not only is it unclear what level of homogeneity we should aim for in selecting constructs for the rows of RDoC, but there are other types of uncertainty as well. In selecting certain features of a particular clinical phenomenon to be modeled by constructs, many other features will be left out. As a result, there may be more than one collection of constructs that can help model the clinical phenomenon in question, and the choice between competing collections will be indeterminate. For example, there is no authoritative manual that dictates that one must include auditory attention or a subjective feeling of arousal in one's explanatory model of panic. Thus, one important challenge for RDoC in its turn to constructs is that it is not objectively clear *which* constructs will most accurately point toward "the" central causal mechanisms underlying psychiatric phenomena.[3] Decisions such as this are part of the pragmatic aspects of successful modeling; RDoC will need to compare models with and without various features to see which ones work best for what purposes.

RDoC and Multiple Realization

Despite the difficulty RDoC faces in selecting which constructs should populate its rows, there may be a potential advantage of RDoC that concerns its *columns*: RDoC may stand a better chance (than the DSM) in correcting a problem with *superficiality*. What is this problem? The problem is that classifying psychiatric distress by "surface features" alone will presumably only reveal one small part of the psychopathological story, and revealing only one part of this story will not bode well for uncovering full causal explanations nor for achieving etiopathological validity.

Consider an analogy with species classification. According to Hyman (2010), constructing a psychiatric classification based upon surface features alone (where "surface features" presumably refer to self-reported symptoms) is like placing all creatures with wings into a single evolutionary taxon. Wings in bats, birds, and bees evolved independently and are not homologous structures. Analogously, the failure to discover objective biomarkers underlying psychiatric symptoms suggests that psychiatry has a superficial picture of what makes certain cases similar or dissimilar.

Acknowledgment of the potential complexity underlying surface features is one advantage of RDoC, and, although not explicitly acknowledged as such by RDoC authors, coheres with both the concept of multiple realization in philosophy of mind and degeneracy in biology. Multiple realization is the idea that mental states can be identical to, or "realized by" one *type* of brain state in some situations, and a *different* type of brain state in other situations. For example, in one person, the mental state of depressed mood could be realized by an alteration in serotonin signaling; in another, it could be realized by an alteration in dopamine signaling (in fact, the efficacy of SSRIs in some instances and atypical antidepressants such as bupropion in others may possibly suggest something along these lines). Degeneracy is virtually the same notion: different structures may perform the exact same function. A classic example is different codons instructing the insertion of the same amino acid. There are several examples of multiple realization and degeneracy actually existing in biology; see Figdor (2010), Price and Friston (2002), and Hoffman (2012) for just a few.

Prima facie, it would seem that acknowledging the depth underlying superficial features would be an important first step to elucidating causal mechanisms. According to Cuthbert, one central goal of RDoC is to furnish mechanistic (i.e., casual) relationships between "RDoC measures" (which presumably include "lower" phenomena like genetic alterations and brain circuit activity) and "presenting signs and symptoms" (which include "higher" phenomena):

> Another issue concerns the relationship of the various RDoC measures to presenting signs and symptoms, since of course the latter are the actual clinical phenomena that bring patients to the clinic. Establishing mechanistic relationships by which disruptions in the functioning of one or more constructs (as assessed by various Units of Analysis [e.g. columns]) result in specified symptoms or impairments is considered as a central task for the RDoC project. (Cuthbert 2014, 32)[4]

Causality may not, however, be the best way to think about the relationships between many of the RDoC columns. Although a mutation in a gene (falling under the column of "genes") could certainly be a causal factor in the production of a new protein (falling under the column of "molecules"), the same would not necessarily hold true for the relationships between brain circuits and self-reports. To see why, note that most research psychiatrists and contemporary philosophers accept that the brain and mind are identical; it is not that some activity in a brain circuit *causes* a mental state; on the contrary, the activity in the brain circuit *is* a mental state (or, in different words, *constitutes* a mental state). If this is right, then RDoC's attempt to correct superficiality may not lead to a greater elucidation of *causal* mechanisms, per se.

RDoC and Multiple Mapping

A proponent of RDoC could respond to our above worry by granting that the relationships between RDoC columns often fail to be causal but could nevertheless maintain that the sort of constitutive relations described above are *equally* helpful in elucidating a comprehensive and cohesive picture of psychopathology. After all, constitutive relations—relations of identity—are certainly capable of providing a clear guide to translation between different columns: an entity in one column would simply be identical to an entity in another.

However, the new problem here is this type of translation does not necessarily follow a "one-to-one" mapping. Indeed, not only may certain members of "higher" columns be identical to (e.g., realized by) more than one entity in lower columns (multiple realization/degeneracy, above), but a given item in a lower column might constitute more than one entity in a higher column. We will call this latter possibility *multiple mapping*.[5] For example, hypothetically, one type of realization at a lower level (e.g., a deficiency of serotonin) may, in different contexts, serve as part of a realization for different types of higher levels, depending on the context (e.g., depressed mood in one person; obsessiveness in another). The possibility of multiple mapping means that, if the psychiatric research governed by RDoC ends up privileging lower levels alone as the fixed reality behind the changing appearances, there may be no systematic way to "climb back up" to higher levels.

Not only does multiple mapping exist as a hypothetical possibility, but there seems to be empirical evidence for it. This evidence is typically presented in the literature on "reverse inference," discussed at length in the context of neuroimaging, most notably by Poldrack (2008). A "forward inference" might be something like this: "If mental state X, then brain state Y." The reverse inference would then be this: "If brain state Y, then mental state X." That is, if we see brain region Y is activated in some individuals, we may be tempted to infer that they are experiencing mental state X. However, this reverse inference does not always follow.[6] Neuroimaging data *alone* cannot necessarily tell us what mental state someone is experiencing since brain region Y could be activated for many different mental states.

Consider the example of the amygdala. Although the amygdala is often activated when people are put in fear-inducing situations (making it a region of interest especially relevant for phobias, OCD, and certain anxiety disorders), it is also active during other emotions and mental states and processes as well: disgust, the experience of emotionally neutral novel information, decision making, and so forth (Kiverstein and Miller 2015, 5; Lindquist et al. 2012, 130–132). And the amygdala is certainly not the only example; a meta-analysis performed by Lindquist et al. (2012) verified that several different brain regions are also each activated during different types of emotions. These include, among others, the anterior insula, the orbitofrontal cortex, the anterior cingulate cortex, the dorsolateral prefrontal cortex, and (perhaps especially surprisingly), the visual cortex: "In all instances where a brain region showed consistent increases in activation during instances of a discrete emotion category (e.g., the amygdala in instances of fear perception), this increase was not specific to that category" (Lindquist et al. 2012, 139). And Anderson provides further evidence that multiple mapping (what he calls "neural reuse") is incredibly widespread: "[T]he question of whether there is significant, widespread, and functionally relevant reuse must be considered closed. In light of all the evidence discussed above, it is clear that there is neural reuse, and there is a lot of it" (Anderson 2010, 263).

However, in order to be sure that multiple mapping is actually a bona fide phenomenon, one must be clear on exactly how to define or individuate the brain states in question. In other words, it might be that the evidence we have for a particular brain state's being multiply mapped is simply an artifact of demarcating its boundaries either too broadly or too narrowly. Consider the latter. Although the problem of multiple mapping asserts itself for brain *regions*, it might be avoided by a focus on brain *circuits*—a focus that RDoC in fact explicitly recommends (after all, the relevant RDoC column is named "circuits"). That is, even though a particular *region* might correspond to more than one mental state, a particular brain *circuit*, as a more complex combination of several regions, may have a unique one-to-one mapping between itself and a mental state.

However, some contend that such a move from regions to circuits (also called "networks") would not be able to dodge the specter of multiple mapping. For example, Pessoa remarks, "I suggest that the attempt to map structure to function in a one-to-one manner in terms of networks will be fraught with similar difficulties as the one based on brain regions ... — the problem is simply passed along to a higher level"[7] (Pessoa 2014, 8; see also Pessoa 2012). Although Pessoa's suggestion remains conjectural, it is at least possible that the problem of multiple mapping will not evaporate by shifting the focus from regions to circuits. Further empirical work will shed more light on the likelihood of this possibility.

Further empirical work can also address the possibility that our currently defined brain regions are too large. For example, the finding that the amygdala seems to realize both fear and disgust may simply be an artifact of not honing in on smaller, specific parts of the amygdala. That is, perhaps one subsection of the amygdala realizes fear, and a different subsection realizes disgust.

Although this may be the case, two things are worth noting. First, Anderson has found that multiple mapping (or "neural reuse") seems to exist for even very small brain regions:

> An empirical review of 1,469 subtraction-based fMRI [functional magnetic resonance imaging] experiments in eleven task domains reveals that a typical cortical region is activated by tasks in nine different domains. The domains investigated were various—action execution, action inhibition, action observation, vision, audition, attention, emotion, language, mathematics, memory, and reasoning ... the observation is not explained by the size of the regions studied ... one gets the same pattern of results even when dividing the cortex into nearly 1,000 small regions. (Anderson 2010, 246)

Second, once we hone in on too small an area (say, ten neurons), the likelihood that this configuration is even going to be preserved from individual to individual is low, given the variation in brain development. Whether or not there is a middle ground—an area precise enough to avoid multiple mapping but large enough to be consistent across most individuals—remains to be seen.

The potential problem posed by multiple mapping/reverse inference has not gone unnoticed by authors of RDoC. For example, in the RDoC working group charged with creating the social processes domain of RDoC, "there was some consideration of the issues of reverse inference arising in fMRI studies" (NIMH 2012). However, a solution to this problem was not detailed. The negative valence working group also pinpointed a possible problem with what we are calling multiple mapping. They noted, specifically, that activation of the hypothalamic–pituitary–adrenal (HPA) axis could be associated with *either* a reaction to threat and/or a reaction to positive stimuli: "[W]orkshop participants noted that HPA axis activation was *insufficiently specific* to negative valence. ..." (emphasis ours) (NIMH 2011, 7).

If there is no one-to-one translation from lower to upper, then knowledge accumulated about brain circuits (and about certain other lower levels, like molecules) will risk remaining uncoupled from facts about patient distress. In other words, wherever multiple mapping obtains, there will be no clear, straightforward, or definitive way to translate from processes in physiology to the signs and symptoms that patients experience.[8]

The Difficulty of Locating Psychopathology at Lower Levels

One possible response from RDoC authors to this problem of "blockage" of translation—either because the relationships between columns are not causal (as discussed in the "RDoC and Multiple Realization" section) or because they are not one-to-one (as discussed in the "RDoC and Multiple Mapping" section)—would be to contend that, as long as researchers can identify *pathology* at a "lower" level, then they need not map it directly to signs or symptoms at a higher level. The idea here, presumably, is that once lower level pathology is detected (e.g., at the level of genes, molecules, cells, or brain circuits), it can be corrected with genetic, biochemical, or physiological (e.g., deep brain stimulation) therapeutic tools. This is, in principle, what medicine does with other disorders. Consider strep throat—we can look at a throat culture and tell if a person has strep throat without gathering any subjective report of symptoms from the patient. Furthermore, once the strep culture is positive, an antibiotic can be prescribed. Neither researchers nor clinicians need fret about whether or how the presence of *Streptococcus* bacterium maps onto "higher" levels like self-reports or behaviors, or about the nature of the bridges between higher and lower: their diagnostic work is complete once the infectious agent is identified.[9] So, we might think that, once we know enough about brain functioning, the case of mental disorder would be similar to the case of strep throat: clinicians would not need to consult the patient about behavior or self-reports and could, indeed, infer disorder by looking at the objective biomarkers alone (perhaps, e.g., during routine "mental health screenings").

However, bracketing the issue of whether "remaining at the lower level" should necessitate biological treatment (biological treatment may not be what is best, all things considered; Hoffman 2013; Biegler 2011), there is another, more conceptually fundamental, issue with this approach. This is that remaining at a lower level might prevent us from learning about mental *disorder* since the relevant psychopathology—the type of distress and impairment that psychiatry deals with—may simply be *undetectable* at lower levels. In other words, we might need information from a higher level in order to tell whether a certain gene, molecule, or pattern of brain activity is a *problem* in the first place. A number of philosophers of psychiatry (Graham 2010; Stier 2013) have argued along these lines that mental or behavioral pathology must be ascertained by referencing specific cultural, social, rational, and other norms of mentation and behavior:

> ... [W]hether something is a mental disorder can only be determined on the mental level. This is so because we can only call a behavior deviant by comparing

> it to non-deviant behavior, i.e., by using norms regarding *behavior*, which simply are not applicable to neurons. (Stier 2013, 1)

Let us explore this further. Even if researchers identify a highly unusual genetic, cellular, or physiological state, this does not in itself mean that it is the basis of some sort of pathology. Wakefield (2014) makes this point regarding "high circuit activation," where "high circuit activation" presumably represents something like especially high activity on an fMRI. Wakefield points out that although particularly high activation might be *unusual*, this does not mean it is a *problem* or a sign of *malfunction*. If an experimental paradigm fails to collect self-reports or behavioral information, or fails to take into account the context in which that person finds himself or herself, it is arguably impossible to ascertain if the brain is *working* properly or not. Wakefield states,

> Particularly pernicious is the lazy notion that disorder is simply high circuit activation. Anyone who has been terrified at imminent danger or experienced an orgasm knows that this can't be right. One might object that RDoC sees atypical or impairing high activation as disordered. But, depending on how you select your dimensions, you can make anything atypical. It is statistically typical to sleep, but the circuit activation during sleep is highly deviant from normative circuit status when awake. ... No RDoC cell will tell you that sleep is a biologically designed condition and not a disorder. (Wakefield 2014, 39)[10]

Now, one might argue that it is possible that *some* pathological brain states can be identified absent consultation of higher levels. For example, if we stimulated part of the brain, and it was completely unresponsive—there were no physiological reactions of any kind—this "deadness" certainly would *seem* to be sufficient for pathology, at least on a number of definitions of *pathology*. However, this is not the type of pathology in which psychiatry is interested. Although this would likely count as cellular or molecular pathology, it would not necessarily be *mental* pathology. One simple reason for this, related to our discussion of multiple realization above, is that there could be compensation from other areas of the brain. If this particular region (call it region D) was "dead," it could in fact be the case that another region, "region E," had "stepped in" to take over the previous function of region D. In fact, depending on the circumstances, it could be that region D was never responsible for the mental function in the first place. Consider the individual case of the bricklayer's assistant who was missing close to his entire cerebellum (as was discovered by an autopsy performed for unrelated reasons). No apparent pathology related to a missing cerebellum—no motor or coordination disorder—was detected during his lifetime (cited in Hicks and D'Amato 1970; see Pascual-Leone et al. 2005 and Price and Friston 2002 for other discussions of compensation).

So in the case of a "dead" brain region D, if we wanted to be certain of a mental pathology by searching exclusively at the level of brain circuits, our search would need to be widened to both regions D and E together. However, if region E seemed a bit physiologically sluggish also, then we should probably look at regions D, E, and F, since F might also be compensating. Ostensibly, in order to understand what is happening mentally, we would need to look across the entire brain [and maybe even the entire body, given the possibility of embodied cognition (see Kiverstein and Miller 2015)]. But since we will certainly note *some* functioning in an entire brain/body of a living person, we need to look back to the mental level to see if this lowered brain activity actually corresponds to lowered mental functioning. In this way, then, the complexity of the brain interferes with our ability to decisively detect pathology at neurological—or other "lower" levels—alone.

Can RDoC Improve Reflective Impact?

Thus far, we have considered whether RDoC can deliver the increase in validity fervently sought by psychiatry at this stage in its history. We argued that such an increase will require pragmatic work on the menu of constructs populating the rows of RDoC, and empirical and conceptual work on the incredible challenge of translating between RDoC columns. These issues deserve attention: an increase in validity could aid psychiatry's ability to develop better therapeutic interventions and, thus, heighten its therapeutic impact. But, as noted in our introduction, psychiatry has not only therapeutic impact but *reflective* impact (Tekin 2014). That is, how psychiatry ultimately chooses to sort, classify, and order people has implications for their well-being beyond whether it provides them with cures for their mental distress (Hacking 1995). Reflective impact describes, among other things, how diagnostic labels can alter patients' reflections about themselves, and how such alterations can subsequently affect many domains in their lives. These domains include their social standing, their future plans and goals, and their vulnerability to stigma.

When advocates of RDoC do address its implications for patients, they focus on its possible therapeutic impact, not its reflective impact. Here, we complement their considerations by briefly outlining how a diagnostic system designed around RDoC might offer promise in improving reflective impact. Of course, since RDoC is officially just a research tool now, it remains to be seen exactly what sort of diagnostic system it would give rise to. Thus, what we surmise here is speculative. However, with this caveat in mind, we think that it is at least possible that RDoC's increased attention on lower levels might actually (to the surprise of some of its critics) support a diagnostic system that could *protect* patients from some of the harmful reflective effects of current psychiatric diagnoses.

The Hyponarrativity of DSM Diagnosis

In order to better understand how RDoC could achieve such a potential benefit, it is helpful to contrast its potential reflective impact with that of its current alternative: the preexisting classification system of the DSM. One long-standing criticism of the DSM is that it fails to treat the patient as a whole person and reduces him or her to a cluster of disjointed symptoms (Sadler 2005; Tekin 2011; Graham 2010). This reductionist tendency of DSM diagnoses has been dubbed "hyponarrativity" by John Sadler. Hyponarrativity, according to Sadler, "means that people's stories and storytelling play only a very small role in the DSMs" (Sadler 2005, 176; see also Tekin 2014).

The problem with hyponarrativity is not just that it focuses on some elements of the patient to the exclusion of others. After all, many diagnoses in other branches of medicine (e.g., cardiology and ophthalmology) focus on select aspects of a patient to the exclusion of others, and this is not *necessarily* a problem.[11] The special problem with hyponarrativity stems from the fact that it may promote the devaluation of a rich life story addressing events, relationships, and social structures to the confines of a more impoverished language of disease. For instance, a patient, by internalizing the label of "OCD," may come to view the majority of his or her feelings, beliefs, and behaviors as "mere symptoms" of his or her obsessive–compulsive disorder.[12] This can certainly happen with nonpsychiatric diagnoses too—imagine a person ascribing his or her profound dissatisfaction at work to "merely" the symptom of lethargy caused by anemia. It all depends on the extent to which the diagnosis causes the patient to see fundamental aspects of his or her life (his or her beliefs, feelings, desires, goals, emotions, values, actions, experiences) as artifacts of a disease.

Hyponarrativity may be detrimental to a patient in a number of ways (see Tekin 2011, 2014, for a greatly extended discussion). As just two examples, it could do the following:

1. Erode self-knowledge and self-trust (relatedly, what Tekin calls "self-insight"). For example, patients may come to view their perceptions (both about themselves and other things) as skewed by their diseases, when in fact those perceptions are accurate.

2. Erode agency. Patients may abnegate responsibility since they may believe their actions, as "simply" symptoms of a disease, are out of their control.[13]

Can RDoC Protect against Hyponarrativity?

Prima facie, it would seem that a diagnostic system based on RDoC would fare far *worse* than DSM with respect to the problem of hyponarrativity. Even though the DSM divorces symptoms from an overarching life story, many of these symptoms still manifest aspects of patient experiences (e.g., "depressed mood most of the day"; APA 2013, 160). RDoC, in contrast, defines disorders as disruptions of brain circuits and devotes five of its seven columns to biological, subpersonal substrates. In fact, many critiques of RDoC have harped on its reductionist tendencies (Berenbaum 2013; Stein 2014; Wakefield 2014; Frances 2014; Jablensky and Waters 2014; Fulford 2014; Fava 2014; Lilienfeld 2014; Phillips 2014; Sartorius 2014). For example, Berenbaum states, "Because RDoC focuses on neural circuits ... , it is likely to neglect quintessentially human phenomena that are remarkably important for understanding humans" (Berenbaum 2013, 897).

However, we wish to propose, perhaps counterintuitively, that a diagnostic system based on RDoC may actually *guard against* the hyponarrativity lurking in the DSM. Although RDoC is reductionist in the specific sense that it places considerable emphasis on "lower levels" of genes, molecules, cells, and brain circuits, it is not necessarily reductionist in other senses. For example, one sense of *reduction* implies taking something at a "higher" level (patient experience) and *transforming* it to a lower level (genes, molecules, etc.). And one of the concerns that we identified above—a lack of bridges between higher and lower levels—may be precisely what prevents RDoC from performing this sort of reduction. Moreover, this sort of transforming reduction presumably depends upon patients' *internalizing* a diagnostic label such that they use it to rewrite events in their life story, for example, coming to see their experiences as "just" symptoms rather than as the consequences of their own or others' actions (see Tekin 2014, 18–19). RDoC may have an advantage over DSM insofar as it may discourage this sort of internalization. The extent to which it does so will depend upon many factors, including how individual patients receive and process a diagnosis based on RDoC, and the meaning and value that the surrounding social matrix ascribes to such a diagnosis (see Hacking 1995). Because of these contingencies, a fuller understanding of the nature and prevalence of this potential effect of RDoC requires further philosophical and empirical investigation. However, here are two potential ways in which

RDoC may discourage internalization and subsequent reduction for some patients.

Less Accessible Language The DSM contains symptoms patients can easily recognize and resonate with, like "feelings of worthlessness," "excessive anxiety and worry," and so forth (APA 2013). However, a diagnostic system based on RDoC may de-emphasize or even eliminate these relatable concepts in favor of empirically derived constructs such as disturbed reward valuation, action perception, and the like. These psychological constructs will also likely be articulated in the language of "lower" columns as revealed by laboratory tests: for example, "decreased activation of the dorsolateral prefrontal cortex" or "upregulation of 5HT1c receptors." If an RDoC-based diagnosis is presented in this sort of psychological, neuroscientific, physiological, and/or biochemical language, then, barring training and special laboratory equipment, patients themselves would have no idea how they fare on each of the different measures, or even what the different measures mean.

In this case, it would be hard to envision how patients would even begin to reductively rewrite their life story in terms of this technical language. At the very least, they would need a translation guide from the data of brain circuits to the language of self-reports. And this relates directly to our above discussion concerning the difficulties of intercolumn translation: namely, that the possibility of multiple mapping will, at best, introduce significant uncertainty into the translation process, or, at worst, completely prevent such translation.

Compare a potential RDoC diagnosis with a diagnosis like thyroid disease. Upon receiving a piece of paper with numerical values for levels of T3, T4, and TSH, this cluster of numbers certainly might mean *something* to patients ("I'm not healthy" or even "This low energy is not my fault"), but it seems difficult to imagine how this numerical lab report could have the sort of pervasive and deep impact that something like "schizophrenia" or "major depressive disorder" would have on their global conception of themselves. For example, knowing that "feelings of worthlessness" is a symptom of major depressive disorder may cause an individual to see his or her feelings of inadequacy following a romantic rejection as "just" a symptom. But if the same patient were to be presented with a symptom of major depressive disorder in the language of numbers, rather than words, he or she may be less likely to see his or her experience in this way since this patient will be less likely to even know what aspects of his or her experience might reduce to a symptom in the first place.[14] Thus, with an RDoC-based diagnostic system, patients may be better able to see their own selves and lives as more or less separate from their diagnoses.

Proliferation of Diagnoses Not only will a diagnostic system based on RDoC likely use technical or numerical language to present aspects of diagnosis, but it will also potentially fragment preexisting syndromes (e.g., depression and schizophrenia) into myriad mix-and-match constructs represented by a matrix of values on the RDoC grid. The more fragmented the characterization of a psychiatric problem is, and the more varieties of "disorder" there are, the more difficult it may be for a patient to internalize a psychiatric label into his or her self-concept.[15] For example, imagine that an individual receives "values" for each of the 287 cells (41 rows × 7 columns in the RDoC matrix). It would be nearly impossible for an individual to *remember* this diagnosis, much less use it to rewrite aspects of himself or herself under its influence. Even if a patient were assigned values for only one row, a conjunct of seven pieces of information would still be a rather cumbersome filter to apply to one's experiences.

Benefits for Reflective Impact? Thus, two potential features of a diagnostic system based on RDoC—the sheer complexity of diagnoses, along with the type of numerical or highly technical language within them—both may prevent internalization of psychiatric diagnostic labels. In addition, what we outlined as a problem for validity above—a problem with translation between columns and thus presumably a problem for therapeutic impact—may be a potential *benefit* for reflective impact. It seems that the more isolated that lower columns are from higher columns, the harder it will be to map changes in brain circuits and genes onto patient experience. As a consequence, the harder it will be to translate advances in science to potential therapies for patients, but the *easier* it will be to insulate the patient's self-concept from reductionist constraints. Whether or not an RDoC-based diagnostic system would have this beneficial reflective impact remains to be seen, but it is worth noting that it may hold promise in this regard.

Conclusions

There is little question that psychiatric research is in a state of crisis, given the variety and persistence of complaints against its principal instrument for psychiatric classification—the DSM. The magnitude of time, care, and consideration that the NIMH is putting into RDoC attests to the urgency of this crisis. Here, in order to assess RDoC's potential in quelling this crisis, we have looked both to its stated intent (a recouping of validity) *and* its possible broader effects on patient flourishing.

RDoC's champions praise its promise regarding the former, arguing that it can indeed offer a much needed increase in validity over the DSM. And its critics bemoan its presumed deficiencies in the latter, citing its seeming tendency to ignore the whole person in favor of subpersonal inhabitants of the lab bench like genes, molecules, and brain circuits. With respect to the champions, we have called attention to the importance of resolving current challenges RDoC faces about the choice of constructs in its rows, and the translatability between its columns. With respect to the critics, we point to a way in which the difficulty in bridging columns can potentially heighten RDoC's reflective impact, protecting a person's subjectivity, self-concept, self-trust, and agency from certain impoverished effects of diagnosis. In doing so, we hope to support further reconstruction and refinement of a research and diagnostic framework that will maximally benefit individuals in multiple dimensions in their lives.

Notes

1. We note that what many consider to be psychopathology or illness, others consider to be forms of neuro- or mental diversity. Our argument does not require us to support one side or the other, and we do not intend to alienate proponents of either side. However, since our arguments concern RDoC specifically, and we endeavor to engage individuals involved in the maintenance and revision of RDoC, we will adopt the preferred terminology of the NIMH and APA.

2. A preliminary understanding of the notion of etiopathological validity may risk obscuring the possibility that two syndromes of the same type may have different causal origins. For example, it may be that two different bona fide instances of depression (perhaps even phenomenologically and behaviorally qualitatively identical to one another) could have been caused by different things. We do not believe that etiopathological validity, as the gold standard of psychiatry, would necessarily be at odds with this possibility. This is because that etiopathological validity pairs the idea of cause ("etio") with the notion of the current nature of the disease ("patho"), and the latter may ultimately carry more weight in classification.

3. Note that RDoC architects admit that the current rows are only an initial pass that is open to revision (Cuthbert and Insel 2013). In fact, the NIMH has even set up a discussion board encouraging participants to "refine the structure of existing matrix components" and "propose and discuss new components of the matrix" (NIMH 2015); the subheading of this forum reads "The Matrix Needs You!" (NIMH 2015). However, our above discussion implies that it is not necessarily obvious *which criteria* should be guiding this type of revision in the first place.

4. Cuthbert's quotation points to many different goals, potentially also including uncovering causal relationships between *rows* in addition to *columns*.

5. Others have called this *multifinality, multiple determinativity* (Haug 2011), or *pluripotency* (Figdor 2010). However, these three terms also have developmental interpretations: a single state at time 1 may *cause* disparate states at time 2. Since it is critical that we avoid any implication that we are talking about causal relations (see the "RDoC and Multiple Realization" section), we have utilized our own term.

6. This is known in logic as committing the fallacy of affirming the consequent—if X, then Y; Y; therefore X (see Poldrack 2008, 224).

7. Bressler and Menon (2010, 286) agree: "[W]e expect that attempts to equate individual brain networks with a set of cognitive functions could prove to be just as inadequate as attempts to equate single brain regions with specific cognitive functions."

8. Of course, some studies collect information about *both* lower *and* higher levels (e.g., they look at both brain circuit activity and self-reports). These studies will not have a problem gleaning information from a higher level since they are already directly collecting it. But note that much of the research that RDoC envisions will *not* collect information at higher levels like self-reports; indeed, a large proportion of it will not use human subjects, but will take place at the level of animals, cell cultures, brain slices, and so forth.

9. Although often self-report is what brings a patient to the doctor in the first place, this need not be the case (medical conditions are discovered all the time via regular preventative diagnostics, or diagnostics for a different purpose—some conditions are asymptomatic).

10. Of course, pathology could be detected from "lower levels alone" if we *first* looked to higher mental levels and then found a robust and reliable one-to-one mapping between a pathological mental state and a particular brain state. But we explained in the previous section why this sort of one-to-one mapping is far from guaranteed.

11. Whether it is a problem will depend upon the type of "focus" here. If the focus on a patient's heart, for example, implies a denial of other aspects of his or her subjectivity (e.g., the patient's comfort, autonomy, and/or ability to consent), then this is certainly a problem (see Miles and Mezzich 2011).

12. This can be *additionally* problematic when this label is coupled with harmful assumptions and stereotypes from a larger stigmatizing society. That is, there are also a myriad selection of harmful consequences that may follow from internalizing a *particular* stereotype associated with a particular diagnosis. For example, people with schizophrenia are often incorrectly stereotyped as being very violent (Stuart 2003). As such, applying the label of "schizophrenic" to oneself may, for some

people, cause them to assume that they themselves are violent and harmful to society and may diminish their self-evaluation. This type of harm is separate from the harm that may arise from internalizing the idea that your experiences and behavior are caused by a disease, in general (whatever that disease is). Here, we focus on the latter type of harm.

13. However, this happens to have advantageous effects on many individuals too. Even though jettisoning responsibility is a way of ceding power, it is also a way of absolving oneself of blame. Many people find the idea that their brains are "simply hardwired a certain way" to be a powerful form of evidence that they are not at fault for their suffering. Thus, there may be some senses in which hyponarrativity is *not* detrimental to individuals.

14. Of course, the absence of particular "entry points" for translation (such as the relatable DSM symptoms) may not block reduction. A given patient, whether provided with a DSM- or an RDoC-based diagnosis, may simply believe that *all* of his or her feelings and experiences reduce to symptoms. But this extreme and global reduction is unlikely to be undertaken by all patients.

15. However, see Spaulding, Sullivan, and Poland (2003) for a potential counterexample: a presentation of a diagnostic and rehabilitative framework that contains multitudinous constructs but is nevertheless designed to aid patients in developing self-narratives.

References

American Psychiatric Association. 2013. *Diagnostic and Statistical Manual of Mental Disorders*. 5th ed. Arlington, VA: American Psychiatric Association.

Anderson, M. L. 2010. Neural reuse: A fundamental organizational principle of the brain. *Behavioral and Brain Sciences* 33 (4): 245–266.

Andreasen, N. C. 1984. *The Broken Brain: The Biological Revolution in Psychiatry*. New York: Harper & Row.

Bentall, R. P., ed. 1990. *Reconstructing Schizophrenia*. New York: Routledge.

Berenbaum, H. 2013. Classification and psychopathology research. *Journal of Abnormal Psychology* 122 (3): 894–901.

Biegler, P. 2011. *The Ethical Treatment of Depression: Autonomy through Psychotherapy*. Cambridge, MA: MIT Press.

Bressler, S. L., and V. Menon. 2010. Large-scale brain networks in cognition: Emerging methods and principles. *Trends in Cognitive Sciences* 14 (6): 277–290.

Chung, M. C., K. W. M. Fulford, and G. Graham, eds. 2007. *Reconceiving Schizophrenia*. Oxford: Oxford University Press.

Clark, L. A., D. Watson, and S. Reynolds. 1995. Diagnosis and classification of psychopathology: Challenges to the current system and future directions. *Annual Review of Psychology* 46:121–153.

Cooper, R. 2012. Progress and the calibration of scientific constructs: A new look at validity. In *Philosophical Issues in Psychiatry II: Nosology*, ed. K. S. Kendler and J. Parnas, 35–40. New York: Oxford University Press.

Cuthbert, B. N. 2005. Dimensional models of psychopathology: Research agenda and clinical utility. *Journal of Abnormal Psychology* 114:565–569.

Cuthbert, B. N. 2014. The RDoC framework: Facilitating transition from ICD/DSM to dimensional approaches that integrate neuroscience and psychopathology. *World Psychiatry; Official Journal of the World Psychiatric Association (WPA)* 13:28–35.

Cuthbert, B. N., and T. R. Insel. 2013. Toward the future of psychiatric diagnosis: The seven pillars of RDoC. *BMC Medicine* 11:126.

Cuthbert, B. N., and M. J. Kozak. 2013. Constructing constructs for psychopathology: The NIMH Research Domain Criteria. *Journal of Abnormal Psychology* 122 (3): 928–937.

Fava, G. A. 2014. Road to nowhere. *World Psychiatry: Official Journal of the World Psychiatric Association (WPA)* 13 (1): 49–50.

Figdor, C. 2010. Neuroscience and the multiple realization of cognitive functions. *Philosophy of Science* 77 (3): 419–456.

First, M. B. 2012. The development of DSM-III from a historical/conceptual perspective. In *Philosophical Issues in Psychiatry II: Nosology*, ed. K. S. Kendler and J. Parnas, 127–140. Oxford: Oxford University Press.

Frances, A. 2014. RDoC is necessary, but very oversold. *World Psychiatry: Official Journal of the World Psychiatric Association (WPA)* 13 (1): 47–49.

Fulford, K. W. M. 2014. RDoC+: Taking translation seriously. *World Psychiatry: Official Journal of the World Psychiatric Association (WPA)* 13 (1): 54–55.

Graham, G. 2010. *The Disordered Mind: An Introduction to Philosophy of Mind and Mental Illness*. London: Routledge.

Hacking, I. 1995. The looping effects of human kinds. In *Causal Cognition: A Multidisciplinary Debate*, ed. D. Sperber, D. Premack, and A. J. Premack, 351–394. New York: Clarendon Press/Oxford University Press.

Haug, M. C. 2011. Natural properties and the special sciences: Nonreductive physicalism without levels of reality or multiple realizibility. *Monist* 94 (2): 244–266.

Hicks, S. P., and C. J. D'Amato. 1970. Motor-sensory and visual behavior after hemispherectomy in newborn and mature rats. *Experimental Neurology* 29 (3): 416–438.

Hoffman, G. A. 2012. What, if anything, can neuroscience tell us about gender differences? In *Neurofeminism: Issues at the Intersection of Feminist Theory and Cognitive Science*, ed. R. Bluhm, A. Jacobson, and H. Maibom, 30–55. New York: Palgrave-MacMillan.

Hoffman, G. A. 2013. Treating yourself as an object: Self-objectification and the ethical dimensions of antidepressant use. *Neuroethics* 6 (1): 165–178.

Hyman, S. E. 2010. The diagnosis of mental disorders: The problem of reification. *Annual Review of Clinical Psychology* 6:155–179.

Insel, T. 2013. Director's blog: Transforming diagnosis. April 29. http://www.nimh.nih.gov/about/director/2013/transforming-diagnosis.shtml.

Insel, T., B. Cuthbert, M. Garvey, R. Heinssen, D. S. Pine, K. Quinn, C. Sanislow, and P. Wang. 2010. Research Domain Criteria (RDoC): Toward a new classification framework for research on mental disorders. *American Journal of Psychiatry* 167:748–751.

Jablensky, A. 2012. The disease entity in psychiatry: Fact or fiction? *Epidemiology and Psychiatric Sciences* 21:255–264.

Jablensky, A., and F. Waters. 2014. RDoC: A roadmap to pathogenesis? *World Psychiatry: Official Journal of the World Psychiatric Association (WPA)* 13 (1): 43–44.

Kendler, K. S., R. A. Muñoz, and G. Murphy. 2010. The development of the Feighner criteria: A historical perspective. *American Journal of Psychiatry* 167 (2): 134–142.

Kiverstein, J., and M. Miller. 2015. The embodied brain: Towards a radical embodied cognitive neuroscience. *Frontiers in Human Neuroscience* 9:237.

Krueger, R. F. 1999. The structure of common mental disorders. *Archives of General Psychiatry* 56 (10): 921–926.

Krueger, R. F., D. Watson, and D. H. Barlow. 2005. Introduction to the special section: Toward a dimensionally based taxonomy of psychopathology. *Journal of Abnormal Psychology* 114 (4): 491–493.

Lilienfeld, S. O. 2014. The Research Domain Criteria (RDoC): An analysis of methodological and conceptual challenges. *Behaviour Research and Therapy* 62:129–139.

Lindquist, K. A., T. D. Wager, H. Kober, E. Bliss-Moreau, and L. F. Barrett. 2012. The brain basis of emotion: A meta-analytic review. *Behavioral and Brain Sciences* 35 (3): 121–143.

Miles, A., and J. E. Mezzich. 2011. Person centered medicine: Advancing methods, promoting implementation. *International Journal of Person Centered Medicine* 1 (3): 423–428.

Morey, L. C. 1991. *The Personality Assessment Inventory: Professional Manual.* Lutz, FL: Psychological Assessment Resources.

National Institute of Mental Health. 2011. NIMH Research Domain Criteria (RDoC) project negative valence systems: Workshop proceedings. http://www.nimh.nih.gov/research-priorities/rdoc/negative-valence-systems-workshop_141983.pdf.

National Institute of Mental Health. 2012. Social processes: Workshop proceedings. http://www.nimh.nih.gov/research-priorities/rdoc/rdoc-social-processes_143400.pdf.

National Institute of Mental Health. 2015. RDoC discussion forum. https://rdocforum.nimh.nih.gov/portal/.

Pascual-Leone, A., A. Amedi, F. Fregni, and L. B. Merabet. 2005. The plastic human brain cortex. *Annual Review of Neuroscience* 28:377–401.

Pessoa, L. 2012. Beyond brain regions: Network perspective of cognition–emotion interactions. *Behavioral and Brain Sciences* 35 (3): 158–159.

Pessoa, L. 2014. Understanding brain networks and brain organization. *Physics of Life Reviews* 11 (3): 400–435.

Phillips, M. R. 2014. Will RDoC hasten the decline of America's global leadership role in mental health? *World Psychiatry: Official Journal of the World Psychiatric Association (WPA)* 13 (1): 40–41.

Poldrack, R. A. 2008. The role of fMRI in Cognitive Neuroscience: where do we stand? Current Opinion in Neurobiology 18: 223–227.

Price, C. J., and K. J. Friston. 2002. Degeneracy and cognitive anatomy. *Trends in Cognitive Sciences* 6 (10): 416–421.

Robins, E., and S. B. Guze. 1970. Establishment of diagnostic validity in psychiatric illness: Its application to schizophrenia. *American Journal of Psychiatry* 126 (7): 983–987.

Russell, J. A. 2003. Core affect and the psychological construction of emotion. *Psychological Review* 110 (1): 145–172.

Russell, J. A. 2012. From a psychological constructionist perspective. In *Categorical versus dimensional models of affect: A seminar of the theories of Panksepp and Russell*, ed. P. Zachar and R. D. Ellis, 79–118. Amsterdam: John Behjamins.

Sadler, J. Z. 2005. *Values and Psychiatric Diagnosis.* New York: Oxford University Press.

Sanislow, C. A., D. S. Pine, K. J. Quinn, M. J. Kozak, M. A. Garvey, R. K. Heinssen, P. S. Wang, and B. N. Cuthbert. 2010. Developing constructs for psychopathology research: Research Domain Critera. *Journal of Abnormal Psychology* 119:631–639.

Sartorius, N. 2014. The only one or one of many? A comment on the RDoC project. *World Psychiatry: Official Journal of the World Psychiatric Association (WPA)* 13 (1): 50–51.

Smith, G. T., and J. Combs. 2010. Issues of construct validity in psychiatric diagnosis. In *Contemporary Directions in Psychopathology*, ed. T. Millon, R. F. Krueger, and E. Simonsen, 205–222. New York: Guilford Press.

Spaulding, W. D., M. E. Sullivan, and J. S. Poland. 2003. *Treatment and Rehabilitation of Severe Mental Illness*. New York: Guilford Press.

Stein, D. J. 2014. An integrative approach to psychiatric diagnosis and research. *World Psychiatry: Official Journal of the World Psychiatric Association (WPA)* 13 (1): 51–53.

Stier, M. 2013. Normative preconditions for the assessment of mental disorder. *Frontiers in Psychology* 4 (611): 1–9.

Stuart, H. 2003. Violence and mental illness: An overview. *World Psychiatry; Official Journal of the World Psychiatric Association (WPA)* 2 (2): 121–124.

Tekin, Ş. 2011. Self-concept through the diagnostic looking glass: Narratives and mental disorder. *Philosophical Psychology* 24 (3): 357–380.

Tekin, Ş. 2014. Self-insight in the time of mood disorders. *Philosophy, Psychiatry, & Psychology* 21:135–137.

Tellegen, A., Y. S. Ben-Porath, J. L. McNulty, P. A. Arbisi, J. R. Graham, and B. Kaemmer. 2003. *The MMPI-2 Restructured Clinical Scales: Development, Validation, and Interpretation*. Minneapolis: University of Minnesota Press.

Wakefield, J. C. 2014. Wittgenstein's nightmare: Why the RDoC grid needs a conceptual dimension. *World Psychiatry: Official Journal of the World Psychiatric Association (WPA)* 13 (1): 38–40.

Widiger, T. A., and D. B. Samuel. 2005. Diagnostic categories or dimensions? A question for the *Diagnostic and Statistical Manual of Mental Disorders—Fifth Edition*. *Journal of Abnormal Psychology* 114 (4): 494–504.

Zachar, P. 2014. *A Metaphysics of Psychopathology*. Cambridge, MA: MIT Press.

Zachar, P., and A. Jablensky. 2014. Introduction: The concept of validation in psychiatry and psychology. In *Alternative Perspectives on Psychiatric Validation, DSM, ICD, RDoC and Beyond*, ed. P. Zachar, D. St. Stoyanov, M. Aragona, and A. Jablensky, 3–24. Oxford: Oxford University Press.

5 Psychopathology without Nosology: The Research Domain Criteria Project as Normal Science

Claire Pouncey

The National Institute of Mental Health (NIMH) introduced the Research Domain Criteria (RDoC) project in 2008 as a novel research initiative intended to address stagnation in psychopathology research. Most research in the United States had until then been organized around the mental disorder taxa identified in the American Psychiatric Association's *Diagnostic and Statistical Manual of Mental Disorders* (DSM) or the World Health Organization's *International Classification of Diseases* (ICD). After three decades of trying to develop a fruitful program of psychopathology research around the DSM, psychiatric scientists recognized that research cohorts defined according to DSM taxa limit the directions new investigations can take, especially with respect to advances in neuroimaging and molecular biology (Kupfer, First, and Regier 2002; Insel et al. 2010; Cuthbert and Kozak 2013). The RDoC program supports psychopathology research that utilizes newer, biologically based investigational methods; avoids preexisting conceptions of mental disorders; and provides insight into the full range of psychological functioning from normal to pathological. The RDoC strategy constitutes a dramatic—to some minds a revolutionary—departure from the nosology-based research efforts that preceded it (Cuthbert and Insel 2013).

The RDoC research guidelines are meant to steer the science funded by NIMH. They do not actually contribute to the content of psychopathological—or as it is now called, "psychophysiological"—theory. The guidelines take the form of a simple matrix, with preferred levels of explanation on one axis, and favored research constructs on the other. The seven "units of analysis"—levels of explanation—RDoC endorses are genes, molecules, cells, neural circuits, physiology, observable behavior, and self-report. The NIMH suggests a number of research constructs to be elucidated at each level of explanation, with the express intention of de-emphasizing the use of currently accepted mental disorders and directly studying the manifestations that emerge in persons with and without those disorders. However, the list of suggested psychophysiological constructs is not exhaustive, and investigators may propose to study others of relevance and interest to psychiatry and psychology (Cuthbert and Insel 2013; Cuthbert and Kozak 2013).

NIMH characterizes RDoC as a "paradigm shift" (Cuthbert and Insel 2013; Insel 2014), but the RDoC project is not a scientific revolution in the traditional Kuhnian sense (Kuhn 2012). In this discussion I demonstrate that RDoC's change in emphasis from discrete mental disorders to psychophysiological constructs does not depart dramatically from prior research strategies although the results and applications of RDoC research may ultimately do so. I argue that RDoC intends to develop existing theory according to well-accepted methodological rules, and thus RDoC research constitutes normal science in the Kuhnian sense rather than extraordinary or revolutionary science.

Kuhnian Paradigms and Normal Science

A Kuhnian paradigm is the collection of laws and generalizations, observable and theoretical entities, experimental practices, instrumentation, methodological rules and values that constitute normal science (Kuhn 2012). For Kuhn, normal science is "business as usual" science, in which the scientific community shares basic commitments to a system of scientific theories, their constituent laws, and the rules that govern research practices within the paradigm. The daily work of normal science is a matter of "puzzle solving," performing experiments, extending methodology and instrumentation, and refining theory and ontology in order to clarify and expand upon the paradigm. As experimental practices are refined by new methods and instruments, scientists better understand their preexisting world view. As normal science progresses, scientific theory becomes both more inclusive and more precise, and investigators are able to understand exceptions to existing laws and why those exceptions exist. The work of normal science is to further develop an existing paradigm.

According to Kuhn, in science "novelty emerges only with difficulty, manifested by resistance, against a background provided by expectation" (Kuhn 2012, 64). Only rarely do scientists encounter experimental findings that the existing paradigm cannot accommodate. Occasionally, however, experimentation produces results that call into question the paradigm itself, both the theory and the rules of puzzle solving. Such "anomalies"—Kuhn's technical term for surprising experimental results that the paradigm cannot explain—can challenge even the most fundamental assumptions of the paradigm. In response, a science may try to adapt the paradigm to the anomaly by developing new technology, shifting or adding concepts, modifying laws and theory, and making internal changes to protect the paradigm itself. According to Kuhn, this is appropriate and expectable. However, when the paradigm cannot be modified to include the anomalous findings, the science experiences "crisis," in which the rules of science, formerly somewhat rigid and widely accepted, begin to loosen (Kuhn 2012, 84).

Kuhn tells us that a crisis can be resolved in one of three ways. First, the paradigm may be adapted to accommodate the anomaly, the process of which Kuhn calls "extraordinary science" (Kuhn 2012). Second, the anomaly may remain refractory to study within the paradigm but be archived as a problem that cannot be accommodated in the present paradigm. Third, a new, rival paradigm may be developed that can account for the anomaly. This third possibility is what Kuhn calls—again, as a term of art—a "paradigm shift" or "scientific revolution" (Kuhn 2012). Paradigm shifts are infrequent and involve dramatic changes in the fundamental assumptions of the science, its methods of experimentation, its concepts, and its rules.

The Normal Science of Psychopathology

It is difficult to formally characterize the science of psychopathology as a strict Kuhnian paradigm. In the first place, the research community is diverse. Psychopathology researchers include psychologists (experimental, cognitive, and clinical), psychiatrists, and neuroscientists and molecular geneticists, among others. Both the theories and the rules for research can differ among these disciplines, making psychopathology an amalgam or an intersection of scientific practices and theories rather than a monolithic, internally consistent body of thought. These may include personality theory, attachment and relational theory, developmental theory, behaviorism, psychodynamic theory, and biological theory, among others. Psychopathology is unified, however, by common puzzle-solving projects and rules for the conduct of research. For instance, it aims to identify and characterize psychological processes and how these underlie behavior. Further, it aims to understand the causes of mental illness and interrupt those processes in order to prevent or eliminate mental illness, or to minimize its effects. These commonalities lead me to characterize psychopathology (or psychophysiology) as a multidisciplinary paradigm.

I do not conflate the science of psychopathology with its classification, nor do I consider classification to be a science in itself. However, the two are related, and often discussed together. For example, many psychopathology textbooks pay as much attention to the classification of mental disorders as they do to the science of mental disorders (for a recent example, see Millon, Krueger, and Simonsen 2010). This is reasonable, since the science usually directs the classification, but discussing psychopathological science and psychopathological classification together risks confusing the two. I want to be very clear that psychopathological science extends beyond what can be encapsulated in a classification or nosology. Psychopathology may or may not lend itself to classification, and our current classifications of mental disorders do not encompass or reflect all of the science of psychopathology.

The ICD and DSM classifications contribute to psychopathological research by focusing research questions and allowing research cohorts to be (ideally) homogeneous so that those specific disorders may be further studied, but the classifications themselves tell us little about the theory behind the disorders they name. Research since DSM-III always has strived to establish systematic theoretical support for mental disorders, and causal explanation for how such disorders develop, so that we can identify treatments. Despite the American Psychiatric Association's insistence that DSM-III and its successors adopt an "atheoretical approach" (American Psychiatric Association 1980, 7), there has never been any pretense that "nosology-based" psychopathology research is anti- or atheoretical.[1] The *DSM-IV Sourcebook* (American Psychiatric Association 1994) and *A Research Agenda for DSM-V* (Kupfer, First, and Regier 2002), as well as much of the psychiatric and psychological literature for the last fifty-plus years, reflect extensive and ongoing research on the theoretical bases for psychopathology that is not reflected in the DSM. In other words, although the DSM is noncommittal about psychopathological theory, psychiatry in general is not. DSM deliberately excludes psychiatric theory from the taxonomy without denying its relevance to psychiatric science. Within the broader psychopathological paradigm, psychiatric science extends well beyond nosology.

Most psychiatric journals publish research that extends beyond or across discrete mental disorders, such as work on environmental, genetic, and relational effects on mental functioning. Psychiatric science may be organized around DSM or ICD diagnostic taxa, but it has never been limited to such "nosology-based" research. For example, one recent psychopathological research project looked at "Brain Structural Abnormalities in a Group of Never-Medicated Patients with Long-Term Schizophrenia" (Zhang et al.

2015). In this study, the research cohort was identified according to DSM diagnostic criteria for schizophrenia, making it nosology based, but the aim of the study was to address the puzzle of whether neuroanatomical changes underlie the psychopathological processes of schizophrenia. Another project, "Defining the Effect of the 16p11.2 Duplication on Cognition, Behavior, and Medical Comorbidities" (D'Angelo et al. 2015), is not nosology based because it is not organized around DSM mental disorder taxa. This study addresses the paradigmatic puzzle of whether specific gene anomalies underlie changes associated with more than one psychiatric diagnosis. Both of these projects exemplify psychiatric science, and as such, both fall under the umbrella of the psychopathological paradigm. One of them is organized around a nosologic taxon, and one is not.

RDoC was introduced because research organized around DSM mental disorders stalled. *A Research Agenda for DSM-V* expressed overt optimism that future DSM editions would be grounded in theoretical connections to neuroscience, molecular biology, and other related scientific fields. The *Research Agenda* anticipated the RDoC departure when it said the following: "[R]esearch exclusively focused on refining existing DSM-defined syndromes may never be successful in uncovering their underlying etiologies. For that to happen, ... [we need] to integrate information from a wide variety of sources and technologies" (Kupfer, First, and Regier 2002, xix). RDoC explicitly proposes to utilize new technologies by deflating the role and importance of DSM mental disorders. RDoC aims to extend existing psychopathological theory while remaining agnostic about mental disorders as disease entities and studying the full range of human psychological functioning. In order to utilize new instrumentation and find etiologic contributors to psychopathology, RDoC narrows its ontology of psychological constructs by eliminating mental disorder constructs as legitimate research foci. In doing so, the project echoes Menninger's view that "the notion that there were disease entities which could be discovered and defined and delimited and confirmed by various tests ... set psychiatrists off on a wild goose chase" (Menninger, Mayman, and Pruyser 1963, 29). RDoC poses a new puzzle for psychiatry: can we understand psychopathology better if we construe it as ranges of functioning across traits or nonsyndromal constructs rather than as discrete disorders?

In describing these objectives, NIMH calls RDoC a "paradigm shift," but the rest of this discussion will demonstrate that RDoC's change in emphasis constitutes a research strategy that can be readily characterized as normal science. RDoC maintains the essential elements of the psychopathological paradigm. It develops and extends the same body of theory as does nosology-based research while establishing some new paradigmatic rules. The continuity of essential paradigm components, theoretical and nontheoretical, makes the RDoC project part of normal science.

Kuhn identifies three tasks of normal science: determination of fact through observation, matching of facts with theory, and articulation and development of theory (Kuhn 2012, 34). The following sections of this discussion will show how RDoC continues these tasks within the existing psychopathological paradigm. Since Kuhn's examples are drawn from physical science rather than psychological or biological science, I use the work of Carl Hempel and Paul Meehl to describe the progression of psychopathological science with respect to Kuhn's three tasks of normal science. Hempel characterizes the first two tasks more fully than does Kuhn and provides a more detailed description of how observations determine scientific facts (task 1) and how facts comprise scientific theory (task 2). Although Hempel's characterization has fallen out of favor in philosophy of science, it is central to our purposes for two reasons. First, Kuhn refers to paradigmatic development over time, and Hempel explains some of what Kuhn seems to presume. Second, Meehl directly builds on Hempel's characterization and provides rules for "observing" unobservable constructs, such as psychological traits and attributes. Meehl's conception of construct validity provides paradigmatic rules for Kuhn's third task of normal science, the articulation and development of theory.

Construct Validity

Construct validity provides rules for puzzle solving in the psychopathological paradigm. Although construct validity is not defined clearly or used consistently by psychiatrists, psychologists, or philosophers of science, it provides the continuity between the RDoC initiative and nosology-based psychopathology research programs. It cannot be defined in terms of either "constructs" in general or a stable concept of "validity" but instead must be understood as a synthetic concept that is only partly related to its component terms. Both the concept and the terminology originate in the philosophy of Hempel, whose work was developed and whose terminology was adopted for psychology by Meehl. In this section I show that construct validity elucidates the three Kuhnian tasks of normal science for both psychology and psychiatry, defines paradigmatic rules of research, and provides a model for understanding how RDoC is consistent with previous research programs.

Hempel's Characterization of Scientific Theory

Psychology's concept of construct validity originates in the philosophy of Carl Hempel. Hempel (1) characterizes theory development as it matures, (2) anticipates RDoC's departure from typological classification, and (3) introduces the terminology for the psychological concept of construct validity. Hempel's description of theory development echoes Kuhn's three tasks of normal science: determination of facts through observation, matching of facts to theory, and articulation and refinement of the theory. In the next section we see that Meehl shares Hempel's view of theory structure and progression and applies it to psychology; Meehl proposes construct validity as a set of rules for the conduct of psychopathological science within the paradigm.

On Hempel's view (Hempel 1965a), sciences evolve from observations of the physical world to explanatory systems of scientific laws and law-like generalizations that provide the meanings of theoretical entities. Hempel identifies three stages of scientific maturity. In the initial stage, theory consists only in simple empirical generalizations that can be tested by prediction. Observation terms provide the preliminary scientific ontology, but even in the first stage there are theoretical terms that have content beyond what a finite set of observations can provide. Hempel calls these theoretical entities "ideal constructs." They are "ideal" and "constructed" in the sense that they are "formed by the synthesis of many diffuse, more or less present and occasionally absent concrete individual phenomena, which are arranged into a unified analytical construct, which in its conceptual purity cannot be found in reality" (Hempel 1965b, 156). Ideal constructs do not exist in nature as such but build additively from serial observations and provide a conceptual richness that extends beyond discrete observations of individual phenomena. The meanings of ideal constructs, the nascent theory's theoretical terms, represent more than the finite number of observations that support them.[2]

Hempel also calls ideal constructs "ideal types" in order to emphasize that constructs can be classes of objects. However, he specifies that constructs are only construed as types or classes during the preliminary phase of theoretical development. This first phase qualitatively establishes what exists in the scientific universe and loosely captures how these entities relate to one another by positing classes and subclasses. For Hempel, however, the classification stage is transient: "[T]he use of ideal types is at best an unimportant terminological aspect, rather than a distinctive methodological characteristic" (Hempel 1965b, 171). Hempel considers classification to be a rudimentary sorting rather than a scientific end point, a conceptual scaffolding that the developing theory eventually disassembles, just as RDoC is doing with respect to DSM mental disorder types.

Hempel's second stage of theory development occurs when the scientific ontology is better established, and empirical work starts to focus on quantitative over qualitative measurement. Whereas the first phase of theory development determines what the ontology is, the second phase compares constructs and measures them along continua, or in Hempel's (and RDoC's) terms, "dimensions," working toward quantitative rankings rather than qualitative distinctions. Generalizations about these comparisons and rankings become preliminary law-like statements that can be empirically tested, which Kuhn calls the matching of fact with theory. In this second phase, the meanings of constructs begin to derive from the nascent, incomplete set of theoretical generalizations that make sense of those features (Hempel 1965b). Construct meanings at this stage are not simply observational, but neither have they obtained full systematic support. This ordering phase eliminates ideal types/constructs and instead posits "extreme types" or "prototypes" in Hempel's terms (Hempel 1965b), which represent the far ends of dimensional scales. This is what we see as RDoC expands psychopathology to psychophysiology, viewing its constructs not as taxa, but as variations that occur along a continuum from normal function to severe dysfunction (Cuthbert and Insel 2013; Cuthbert and Kozak 2013).

In Hempel's third and final phase of scientific maturity, constructs derive full meanings from observations as well as the developing system of causal laws that comprise the mature theory. In this final stage, the laws of the theory have both predictive and explanatory power, and construct meanings are provided by their roles in the entire scientific system. In a mature science with explanatory laws, regularities, and generalizations, the dimensional rankings and "prototypes" of the second phase are obviated by the full theoretical system, giving mature constructs import and meaning that derive both from observation and from the laws in which they appear (Hempel 1965a).

Hempel's three phases of theory development thus correspond with Kuhn's three tasks of normal science. The scientific ontology at Hempel's preliminary stage exists as ideal types that are synthesized from discrete observations. This corresponds to Kuhn's task of establishing facts through observation. Hempel's secondary stage of maturity replaces typological constructs with dimensional constructs to provide both more substance and more subtlety. In this stage, corresponding to what Kuhn calls the "matching of facts with theory," construct meanings begin to be determined by both observation and rudimentary theoretical content. Hempel's final stage is what Kuhn calls the task of theory articulation and development. Here, mature construct meanings are fully defined by their roles in the theoretical network, and theory has developed to be explanatory as well as predictive. We will see next that Meehl adopts this progressive view of theory development and construct meaning for psychology's construct validity.

Meehl's Conception of Construct Validity in Psychology

Paul Meehl was a professor of psychology at the University of Minnesota and a member of its Center for the Philosophy of Science. Drawing on Hempel's view of progressive theory maturity, and his conceptions of "constructs" and of systematic "validity," in the early 1950s Meehl, Lee Cronbach, and others developed the American Psychological Association's formal conception of "construct validity" (Committee on Psychological Tests, American Psychological Association 1954). In 1955 Cronbach and Meehl published the seminal paper on construct validity (Cronbach and Meehl 1955). Construct validity continues to be a central concept in the psychopathological paradigm because it promulgates Kuhnian methodological rules for ascribing meaning to unobservable constructs in psychopathology.

Meehl proposed construct validity in response to psychological functionalism, which does not acknowledge scientific entities (psychological constructs) that cannot be directly observed—for example, thoughts, fears, personalities, and tendencies—the basic stuff of psychological research at the time. Construct validity provides epistemic license to extend psychological ontology beyond what can be directly observed and operationally defined (Cronbach and Meehl 1955). In Kuhn's terms, construct validity provides a methodological rule within the paradigm. For Meehl, like Hempel, constructs can be described in both observational and theoretical terms:

> Constructs may vary in nature from those very close to "pure description" (involving little more than extrapolation of relations among observation-variables) to highly theoretical constructs involving hypothesized entities and processes. (Cronbach and Meehl 1955, 201)

Also with Hempel, observations contribute partial meanings of constructs. The full meanings of constructs are imparted by the system of laws, or "network of associations" (Cronbach and Meehl 1955), that constitute the theory. As the theoretical network develops over time, construct meanings change. Initially, a construct may be defined purely operationally, according to a few observation statements. As the theory develops and the construct becomes linked to other constructs, the construct comes to be defined by the system as a whole, and not just the observations from which it was first posited. Meehl thus adopts Hempel's view that construct meanings change as the theory matures (Cronbach and Meehl 1955; Meehl 1977).

Meehl calls a theoretical construct "valid" when its meaning derives from mature theory with causal, explanatory laws. Hempel described theoretical maturity as "validity," borrowing the same term that describes truth and legitimate inference in logic and mathematics (Hempel 1965b). Hempel does not explain how or why "validity" extends to theoretical maturity, but Meehl adopts the same terminology while adjusting the meaning. Whereas Hempel applied the term "validity" to mature nomological systems, Meehl uses it to describe the theoretical endorsement of constructs. This shift is subtle and misleading, for Meehl's "construct validity" sounds like a property of constructs. Construct validity is not a property, but rather a methodological rule for imbuing unobservable objects in a scientific ontology with meaning provided by systematic support rather than purely observational meaning. For Meehl, a construct is more or less "valid" with respect to the sophistication of the theoretical network in which it appears:

> The richer such a nomological network becomes, the more the network contributes to the contextual or implicit definition of the theoretical entities that occur in it, despite the fact that each of the single sentences attempts to make its own separate factual claim. (Meehl 1977, 37)

The term "construct validity" creates a temptation to misconstrue constructs as more or less "real," "true," or "accurate" rather than "supported" by the mature theoretical system.

With Kuhn, both Meehl and Hempel expect mature theory to provide causal explanation. Meehl writes,

> We expect a disease entity [construct] to become defined jointly by the pathology and etiology when these become known, and we recognize that it cannot be defined explicitly … until that advanced state of knowledge has been achieved (Meehl 1977, 51).[3]

In other words, Meehl expects constructs with full theoretical support to exhibit causal explanatory power. Now compare Hempel:

> The emphasis on systematic import in concept formation has been clearly in evidence in the development of classificatory systems for mental disorders. The concepts determining the various classes or categories distinguished now are no longer defined just in terms of symptoms, but rather in terms of the key concepts of *theories* which are intended to *explain* the observable behavior, including the symptoms in question. (Hempel 1965a, 149, original emphases)

Both authors believe that mature psychopathological theories provide causal explanation.

Meehl also expects that mature theories will exhibit the epistemic virtue of consilience. "Construct validation" is the process of enriching a construct's meaning by discovering other tests and procedures to support it within the paradigm (Cronbach and Meehl 1955). Validation thus requires the accrual of more *kinds* of evidence for a construct as the theory is improved and refined, which presumably provides greater doxastic support. In other words, the process of construct validation endorses the view that converging evidence from a variety of sources supports the theory and provides greater reason for belief in its unobservable entities. We will see that consilience is an important goal of the RDoC project, as is the search for causal explanation.

To summarize, Meehl's construct validity provides methodological rules for inferentially supporting unobservable theoretical psychological entities within a Kuhnian paradigm of psychopathology. Meehl applies to psychology a Hempelian view of progressive theory development, his description of how theoretical entities derive meaning over time, and his terminology. All theoretical entities are "constructs," and "valid" constructs derive meaning from the mature network of explanatory, causal laws.

Kuhn's Third Task for the Psychophysiological Paradigm: RDoC as Theory Articulation and Development

Together, Hempel and Meehl describe Kuhn's three tasks of normal science for psychology and psychiatry. Hempel and Meehl both treat the initial task, the determination of fact, as a matter of (1) making and ordering observations and then (2) positing simple law-like regularities and typologies from them. Hempel describes theory development as entailing a progression from ideal constructs/types (nominal measures) to dimensional (ordinal) measures and then, as the theory matures, to theoretical constructs whose meanings are given by the theory as a whole. Meehl uses a view of theory development similar to Hempel's to establish methodological rules for providing meaning to unobservable, psychological entities so that these can be measured and studied empirically. As theories mature, both Hempel and Meehl expect them to show explanatory as well as predictive power, and Meehl expects mature psychopathological theory to show consilience with related theories and disciplines, utilizing new instrumentation as it develops. What Kuhn calls the third task of normal science, the development and articulation of theory, also is meant to demonstrate consilience and explanatory power. RDoC takes on this task for psychopathology.

Kuhn's third task of normal science is the articulation and refinement of the paradigm under new and more stringent experimental conditions. Puzzle solving starts to integrate the instrumentation and theory of related sciences. We see this third task first being addressed in 2002 when *A Research Agenda for DSM-V* called for more advanced and cross-disciplinary puzzle solving: "It is our goal to translate basic and clinical neuroscience research relating brain structure, brain function, and behavior into a classification of psychiatric disorders based on etiology and pathophysiology" (Kupfer, First, and Regier 2002, 70), thus pushing for expanded efforts toward explanatory power and consilience, even while recognizing that nosology-based research would limit those efforts. As the paradigm developed further, it became clear that the DSM taxonomy interfered with puzzle design and puzzle solving.

RDoC makes two strategic moves. First, it continues the process of theory development and articulation but—as Hempel anticipates—it gives up both the centrality of DSM nosology and efforts toward classification in favor of dimensional, ordinal characterization of psychopathology.[4] RDoC recognizes typological mental disorder constructs in its ontology but does not prioritize them. RDoC utilizes Meehl's concept of constructs, which NIMH conceives as functional dimensions of behavior that are subject to continual refinement with advances in science (Cuthbert and Insel 2013). This move to dimensional constructs accords with Hempel's second stage of theory development:

> The advantages of ordering over classification can be considerable. In particular, ordering allows for subtler distinctions than classification; furthermore, ordering may take the special form of a quantitative procedure, in which each dimension is represented by a quantitative characteristic. And quantitative concepts not only allow for a fineness and precision of distinction unparalleled on the levels of classification and of nonquantitative ordering, but also provide a basis for the use of the powerful tools of quantitative mathematics. (Hempel 1965a, 153)

Like Hempel, RDoC explicitly moves to dimensions as an advance from the preliminary stage of psychopathological theory: "A key goal is to achieve ratio or interval scales for as many constructs and units of analysis as possible, as opposed to the leaner ordinal scales of the DSM" (Cuthbert and Kozak 2013, 930).

RDoC's second move—predicted by both Hempel and Meehl—is to develop theory with explanatory power and consilience with other sciences

(Kupfer, First, and Regier 2002; Cuthbert and Kozak 2013; Cuthbert and Insel 2013). The RDoC program utilizes new theoretical sources, investigational approaches, and technologies in order to understand both normal and anomalous psychophysiology. RDoC aims to "maximize the potential for cross-fertilization of multiple research disciplines, which will stimulate new and creative approaches to integrating their findings" (Kupfer, First, and Regier 2002, xxii). However, RDoC intends to develop paradigmatic theory, not replace it.

The RDoC program maintains the essential elements of the existing psychopathology paradigm. It also utilizes construct validity as it was proposed by Meehl. It develops the same body of psychophysiological theory as was pursued by nosology-based research. In Kuhnian terms, this continuity of paradigmatic theory and rules makes RDoC normal science.

Cuthbert and Kozak specify that RDoC research does not start from scratch but rather develops existing theory and the dimensional constructs within it:

> The business of RDoC is to concentrate on developing new measures to characterize constructs with respect to the various units of analysis, and then to validate the constructs using the nomological net approach that has classically been used for construct validation in psychology. (Cuthbert and Kozak 2013)

Other authors similarly view RDoC as a process of ongoing theory development utilizing constructs as "imperfect representations" that are intended to be refined indefinitely as the theory continues to mature (Sanislow et al. 2010, 637). Calling it the "construct network approach," one research group specifically invokes construct validity to explain how familiar clinical constructs derive meanings not just from observational generalizations, but from a theoretical network that integrates existing psychopathology theory with neuroimaging, electrophysiology, and genetics. These investigators describe the RDoC project as expanding preexisting theory by adding generalizations from new research in neural circuitry and thus "bridging between clinical problems as indexed by standard assessment methods (clinical interview or self-report) and activity in neural systems as indexed by brain response measures" (Patrick et al. 2013, 903). RDoC research strives to broaden the theoretical network for some constructs already in use, as well as to introduce new constructs that may be posited as a result of further study using genetic, molecular, cellular, and physiological techniques.

According to Kuhn, this is the work of normal science. The pathophysiological paradigm has progressed from Hempel's preliminary, pretheoretical phase of development, in which ideal types constitute the limited theoretical ontology, to Hempel's second, dimensional phase, which favors quantitative relationships over qualitative ones. The methodological rules of meaning provided by Meehl's construct validity explicitly apply, and psychophysiology is working toward Kuhn's third task of normal science, theory articulation and development. It does so by utilizing new theory and investigational techniques in molecular biology, electrophysiology, and neuroimaging (among others) to provide consilience and expand existing theory for better explanatory power. RDoC has not altered most of the commitments of the psychopathological paradigm. What it has done is de-emphasize mental disorder constructs in hopes of furthering psychophysiological science. RDoC changed the paradigmatic rules in order to further articulate and develop the paradigmatic theory.

Conclusion

I have argued that because the RDoC research program is grounded in construct validity and aims to develop existing theory, it does not constitute a paradigm shift in the technical, Kuhnian sense but simply favors other constructs over mental disorder syndromes as research foci. I traced the concept of construct validity from Hempel to Meehl, along with the attendant philosophy of theory maturation over time, and the replacement of qualitative types with dimensional constructs. I argued that RDoC explicitly assumes the centrality of construct validity and thus takes itself to be developing a preexisting and already developing body of theory. I now conclude that NIMH misdescribes the RDoC project as a paradigm shift. The advancements RDoC introduces to puzzle solving within the existing paradigm may well generate anomalies in the future, and perhaps eventually lead to extraordinary science or even crisis, but the RDoC program itself, as Kuhn would say, is business as usual.

Notes

1. DSM-III's "operational" diagnostic criteria reflect agnosticism about what the admittedly immature psychopathologic theory will eventually show rather than a disavowal of explanatory theory generally (American Psychiatric Association 1980; Pouncey 2001). Meehl agrees: "Since neither psychodynamics, classical psychometrics, taxonometrics, organic medicine, genetics, learning theory, or trait theory has proceeded by explicit identification between theoretical entities and their indicators, it would be strange to hold that rational use of DSM-III requires us to consider its syndromes as literally definitive and totally noninferential" (Meehl 1986, 223).

2. The DSM literature seldom recognizes Hempel's position on ideal constructs, and much of it construes "construct" with the antirealism of the social constructionist movement in philosophy of science (cf. Barnes and Bloor 1977). With respect to DSM, mental disorders are sometimes called "constructs" to suggest that, in contrast to unobservable, abstract terms in the rest of medicine, they are invented rather than discovered and thus have lesser ontic status (Cooksey and Brown 1998). However, it is important to recognize that in psychophysiological science, constructs are no more or less invented than are abstract entities in other fields. In Hempel's view of theory development, there is no suggestion that constructs are not real or legitimate. Calling theoretical entities "constructs" alerts us to their idealized status without entailing a commitment to antirealism.

3. In the original 1955 formulation of construct validity, Meehl limits the application of "construct" to the postulated attributes of persons that a psychological test is meant to detect or measure. In 1959, he expands "construct" to apply to disease entities and "nosological labels" (Meehl 1959).

4. Although NIMH initially describes the RDoC project as a means to a new classification, this is not one of the project's aims (Insel et al. 2010; Cuthbert and Kozak 2013).

References

American Psychiatric Association. 1980. *Diagnostic and Statistical Manual of Mental Disorders*. 3rd ed. Washington, DC: American Psychiatric Association.

American Psychiatric Association. 1994. *DSM-IV Sourcebook*. vol. 1–5. Washington, DC: American Psychiatric Association.

Barnes, B., and D. Bloor. 1977. *Interests and the Growth of Knowledge*. Boston: Routledge & Kegan Paul.

Committee on Psychological Tests, American Psychological Association. 1954. Technical recommendations for psychological tests and diagnostic techniques. *Psychological Bulletin* 51 (2, part 2 Suppl.): 1–38.

Cooksey, E. C., and P. Brown. 1998. Spinning on its axes: DSM and the social construction of psychiatric diagnosis. *International Journal of Health Services* 28 (3): 525–554.

Cronbach, L. J., and P. E. Meehl. 1955. Construct validity in psychological tests. *Psychological Bulletin* 52 (4): 281–302.

Cuthbert, B. N., and T. R. Insel. 2013. Toward the future of psychiatric diagnosis: The seven pillars of RDoC. *BMC Medicine* 11 (126).

Cuthbert, B. N., and M. J. Kozak. 2013. Constructing constructs for psychopathology: The NIMH Research Domain Criteria. *Journal of Abnormal Psychology* 122 (3): 928–937.

D'Angelo, D., S. Lebon, Q. Chen, S. Martin-Brevet, L. G. Snyder, L. Hippolyte, E. Hanson, et al. 2015. Defining the effect of the 16p11.2 duplication on cognition, behavior, and medical comorbidities. *JAMA Psychiatry*. Published online December 02, 2015.

Hempel, C. G. 1965a. Fundamentals of taxonomy. In *Scientific Explanation: Essays in the Philosophy of Science*, edited by C. G. Hempel, 137–154. New York: Free Press.

Hempel, C. G. 1965b. Typological methods in the natural and social sciences. In *Scientific Explanation: Essays in the Philosophy of Science*, edited by C. G. Hempel,155–171. New York: Free Press.

Insel, T. R. 2014. RDoC research framework will help guide the classification of patients in clinical studies [Press release]. Accessed October 30, 2014. http://www.nimh.nih.gov/news/science-news/2014/nimh-creates-new-unit-to-support-its-research-domain-criteria-initiative.shtml.

Insel, T. R., B. N. Cuthbert, M. A. Garvey, R. Heinssen, D. S. Pine, K. Quinn, C. Sanislow, and P. Wang. 2010. Research domain criteria (RDoC): Toward a new classification framework for research on mental disorders. *American Journal of Psychiatry* 167 (7): 748–751.

Kuhn, T. 2012. *The Structure of Scientific Revolutions*. 4th ed. Chicago: University of Chicago Press.

Kupfer, D. J., M. B. First, and D. A. Regier, eds. 2002. *A Research Agenda for DSM-V*. Washington, DC: American Psychiatric Press.

Meehl, P. E. 1959. Some ruminations on the validation of clinical procedures. *Canadian Journal of Psychology* 13 (2): 102–127.

Meehl, P. E. 1977. Specific etiology and other forms of strong influence: Some quantitative meanings. *Journal of Medicine and Philosophy* 2 (1): 33–53.

Meehl, P. E. 1986. Diagnostic taxa as open concepts: Metatheoretical and statistical questions about reliability and construct validity in the grand strategy of nosological revision. In *Contemporary Directions in Psychopathology: Toward the DSM-IV*, ed. T. Millon and G. Klerman, 215–231. New York: Guilford Press.

Menninger, K., M. Mayman, and P. Pruyser. 1963. *The Vital Balance: The Life Process in Mental Health and Illness*. New York: Viking Press.

Millon, T., R. F. Krueger, and E. Simonsen, eds. 2010. *Contemporary Directions in Psychopathology: Scientific Foundations of the DSM-V and ICD-11*. New York: Guilford Press.

Patrick, C. J., N. C. Venables, J. R. Yancey, L. D. Nelson, B. M. Hicks, and M. D. Kramer. 2013. A construct-network approach to bridging diagnostic and physiological domains: Application to assessment of externalizing psychopathology. *Journal of Abnormal Psychology* 122 (3): 902–916.

Pouncey, C. 2001. *The Validity of Psychiatric Nosology*. Ph.D. Dissertation, Philosophy, University of Pennsylvania.

Sanislow, C. A., D. S. Pine, K. J. Quinn, M. J. Kozak, M. A. Garvey, R. K. Heinssen, P. S. Wang, and B. N. Cuthbert. 2010. Developing constructs for psychopathology research: Research Domain Criteria. *Journal of Abnormal Psychology* 119 (4): 631–639.

Zhang, W., W. Deng, L. Yao, Y. Xiao, F. Li, J. Liu, J. A. Sweeney, S. Lui, and Q. Gong. 2015. Brain structural abnormalities in a group of never-medicated patients with long-term schizophrenia. *American Journal of Psychiatry* 172 (10): 995–1003.

6 The Promise of Computational Psychiatry

Jeffrey Poland and Michael Frank

This chapter begins with the assumptions of the present volume that a crisis exists in psychiatric research and that research concerning mental illness has entered a period of "extraordinary science." After clarifying certain key features of both the crisis and extraordinary science, we examine the reasons for the crisis so as to identify some major challenges facing mental illness research during this period. We identify four broad classes of challenge: ideological, methodological, clinical, and transitional. We then articulate a version of the innovative research program of computational psychiatry that introduces novel representational and methodological resources and holds promise for meeting some of the various challenges. Finally, we demonstrate this promise using some concrete examples of research in this area.

The Crisis in Psychiatric Research

It is now widely recognized that a crisis exists in psychiatric research based upon conventional psychiatric diagnostic categories as characterized in the American Psychiatric Association's *Diagnostic and Statistical Manual of Mental Disorders* (DSM). More specifically, it is widely recognized that (1) there is a lack of validation of diagnostic categories, (2) there is substantial heterogeneity of the categories at many levels of analysis (e.g., symptoms, causal processes), (3) there are confounding rates of comorbidity, (4) DSM categories are not well-defined phenotypes, and (5) in general the record of research employing DSM categories has been disappointing.

Several issues make these problems of classification and research impossible to ignore: concerns about apparent overdiagnosis and overmedication in conventional psychiatric practice; a complementary concern that research concerning psychiatric medications appears to have stalled (Hyman 2012); and a growing concern that conventional psychiatric practice is not suitably responsive to the needs of those in need of services, something echoed recently by the director of the NIMH (Insel 2013). The bottom line is that there has been an increasing loss of confidence in psychiatric clinical and research practices, thereby amplifying the seriousness of the current crisis in research.

Extraordinary Science

According to Kuhn (2012, chapter 8), mature sciences in crisis enter a period of extraordinary research characterized by a loss of confidence in the dominant research paradigm(s), as well as by an expanded range of research activities beyond those of "normal science," including a return to debate over fundamentals, relaxation of the "rules" of research, attempts to save the dominant paradigm, exploration of alternatives, and a role for philosophical analysis. Although not a mature science, current mental health research is arguably in such a period given the crisis and the recently shifting landscape of such research. For example, there are vigorous efforts under way to resolve some of the problems with psychiatric diagnostic categories and associated research by exploring subtypes and spectrum disorders, grouping and locating DSM disorders in a higher order diagnostic metastructure, searching for endophenotypes, postulating symptom-based dimensional approaches, focusing on transdiagnostic individual symptoms, and introducing novel research programs such as "computational psychiatry" (see below). Most visible among these various efforts is the NIMH RDoC initiative (Insel et al. 2010), which explicitly aims at relaxing the requirement that psychiatric research be conducted in terms of DSM diagnostic categories.

Why the Crisis Exists

In the present context of crisis and extraordinary science, it is important to get a line on why the crisis in psychiatric research exists, both to better understand why the DSM-based framework encounters the problems it does but, more importantly, to identify the challenges to be met if novel approaches are to be successful.

The stock explanation for why the crisis exists is that the brain sciences (e.g., genetics, neuroscience) are too immature to support an etiologically based classification system and that a symptom-based approach is all that is currently possible (Hyman 2010; Insel et al. 2010). On this view, as brain science matures, this symptom-based approach will be replaced by one based on etiology and pathophysiology. Hyman (2010) augments this explanation by claiming that, in addition, clinicians and researchers inappropriately "reified" DSM categories and expected more from them than was reasonable. Although it is true that the brain sciences are relatively immature and that the developers/adopters of the DSM were very likely guilty of inappropriate reification, we think a deeper explanation of the shortcomings of the DSM-based research program is required for clarifying the challenges ahead. This explanation is that, in fundamental ways, the DSM approach is simply not up to the job of scientifically describing and explaining mental illness; it does not "fit" the domain of mental illness (Poland 2014; Poland and Von Eckardt 2013). This lack of fit is based not only on the features of the DSM approach and the immaturity of brain science but also on the complexity of the domain. Informally, this domain consists of human suffering, distress, impairment, and deviance in which behavioral, cognitive, affective, and psychosocial capacities and processes are centrally involved. More formally, the domain can be described in terms of various critical features listed in table 6.1. See Poland (2014) for fuller discussion of these features.

The best way to understand the shortcomings of the DSM approach is that it is inadequate relative to those features. More specifically, because its representational resources are impoverished (viz., atheoretically and polythetically conceived criteria concerning clinically identifiable symptoms) and some of its assumptions (e.g., individualism, "mental disorder") are questionable, it cannot represent and manage critical features of the domain of mental illness. As a result, DSM-based research has been disappointing: its categories have not been validated and its research findings have not been robust because of unrepresented and uncontrolled sources of error,

Table 6.1
Features of the Domain of Mental Illness

Causal ambiguity
Multidimensional causal complexity
Hierarchical organization
Dynamics (on many scales)
Context sensitivity and nonlinear interactivity (within and across levels of organization)
Individual variability
Personal perspective and agency
Relational problems and processes (i.e., an assumption of individualism is problematic)
Normative pluralism and normative diversity (multiple types of norms can be applied; normal and abnormal processes are relevant)

problematic sampling and subject grouping, heterogeneity at multiple levels of analysis, and poorly conceived research questions. As a consequence, DSM-based research does not hold out much promise for responding to the current crisis. The upshot for present purposes is that during this period of extraordinary science, the mental health field is facing a major challenge: to develop an alternative approach to mental health research that is responsive to both the current crisis and the critical features of the domain. More specifically, this "big" challenge can be broken down into several subchallenges, as outlined in table 6.2.

Table 6.2
Challenges for Extraordinary Science

	Ideological/Conceptual Challenges (IC)
IC1	Development of conceptual and theoretical resources sufficient for representing and managing features of the domain of mental illness
IC2	Development of accurate and fruitful substantive assumptions concerning the domain of mental illness
IC3	Development of an appropriate approach to understanding norms concerning aspects of the domain of mental illness
	Methodological Challenges (MC)
MC1	Development of tools, techniques, and strategies for investigating phenomena exhibiting the various features of the domain (see table 6.1) and for serving various research purposes (e.g., sampling, subject grouping, measurement, design, analysis, interpretation)
MC2	Development of progressive exemplars (see table note) for research
MC3	Strategies/techniques for identifying and developing relevant norms
MC4	Appropriate incorporation of personal perspectives and agency of subjects in research programs
	Clinical Challenges (CC)
CC1	Responsiveness to the needs, interests, goals, and values of clinical practice centered around the management of clinical uncertainty: (1) provision of assays and strategies for disambiguating clinical presentations and identifying problems (assessment); (2) provision of etiologically based understanding of individual problems, processes, capacities, impairments, and so forth (understanding); (3) provision of a clinically useful taxonomy of problems (classification); (4) provision of a rational basis for clinical interventions (intervention); and (5) provision of a rational basis for preventative strategies and techniques (prevention)
CC2	Responsiveness to the needs, interests, and values of those seeking and receiving help
CC3	Responsiveness to the needs, interests, and values of society

Table 6.2 (continued)

CC4	Development of appropriate strategies for integrating scientific research findings with the realities and needs of the clinic, individuals, and society
	Transitional Challenges (TC)
TC1	Answering the question: how should research during this period of extraordinary science proceed? What sorts of bootstrapping strategies should be entertained? What practices and assumptions of existing psychiatric research and practice should be retained or suspended or rejected? Along these lines, three specific questions arise: (1) How should the existing DSM-based research record be interpreted and used, given the recognized problems with the DSM? (e.g., is it usable?; and if so, how?); (2) What role, if any, should DSM categories play in research going forward? (e.g., a cautious and modest role?; a clean break from their use?); and (3) What should be the exemplars of research during this period of extraordinary science?
TC2	Answering the question: What kinds of science should be pursued, and with what priorities? (i.e., what should the scientific research agenda look like?). Should there be a relative focus on any of the following: genetics, neuroscience, physical interventions, cognitive/psychological/social processes, developmental processes, prevention? Alternatively put: how should the various interests, needs, goals, and values of various stakeholders, combined with an understanding of the domain of mental illness, influence the character of the research agenda? (These points draw on Kitcher's idea of "well-ordered science"; Kitcher 2011.)

Note. We use the term "exemplars" in the Kuhnian sense of a concrete scientific achievement that incorporates theory, methods, findings, and standards and is productive.

The four sets of challenges listed in table 6.2 provide both substantial constraints on research as well as a fair amount of latitude. In other words, although the demands of the various challenges are severe, different researchers and research programs can position themselves in a wide variety of ways in relation to both these challenges and the assumptions and practices of conventional psychiatric clinical and research practice.

In the remainder of this chapter, we will focus on a subset of these challenges—namely, ideological/conceptual challenges (ICs) 1 and 2, methodological challenges (MCs) 1 and 2, clinical challenge (CC) 1, and transitional challenge (TC) 1—as engaged by a version of the emerging research program of "computational psychiatry." Specifically, we will outline core thematic ideas, substantive and methodological assumptions, and some specific techniques and findings so as to articulate a version of the research framework and to demonstrate its promise for meeting the various challenges identified above.

Computational Psychiatry: Assumptions and Research Paradigms

The central thematic idea underlying computational psychiatry is to bring to bear the concepts, theoretical ideas, findings, and methodological tools, techniques, and strategies of computational cognitive neuroscience on the domain of mental illness to address associated research and clinical questions and practices. The goals are that, in addition to promoting scientific research concerning mental illness, such research will also likely promote the more fundamental research agenda of computational cognitive neuroscience insofar as the study of abnormal conditions can shed light on basic science questions concerning neural, cognitive, and behavioral functioning. Further, a research program based on this strategic idea will also contribute to the development of improved clinical practices of assessment, classification, causal understanding, intervention, and prevention. The achievement of these goals will likely require more or less radical reconceptualization of clinical phenomena and more or less radical reconstitution of clinical practices. For representative expressions of versions of the thematic ideas, goals, and related assumptions and practices of computational psychiatry, see Maia and Frank (2011); Montague et al. (2012); Huys, Moutoussis, and Williams (2011); Stephan and Mathys (2014); Wiecki, Poland, and Frank (2015); Wang and Krystal (2014); and Friston et al. (2014).

A number of substantive and methodological assumptions further articulate this central thematic idea. See table 6.3 for a summary.

These substantive and methodological assumptions structure a research program aimed at explaining and understanding mental illness and informing and refining related clinical practices. To accomplish these goals, the assumptions of the program require articulated research paradigms (exemplars) for their implementation in actual research practice. Such exemplars involve concrete successful applications of methods, standards, theoretical ideas, and empirical findings designed to address specific research questions and to perform various research tasks that include the following.

Data generation and data mining (Montague et al. 2012) involves the assembling and utilization of existing or new data sets for analytic purposes. Computational modeling research practices are dependent on the existence of such data sets to both inform and constrain the construction of models and provide a basis for the subsequent testing of those models

Table 6.3
Assumptions of Computational Psychiatry

	Substantive Assumptions (SA)
SA1	The (embodied and embedded) brain is an information processor that can be understood in terms of representations and computational processes, objectives, and trade-offs at many levels of analysis.
SA2	Mental health problems are at least partly the result of normal and abnormal variants of these processes (e.g., clinical symptoms, measureable impairments, problematic interpersonal relationships).
	Methodological Assumptions (MA)
MA1	Human cognitive processes and capacities can be decomposed and understood in terms of computational models that are fit to behavioral, physiological, and other sorts of data.
MA2	The tools, techniques, and strategies of computational cognitive neuroscience are well suited for managing many of the features of the domain of mental illness (viz., complexity, hierarchical organization, dynamics, context sensitivity, nonlinear interactivity, and causal ambiguity), as well as for representing individual variability, identifying meaningful clusters, managing the heterogeneity of groups, and filling a variety of "explanatory gaps."
MA3	Clinical practices concerning mental illness (viz., assessment, classification, understanding, intervention, prevention) will be well served by the theoretical ideas, models, and techniques of computational cognitive neuroscience: for example, they will contribute to the development of: clinical assessment tools, techniques, and strategies; models of causal processes leading to deepened understanding of clinical presentations, processes, and problems; a refined approach to clinical classification that will better fit the domain of mental illness; and more effective and rationally based prevention and intervention tools, techniques, and strategies.

against novel data that have been strategically developed. The types of data collected can include data from behavioral tasks (or batteries of such tasks) aimed at probing neurocognitive capacities and processes (Wiecki et al. 2015), neurophysiological measurements (e.g., functional magnetic resonance imaging, EEG, optogenetics), genotyping, and so forth.

Computational modeling is the centerpiece of computational psychiatry aimed at using various data sets to create models of brain function at various levels of analysis. There are two general sorts of model that are widely employed in computational psychiatry: (1) biophysical models that are neural network models of interacting brain areas, neurotransmitters, pathways of connectivity, and so forth, that have a number of free parameters, and that are constrained by a variety of data, and (2) more abstract algorithmic mathematical models of cognitive processes summarizing the functional properties of brain mechanisms with only a few free parameters, which can be quantitatively fit to behavioral data, and which can be used to probe neural data (e.g., to examine whether computations and internal variables of these models are reflected in neuroimaging measurements). The employment of both sorts of model highlights computational psychiatry's commitment to engaging the hierarchical nature of human functioning and to the importance of both lower level neural processes and higher level cognitive processes in the understanding of normal and abnormal functioning (Maia and Frank 2011; Frank and Badre 2015; Wang and Krystal 2014).

Parameter extraction and computational phenotyping involve the extraction of clinically and scientifically meaningful parameters from computational models and employing them in a variety of contexts. For example, parameter estimates can provide both group- and individual-level estimates of key performance variables, thereby allowing for the scientific study of significant groups (e.g., to identify possible neural or genetic correlates) as well as the assessment of an individual's functional capacities and a study of sources of individual differences. Computational parameters can also be extracted and studied singly, or several parameters can be combined into computational functional profiles (Wiecki et al. 2015) that may help identify important subtypes within some grouping or be indicative of some deeper causal process. Finally, it may be possible to relate such parameters to components of lower level or higher level models in a hierarchically organized system, thereby possibly identifying a function of a lower level mechanism or identifying a mechanism for a higher level state or function (cf. Frank 2015 and see "linking of levels" below).

Grouping and classification of individuals can be achieved through the use of supervised or unsupervised learning algorithms applied to parameter estimates (e.g., single parameters, parameter profiles), as well as to data gleaned from behavioral tasks, genetic assays, or neurophysiological measurements. Such groupings may represent neurocognitively meaningful clusters that can be useful research targets, or they can provide the basis for clinical assessment and classification related to intervention, prognosis, or other clinical purposes. Wiecki et al. (2015) present a demonstration of this approach as applied to two existing data sets.

The *linking of levels* in a hierarchical system of computational models is an especially important task to enable identification of (1) lower level mechanisms that implement higher level functions and processes, (2) higher level functions of lower level processes, (3) mutual constraint relations between higher level and lower level processes, and (4) means for generating and testing novel hypotheses concerning any aspect of the hierarchical system and its functioning. Frank (2015) outlines a stepwise procedure for linking neural network and algorithmic models in contexts in which both sufficient knowledge about basic mechanisms that can be implemented in a neural network and candidate algorithmic models are available. In such cases, linking of levels can lead to any of 1–4 above. Further, such coordinated levels may provide constraints and predictions regarding how component processes are altered in various forms of mental illness. In other cases, however, where much less is known about basic mechanisms, it makes sense to proceed by starting at the higher algorithmic level which can characterize behavior. Such algorithmic modeling can then motivate the search for implementational mechanisms that can then be tested and used to refine the higher level models and eventually to enable more precise linking of levels.

Inferential practices concerning specific forms of pathology are often grounded in research designs that trade on models of normal functioning. Maia and Frank (2011) have articulated four such research designs (see figure 6.1) employed in computational psychiatry that underwrite different sorts of inferential practice concerning pathology: deductive, abductive, quantitative abductive, and trial-to-trial tracking of individual parameter values. Such practices are based on the use of models of normal neural or neurocognitive functioning in order to test neural or neurocognitive hypotheses regarding identifiable clinical conditions or to identify neural correlates of model-based parameters associated with some form of pathology. Such modeling can be pitched at both a group level of analysis and at the level of individual subjects. Maia and Frank proceed to demonstrate how such research designs have been applied to various clinical groups (e.g., Parkinson's disease [PD], Tourette's syndrome, schizophrenia [SZ], attention deficit/hyperactivity disorder [ADHD], substance abuse).

This overview of assumptions, tasks, and research practices characteristic of computational psychiatry provides a framework within which specific research programs and activities become articulated and pursued. In the next two sections we will provide a detailed case study of research in computational psychiatry. We begin with an overview of multilevel modeling of normal function with respect to two cognitive capacities (viz., action selection/choice and reinforcement learning; RL) and associated neural circuitry involving the cortex and the basal ganglia. We then turn to the application of this modeling activity to the study of PD and SZ.

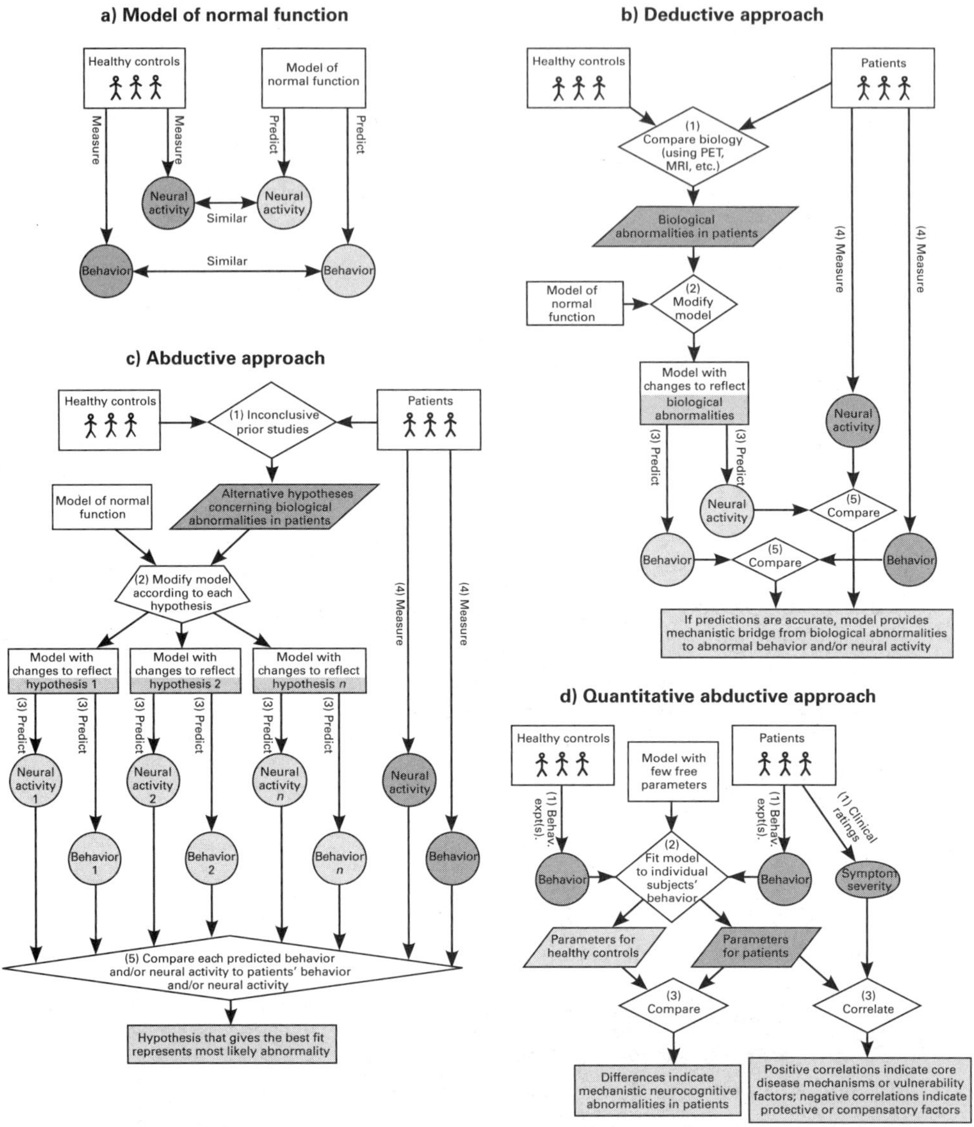

Figure 6.1

Patterns of inference in computational psychiatry. (a) The starting point is a model of normal function that captures key aspects of processing at some level of analysis (e.g., neural, algorithmic). (b) The deductive approach uses a detailed neural network model of normal function to simulate pathophysiological processes by making changes to the model that correspond to biological alterations in the disorder under consideration (e.g., alterations in striatal dopaminergic innervation). The neural and

Neural Network and Algorithmic Models of Choice and Learning

Over the past decade, evidence has accumulated (for a review, see Collins and Frank 2014) to support a neural circuit model of normal neurocognitive functioning concerning the capacities for choice (action selection) and learning. The critical circuitry involves cortico–basal ganglia–thalamo–cortico (CBGTC) loops. The basal ganglia are a collection of anatomically, neurochemically, and functionally linked subcortical structures that are part of a network of interconnected loops with the frontal cortex. Such loops modulate motor, cognitive, and affective functions, depending upon which cortical regions are involved (Frank 2011). On the basis of developments in neuroscience concerning this circuitry, neural network models have been developed to simulate the relevant processes (see figures 6.2 and 6.3).

More specifically, these CBGTC loops perform a gating function in which (1) the frontal cortex generates candidate options based on prior history of execution in the current sensory/cognitive context and (b) the basal ganglia facilitates selection of one of the candidates given their relative learned reward values. To accomplish this, there are two main projection pathways

behavioral implications of these changes can then be explored, leading to testable predictions. (c) The abductive approach uses a model of normal function to try to infer the causes of observed abnormalities in neural activity or behavior by reasoning from consequences (in behavior or neural activity) to their possible causes (e.g., underlying biological abnormalities). Specifically, alternative hypotheses concerning possible biological abnormalities in a given disorder are used to make alterations in the model of normal function, and they can be compared to determine which, if any, produce the same abnormalities in behavior and neural activity that are found in the disorder. (d) The quantitative abductive approach involves reasoning from behavior to its mechanistic causes and is used more often with algorithmic than with neural models. It involves fitting a model's parameters to the behavior of individual subjects on a suitable task or set of tasks and then determining whether there are either parameter differences between patient and healthy subject groups or correlations between parameters and disorder severity. A fourth approach (not shown) involves fitting a model to subjects' behavior, but the goal is to estimate, on a trial-by-trial basis, each subject's putative internal representation of the quantities embedded in the model (e.g., state values or prediction errors). These predicted internal representations are then used as regressors in functional imaging (e.g., functional magnetic resonance imaging, EEG), to find their neural correlates, which are then compared across the patient and healthy groups. PET, positron emission tomography; MRI, magnetic resonance imaging; Behav. Expt(s), behavioral experiment(s). (Based on Maia and Frank 2011.)

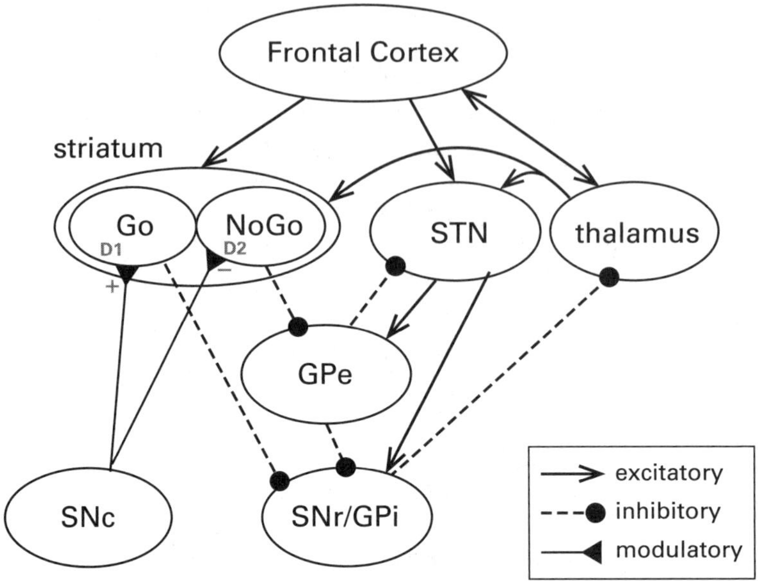

Figure 6.2
Functional architecture of the cortico–basal ganglia–thalamo–cortico circuitry. STN, subthalamic nucleus; GPe, globus pallidus external segment; SNc, substantia nigra pars compacta; SNr/GPi, substantia nigra pars reticulata and globus pallidus internal segment; D1, dopamine receptor subtype D1; D2, dopamine receptor subtype D2.

from the striatum through different nuclei to the thalamus and back to the cortex. The first direct ("Go") pathway provides evidence in favor of facilitation of a cortical action by disinhibiting thalamocortical activity for the action with the highest reward value. The second indirect ("NoGo") pathway provides evidence that an action is maladaptive and should not be gated by actively making it more difficult to disinhibit relevant thalamocortical activity. In general, for any given choice, direct pathway neurons convey the positive evidence in favor of that action based on learned reward history (i.e., its likelihood of leading to a positive outcome) whereas indirect pathway neurons convey the negative evidence concerning that action (i.e., its likelihood of leading to a negative outcome). The action most likely to be gated is a function of the relative difference in Go/NoGo activity for each action.

Some further clarifications are called for concerning the neural network model that simulates these biophysiological processes. First, dopamine (DA), supplied by projections from the substantia nigra pars compacta

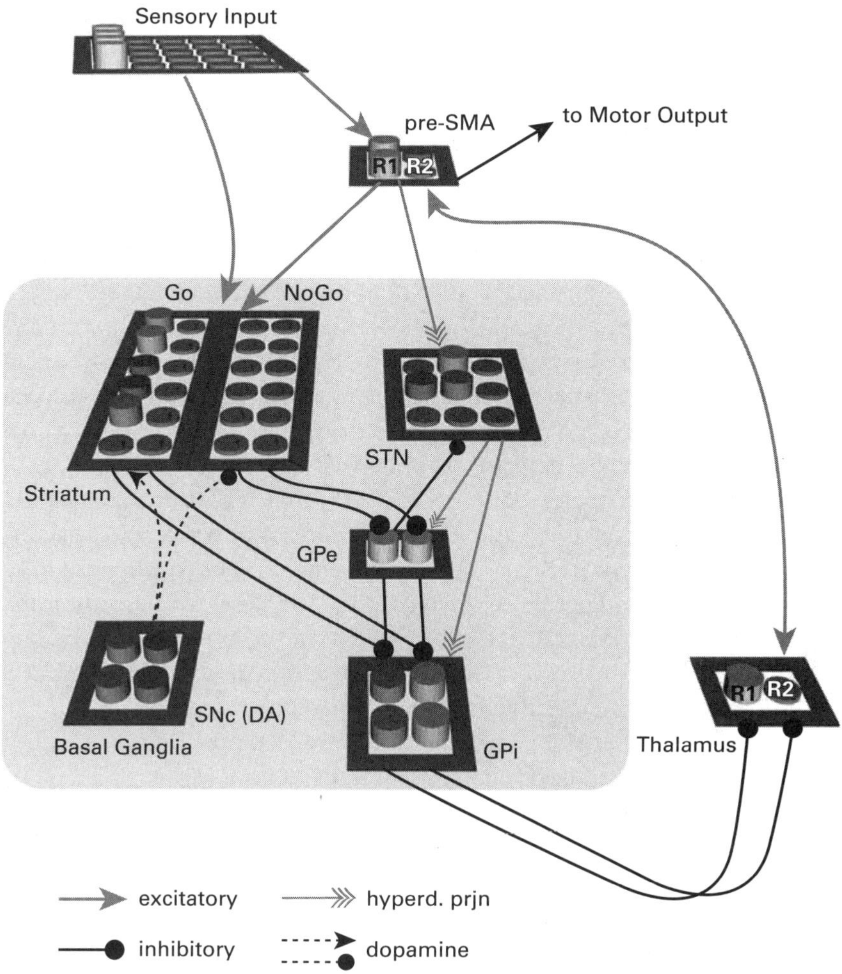

Figure 6.3

Neural network model of the cortico–basal ganglia–thalamo–cortico circuitry. The cylinders in the neural network figure represent neurons, with height and shading representing instantaneous firing rate. pre-SMA, pre-supplementary motor area; STN, subthalamic nucleus; GPe, globus pallidus external segment; SNc, substantia nigra pars compacta; DA, dopamine; GPi, globus pallidus internal segment; hyperd. prjn, hyperdirect projection; R1, response option 1; R2, response option 2.

(SNc) to the striatum, plays a major role in the operations of this circuitry. Specifically, DA influences the cost/benefit trade-off by modulating the balance of activity in the Go and NoGo pathways by differential effects on D1 and D2 receptors, respectively. Thus, even if the system has properly learned the positive and negative evidence for each action, encoded in the corticostriatal synaptic weights in Go and NoGo populations, the level of DA can then modulate which of these systems is predominantly active during choice, thereby modulating choice incentive, that is, whether choices are determined by prospective positive or negative potential outcomes. Second, as noted above, the CBGTC loops perform gating functions for motor, cognitive, and affective processes depending on what regions of frontal cortex are involved. The same principles apply to action selection with respect to all such functions (e.g., working memory [WM] gating; O'Reilly and Frank 2006). Finally, this basic model of normal function provides for a role for the subthalamic nucleus (STN), a structure that is part of the so-called "hyperdirect" pathway (see figure 6.3). In situations in which there is conflict between competing choices (e.g., due to equivocal or equally weighted evidence or to prepotent biases), such conflict is represented in mediofrontal or premotor cortices that activate the STN via the hyperdirect pathway. The role of the STN in such cases is to delay action selection by issuing a "global NoGo" signal, effectively raising the decision threshold, making it more difficult for striatal Go signals to facilitate a choice and thereby buying time to settle on an optimum choice (Frank 2006).

As mentioned above, this CBGTC model provides mechanisms for both choice (action selection) and learning. With respect to the latter, the model simulates phasic changes in DA levels that occur during positive and negative reward prediction errors (the difference between expected and obtained reward) and their effects on plasticity in the two striatal (Go, NoGo) pathways. On the one hand, phasic bursts of DA cell firing during positive prediction errors (better than expected outcome) act as teaching signals that drive Go learning of rewarding actions via D1 receptor stimulation. On the other hand, negative prediction errors (worse than expected outcomes) lead to pauses in DA firing, supporting NoGo learning to avoid unrewarding choices via D2 receptor disinhibition.

This base dynamical model of corticostriatal circuits and their effects on choice and learning can be extended in at least two ways. First, variants of the neural network model can build on this one to include multiple circuits and their interactions. For example, Doll et al. (2009) extended the basic model by incorporating units simulating prefrontal cortex/hippocampal (PFC/HC) structures and processes involved in learning and representing "rules" that might influence striatal learning processes or output choice functions; two models were created, one with PFC/HC projections to the striatum and one with projections to the motor cortex. In their investigation, they collected evidence suggesting that, in addition to a direct override of motor outputs, it is likely that there is also a top-down influence of the rules on learning processes constituting a "confirmation bias" that distorted the processing of evidence in the learning process.[1]

Second, one limitation of this sort of neural network model is that, because such models simulate internal neural dynamics consistent with a wide range of electrophysiological and neuroanatomical data, they require many more parameters than are necessary to fit to behavioral data in order to represent higher level cognitive processes. In addition, such models require many more parameters than can be identified on the basis of behavior alone. High-level computational models, on the other hand, require fewer parameters and allow abstraction away from the details of a neural implementation. Thus, a different way to extend the basic model is to add an algorithmic model that captures high-level cognitive processes implemented by the neural network model.

For example, researchers have drawn on the RL traditions in psychology and computer science to develop abstract models of normal learning from the outcomes of actions. Such models capture the tendency to incrementally learn from reward prediction errors and to select from among multiple candidate options. In one version of this approach a key parameter is a Q value that summarizes the valuation of options incremented or decremented as a function of reward prediction errors. Choice functions are then implemented via a comparison of Q values across all options and a selection of the option with the highest predicted value. Another key parameter, learning rate, captures how rapidly individuals learn from feedback, and asymmetries in learning from positive or negative outcomes can be captured by different learning rates associated with the different types of learning, or better, by refinements to include separate Q values and associated learning rates within each one that capture the functional properties of the D1/D2 system (Collins and Frank 2014). There is a clear mapping from the RL model to the neural network model, and evidence for this multilevel model mechanism is drawn from animal and human studies.

With respect to any given cognitive capacity, either sort of model (neural network, algorithmic) might or might not be available at a given stage of research. Each type has advantages and limitations, and hence each can supplement the other (i.e., focusing on one level of modeling may blind one to processes and findings available to the other). For example, high-level algorithmic models are simpler and more readily usable for quantitative behavioral fits. Further, they can include relevant processes that are out of the scope of an available neural network. An important example of this for our purposes arises with respect to the task impurity problem (TIP): the problem that variance in performance on a task is due to contributions from a variety of capacities engaged by the task, and not exclusively from a target capacity for which the task is introduced (e.g., a "reinforcement learning" task, a "working memory" task, etc.). In such cases, it might be possible for researchers to augment an algorithmic model with a key parameter even while available neural network models lack the resources for simulating the relevant processes at the neural level. Strategies for managing this problem are especially important for computational psychiatry since one major long-term objective is to develop clinical assessment tools that can identify and measure impairments in specific functional domains. Any proposed assessment tool is potentially vulnerable to the TIP and, hence, liable to provide misleading information. The following is one example of both the problem and a proposed solution.

In an RL task, Collins and Frank (2012) showed that subjects are not simply incrementally learning stimulus–action–outcome associations and choosing among them. To perform the relevant task, cognitive strategies involving hypothesis testing and WM were also engaged. Hence, when fitting behavior with the RL model alone, variance due to WM capacity was absorbed into the learning rate parameters of the RL process. Task manipulations (e.g., of stimulus set size and stimulus delay) revealed these effects; thus, the RL model required different learning rates for different stimulus set sizes, and a gene (COMT) related to the PFC (not the striatum) was predictive of the learning rate. As a consequence, an augmented RL and WM model was developed by including a module exhibiting the properties of WM (viz., with information immediately available but capacity limited and subject to decay/forgetting) that allowed for an improved fit to the data. Nevertheless, the WM process alone was not sufficient either, and indeed behavior was better accounted for by a hybrid WM–RL model (now allowing for just a single learning rate within the RL module), and where the degree to which each module governed choices was itself dynamically adjusted (i.e., WM dominated early during learning but gave way to RL as information was accumulated). Convergent genetic evidence suggested that learning rate was correlated with striatal genetic function (GPR6) whereas the PFC gene mentioned above (COMT) was no longer predictive of learning rate but instead, in this better fitting model of behavior, related to WM capacity. Thus, even in the absence of an appropriately detailed neural network model, computational methods can be deployed to isolate separate sources of variance in performance on a behavioral task, thereby addressing the TIP in research and providing a possible assessment strategy for use in clinical contexts.

The foregoing discussion provides some examples of modeling in computational cognitive neuroscience with respect to capacities for choice and learning, and it clarifies two distinct levels of modeling, both of which are important and complementary. In addition, the discussion identified a strategy for engaging the TIP and findings concerning the genetic context of circuitry function.

Computational Psychiatry: A Tale of Two Diseases

In this section, we demonstrate why computational psychiatry holds out promise for meeting many of the challenges currently confronting researchers by looking at how the above-described computational methods and models have been applied to PD and SZ.

Parkinson's Disease

Parkinson's disease is a brain disease associated with a typical symptom profile of motor impairments (e.g., bradykinesia, akinesia, hypokinesia, rigidity, tremor, and progressive motor degeneration) and with a core brain pathology: namely, cell death in the SNc, which leads to a reduction of DA in the striatum. It has also been discovered that there are associated cognitive impairments and typical treatment effects (for a review of these findings, see Wiecki and Frank 2010). Cognitive impairments associated with PD include (1) a RL bias favoring learning from negative feedback over learning from positive feedback (i.e., a bias toward avoidance learning and behavior), (2) WM impairments involving impaired updating leading to reduced tendency to maintain information such that most information is treated as irrelevant, and (3) a cognitive control impairment characterized by excessive global inhibition in high-conflict situations requiring dynamic modulation of behavior.

PD is also associated with a number of treatment effects involving DA replacement therapy and deep brain stimulation of the subthalamic nucleus (DBS/STN). With respect to DA replacement therapy, administration of the drug is associated with improved motor function and reduction of motor symptoms, a reduction in avoidance behavior, a reversal of the RL bias (i.e., increased sensitivity to positive outcomes and decreased sensitivity to negative outcomes), an increase in WM updating, increased susceptibility to distracters, impaired reversal learning, induction of dyskinesias, and a proclivity in some patients to "pathological gambling." DA replacement has no impact on impairments in the capacity to slow down in high-response-conflict situations (i.e., patients continue to exhibit excessive global inhibition in such contexts). With respect to DBS/STN, while effective for the cardinal motor symptoms of PD, there is no impact on either RL impairments or WM impairments, and the procedure does tend to induce impulsivity in high-response-conflict situations. There is, therefore, an apparent double dissociation involving DA replacement therapy and DBS/STN with respect to the cognitive impairments seen in PD.

Given this profile of symptoms, impairments, and treatment effects, we are in a position to see how computational methods can play a variety of roles in interpreting this profile and demonstrating the value of computational psychiatry in meeting some of the challenges of extraordinary science. As represented in the model, cell death of DA neurons in the SNc leads to a reduction of DA in the striatum. As can be seen in figure 6.3, which illustrates the CBGTC neural network (which includes projections from SNc to the striatum), this pathology is at the base of neural circuitry that extends throughout many components of the neurocognitive system and produces in individuals a pathogenic cascade leading to a specific deficit structure and associated symptoms, as well as a variety of treatment effects. Thus, in unmedicated PD, given the CBGTC circuit structure and the key role of DA, the diverse symptomatology and associated impairments of PD are caused by a lack of DA in the striatum which impacts on both action selection and RL. More specifically, reduced striatal DA leads to increased NoGo pathway activation (since DA normally inhibits this pathway), leading to motor suppression. This increased activation also leads to increased avoidance learning, leading to progressive motor decline and reduced updating of WM. In addition, reduced striatal DA leads to a hyperactive STN (i.e., increased NoGo excitability results in inhibited globus pallidus external segment activity and hence disinhibited STN; see figure 6.3), causing excessive global inhibition in high-conflict situations.

On the other hand, in medicated PD, DA agonists increase striatal DA, leading to inhibition of the NoGo pathway and increased activation and learning in the Go facilitatory pathway, which, in turn, account for initial alleviation of motor symptoms, later excesses of motor function (i.e., dyskinesias), increased anticipatory learning, and a consequent reversal of the RL bias exhibited in unmedicated PD. Further, medications that increase striatal DA lead to an increased (excessive) updating of WM and a related vulnerability to distracters. Finally, the model gives some insight into why it is that some PD patients exhibit a vulnerability to "pathological gambling" consequent to DA agonist therapy: namely, such behavior may be due to a positive RL bias (i.e., learning more from positive outcomes than from negative outcomes) and a consequent misjudgment of risk. Here rash or impulsive behavior is a problematic side effect of treatment that enhances available DA, and the model provides a possible mechanism for understanding why it arises.

An alternative treatment for PD involves deep brain stimulation of the STN, a treatment that initially alleviates symptoms by interfering with the hyperactive STN and reducing the associated global NoGo signal. As noted above, this treatment does not impact the RL bias and WM impairments exhibited by unmedicated patients, presumably because it has less impact on striatal DA levels. Further, chronic use of this treatment leads to increased impulsivity because disabling the STN prevents adaptive slowing in the face of response conflict (i.e., there is no dynamic braking mechanism to enable slowing down in high-conflict situations). Note that this is a separate mechanism underlying impulsivity from that which is influenced by medications. Here, in addition to a model-based explanation of treatment effects, we also have a nice example of how a clinical symptom (viz., impulsivity) can exhibit causal ambiguity requiring precise measurement for its resolution. Finally, this explanatory framework provides both a mechanistic explanation for the double dissociation between treatment modalities mentioned above and a rational foundation for treatment development and selection.

In addition to exemplifying the descriptive and explanatory resources of computational psychiatry, there are a number of other important features of this first example of computational psychiatry that highlight the strengths of the approach. To begin, PD is distinctive because it is defined by a core pathology (cell death in the SNc) which is at the head of a pathogenic cascade that propagates through the neurocognitive system given prevalent circuitry and other contextual factors (e.g., genetics). As we will see below, not all currently recognized disorder categories exhibit this feature (i.e., a core pathology at the head of a pathogenic cascade), a fact that may limit their value as research targets. The discussion above also brings to the fore the importance of a background model of normal functioning (cf. Maia and Frank 2011) for understanding the pathology of PD and how it manifests itself with respect to symptoms, impairments, and treatment effects. Thus, in this case, computational modeling of the disorder based on a model of normal function provides an explanatory framework that has led to a deeper causal understanding of how a core pathology manifests itself in a hierarchical and dynamically interactive neurocognitive system.[2] Further, as we saw, the employment of modeling techniques enables the causal disambiguation of a clinical symptom (viz., impulsivity) that can be the result of distinct causal processes. And, given the productivity of this research, this application of modeling techniques provides a possible exemplar (but not the only one) for how research in computational psychiatry can be conducted going forward.

Another aspect of this example is that computational modeling has led to a reconceptualization of the nature of the disorder (Wiecki and Frank 2010): PD is not only a motor disorder due to cell death in the SNc, but rather it is a more general disorder of the capacity for action selection, exacerbated by a learning process that induces a bias in the system to avoid selecting actions (i.e., both poverty of movement and of cognitive actions). The significance of this reconceptualization is substantial, as it both expands the scope of related (i.e., not independent) impairments and enriches understanding of the relevant causal processes. With respect to the latter, Wiecki and Frank (2010, 286) observe,

> The progressive worsening of symptoms in PD is generally attributed to the progressive cell death of dopaminergic neurons. However, the data reviewed above, along with modeling results, let this symptom progression appear in a different light. Even though it might sound counter intuitive, it seems that motor (and cognitive?) symptoms in PD are, at least partially, learned.

As they go on to point out, this opens up the question of how much of the manifest symptomatology and measureable impairments in a given case are learned due to a dysfunctional learning signal, and this reconceptualization suggests the possibility of alternative modes of intervention aimed at unlearning the symptoms (cf. Beeler et al. 2012).

Finally, computational modeling approaches provide insight into how a certain condition (e.g., modulation of striatal DA) and an associated neurocognitive structure (e.g., CBGTC action selection/learning circuitry) might crosscut crude clinical or demographic categories and yield more productive research and clinical targets. Thus, similar processes can be found in the elderly (Frank and Kong 2008; Eppinger et al. 2013) and in individuals within any number of clinical categories (cf. Maia and Frank 2011: ADHD, Tourette's syndrome, SZ, substance abuse), as well as being a part of the normal variance across individuals within the general population. As such, the model-based conditions will likely be more productive research targets than the crude clinical/demographic categories. As a consequence, this example again has implications for transitional challenges concerning how to conduct research during this period of extraordinary science, as it suggests the need for improved sampling and subject grouping strategies and techniques.

In light of the above discussion, we conclude that PD is a researchable target that, although it likely requires reconceptualization, provides a robust example of how computational assumptions and methods can lead to a productive research program that promotes the goals of computational psychiatry and meets many of the challenges of extraordinary science. We turn now to a second example that will provide a somewhat different set of conclusions.

Schizophrenia

"Schizophrenia" (or its predecessor "dementia praecox") is a psychiatric diagnostic label that has been employed in clinical and research contexts for over a century, with varying conceptualizations and diagnostic criteria including those of Kraepelin, Bleuler, Schneider, and various iterations of the DSM. Current criteria include a disjunctive mix of symptoms drawn from the following symptom categories: "positive" (e.g., the presence of unwanted psychotic symptoms such as hallucinations, delusions), "negative" (e.g., the lack of adaptive motivation, thus avolition, anhedonia, alogia, flat affect), and "disorganized" speech and behavior. In addition, cognitive impairments of attention, memory, judgment, and cognitive control, although not among the diagnostic criteria, are typically viewed as associated with the condition.

There is controversy over whether "schizophrenia" is a meaningful disorder category given its widely varying conceptualization over the past century, its generally acknowledged heterogeneity, and its somewhat disappointing research history. This is not to say that there is no such thing as severe mental illness (SMI) or that there has not been valuable research in this area (see below); it is to say that the concept of SZ writ large might not be the most useful conceptual resource for understanding SMI for either clinical or research purposes. That said, there is, nonetheless, much to be learned from a review of research in computational psychiatry on "schizophrenia." This research has targeted, in addition to the diagnostic category, clinical symptom types (e.g., positive, negative), specific clinical symptoms within these types (e.g., delusions, anhedonia, avolition), and measureable cognitive impairments in individuals (e.g., WM, RL). Researchers have also deployed both biophysical and algorithmic models useful for probing and understanding these various research targets, and for teasing apart differential contributions of various mechanisms.

Of special relevance here are findings that suggest an important role for DA and frontostriatal circuitry in the production of various symptoms and impairments associated with the diagnostic category. Although appropriate caution should be observed with respect to DA hypotheses of SZ (Kendler and Schaffner 2011), the following are working assumptions for our discussion:

Hypothesis (H) 1: SZ is associated with DA dysregulation in frontostriatal circuits (an excess of striatal DA, a deficit of prefrontal DA).

H2: Positive symptoms in SZ are associated with excess striatal DA (and D2 receptors) (cf. Abi-Dargham et al. 1998; Howes et al. 2009).

H3: Negative symptoms in SZ are associated with dysregulated DA and NMDA in PFC (cf. Weinberger 1987).

H4: Negative symptoms in SZ are also associated with reduced PFC functional integrity, and they correlate with the types of deficits exhibited in patients with orbitofrontal cortex (OFC) lesions (cf. Gold et al. 2012; Waltz and Gold 2007; Strauss, Waltz, and Gold 2014).

To the extent that reduced PFC/OFC functional integrity and DA dysregulations in frontostriatal circuits are present, computational models of frontostriatal circuits in which DA plays a critical role are worthy of exploration. Table 6.4 identifies various findings for which explanatory hypotheses exist based upon the CBGTC model, H1–H4, and specialized algorithmic models introduced to probe the findings more deeply.

As with PD, explanations of such empirical findings can be developed in terms of CBGTC circuitry, the various neurocognitive functions and processes realized by that circuitry, and DA modulation thereof. Thus, the identified "Go bias" in SZ subjects (finding [F] 1) is plausibly due to an excess of tonic DA in the striatum leading to a prepotent tendency for activation of the Go pathways in action selection; indeed, the same patterns are seen as a function of medications that elevate striatal DA in PD patients and healthy participants (Moustafa, Sherman, and Frank 2008; Frank and O'Reilly 2006). The same mechanism also predicts too much attention to irrelevant thoughts (Kapur 2003) and an associated excessive updating of WM contents. On the other hand, explanations of the identified RL bias (viz., impaired Go learning, spared NoGo learning) (F2), as well as reduced learning to speed up to maximize rewards (F6), have undergone revision. These findings were initially hypothesized to be due to either faulty phasic DA signals (e.g., reduced striatal phasic DA) or faulty striatal D1 receptor

Table 6.4
Research Findings Concerning Schizophrenia

F1	SZ is associated with a Go bias (i.e., an overall tendency to respond more in a Go/NoGo task) (Waltz et al. 2011).
F2	SZ is associated with impaired Go learning and spared NoGo learning (Waltz et al. 2007; Waltz et al. 2011; Gold et al. 2012).
F3	SZ is associated with reduced WM capacity (Collins et al. 2014).
F4	In RL tasks, SZ is associated with impaired reversal learning (Waltz and Gold 2007) and a decreased capacity to rapidly adapt choices on a trial-by-trial basis (Waltz et al. 2007); this impairment is correlated with NS severity (Strauss et al. 2011a).
F5	SZ is associated with reduced uncertainty-driven exploration of the environment (i.e., a reduced tendency to explore actions that have unknown outcomes but could potentially improve the status quo); this impairment is correlated with anhedonia (Strauss et al. 2011a).
F6	SZ is associated with failure to show normal tendency to speed responses when faced with high reward incentives (i.e., reduced likelihood of learning to speed up to maximize rewards) (Strauss et al. 2011a).
F7	SZ is associated with reduced tendency to select actions requiring physical effort particularly as the reward benefit increases; this impairment is correlated with negative symptoms (Gold et al. 2013).
F8	High NS in SZ is associated with a reduced tendency to rely on expected value when making choices between potential gains, losses, and loss avoiders (Gold et al. 2012), and patients are intransitive in their reward-based choices (Strauss et al. 2011b).

Note. F, finding; SZ, schizophrenia; WM, working memory; RL, reinforcement learning; NS, negative symptoms.

function (e.g., reduced neural responses to positive prediction errors), both of which would lead to impairment in learning from positive prediction errors (Frank 2008; Waltz et al. 2011). However, using computational approaches and refined tasks to disentangle various processes, subsequent research has suggested the identified RL impairments are due to degraded cortical functionality (e.g., disruption of WM; failure to properly represent expected value) rather than disrupted prediction error learning per se (Gold et al. 2012). Further, along the same lines, impairment in trial-to-trial adaptation of responses (F4) is plausibly the result of primarily dysregulated cortical DA function and associated functional impairments, possibly the result of frontocortical degradation (indeed similar patterns are seen in healthy volunteers with reduced PFC DA according to their genetic background; Frank et al. 2007). Finally, a similar mechanism is currently favored for explaining the findings F3, F5, F7, and F8.

We note that the association of some of these findings with specific clinical symptoms or symptom types (viz., F4, F5, F7, F8) provides a starting point for identification of mechanisms for these symptoms or for reinterpreting their significance. Thus, the discussion above has identified two broad classes of mechanisms: the first related to DA function in the basal ganglia (e.g., associated with action selection and RL), and the second related to the PFC/OFC and related DA function (e.g., associated with the representation of value during decision-making, trial–trial learning, and WM capacities). These mechanisms provide resources for explaining impairments and clinical symptoms, identifying meaningful symptom clusters and patterns, and providing productive model-based targets for research such as model parameters, clusters of such parameters, and factors that modulate circuitry functioning (e.g., genes, drugs).

In addition to the findings outlined in table 6.4, two more lines of research provide context for making sense of the various findings and demonstrating the strengths of a computational modeling approach. The first is a study demonstrating the value of modeling and task design in resolving causal ambiguity with respect to measured impairments. Collins et al. (2014), building on the work of Collins and Frank (2012) reviewed above, address the problem of task impurity in order to identify sources of impairment in SZ subjects compared to healthy control (HC) subjects when performing a "reinforcement learning" task (i.e., finding F2). At issue is whether impaired performance is due to impairment of RL processes or WM processes required for successful task performance. As a consequence of task manipulations (viz., varying the WM load across trials) and associated modeling techniques (e.g., extension of the basic model of RL to include a WM component), Collins et al. were able to tease apart contributions to task performance from both learning processes and WM processes. They concluded that the previously identified impaired performance of SZ subjects compared to HC subjects was due to impaired WM processes and not impairment of specific RL processes. This converges with the points made above which effectively conclude that a lot of the RL impairments we see in negative symptoms and previously attributed to Go learning are related to impairments of PFC/OFC in computations of expected value (Gold et al. 2012). Thus, in SZ subjects, the WM system contributes strongly to measured impairments on "RL tasks," and specialized assessment techniques are required for isolating specific sources of impairment. These findings have significance for both research and clinical practice since the TIP is a quite general problem in research concerned with mental illness, and, in clinical settings, disentangling diverse contributions to behavioral deficits is critical for assessment, causal understanding, and rational intervention planning.

One final example of how computational methods can promote the aims of computational psychiatry and respond specifically to the clinical challenges involves the impact of antipsychotic medications that operate via D2 receptor blockade. It is widely assumed that such drugs are useful for management of the positive symptoms of SZ but ineffective for the management of negative symptoms. It is also recognized that, for the most part, although the mechanisms of drug action are understood, the mechanisms by which symptoms are produced and reduced (or not) are not well understood. As a consequence, there is little rational basis for drug design or clinical use. Further, a recent paper by Wunderink et al. (2013) presents evidence that there are increased negative symptoms and dramatically reduced functional recovery at seven-year follow-up with increased antipsychotic treatment load early in the course of psychosis. This suggests (but does not prove) that antipsychotic medications have unrecognized toxic effects.

Focusing in on the impact of drugs that establish a D2 blockade, insight might be gained from computational models of corticostriatal function that postulate an important role for DA. Beeler et al. (2012), pursuing this strategy, make two model-based predictions: (1) in the presence of D2 blockade, learning from negative prediction errors (i.e., avoidance learning) will be enhanced, thereby generating context-dependent corticostriatal plasticity via the NoGo pathway and ultimately leading to suppressed motivation as a consequence of this enhanced avoidance learning (i.e., motivation is partially shaped by learning processes); (2) because this suppression is learning dependent, motivational deficits will persist even after D2 blockade has ceased. The aim of subsequent and ongoing research is to test these predictions by identifying their behavioral and neural signatures, using a combination of behavioral, optogenetic, electrophysiological, and computational tools directed upon various targets at multiple levels of analysis.

We note there is evidence that antipsychotic drugs (i.e., D2 blockers), while being ineffective in reducing negative symptoms in those diagnosed with SZ, induce "negative symptoms" in healthy subjects (Artaloytia et al. 2006). In addition, the finding of effort avoidance (viz., F7 in table 6.4; Gold et al. 2013) is something that is well established to result from D2 blockade in rodents (Salamone and Correa 2012). Thus, the model-based predictions outlined above are not specific to the SZ diagnostic grouping, but rather they likely pertain to any clinical or nonclinical target group or individual. Finally, a further model-based prediction is that the impact of D2 blockade on corticostriatal circuits (viz., increased learning from negative prediction errors) should also impact other cognitive functions (e.g., WM updating) in addition to causing biases toward avoidance learning and consequent suppression of motivation.

This line of research grounded in model-based predictions, along with the research discussed earlier, demonstrates the robustness of the model-based approach and suggests lines of research that promise to flesh out the various features of the targeted neural circuitry and the capacities it implements. Note that it also promises to inform a reconstitution of clinical practices such as the following:

- *Assessment*: For example, by identifying important dimensions of functional capacity and by providing strategies for resolving ambiguous symptom pictures and isolating specific impairments,
- *Classification*: For example, by identifying more precisely the kinds of impairments people can exhibit,
- *Individualized causal modeling*: For example, by making possible the identification of both mechanisms for specific symptoms and the causal basis of a given deficit structure in an individual, and
- *Intervention*: For example, by providing a rational basis for intervention planning and by identifying untoward consequences of current intervention practices.

In light of the above, what can be concluded regarding this research in computational psychiatry concerning the diagnostic category of SZ? Unlike the case of PD, SZ does not, as far as is currently known, have a well-established core pathology definitive of the condition and shared by all members of the diagnostic group. Rather SZ is broadly defined in terms of polythetic, atheoretical, and causally ambiguous clinical features that generate heterogeneous groupings. Hence, although some of the research reviewed above identifies some sources of this heterogeneity (e.g., genetic variation; independent processes and impairments that can lead to similar symptoms), the research findings cannot be confidently generalized with respect to the diagnostic category.

All of the findings and theoretical elaborations reviewed above trade on features of the computational model and various manipulations of that model (e.g., drugs or other factors impacting on DA function in various parts of the CBGTC circuitry) to generate predictions and explanations of clinical features or other measureable impairments. That is, processes involving DA dysregulations, modulations, and manipulations underlie pathogenic cascades throughout the circuitry represented in the models. The model helps to clarify the deficits, causal dynamics, impacts of contextual factors, and the normal/abnormal processes at work. As a consequence, the findings are of considerable value for understanding SMI and for meeting the challenges of extraordinary science, but it remains to be seen—as would be predicted—whether the very same processes generalize to other forms of SMI because of overlapping neural pathology or other factors, in which case they may not really be specific to a well-defined condition called "schizophrenia."

Further, clinically defined symptoms, more rigorously measured impairments, or model-based processes and parameters might turn out to be better research targets than the diagnostic category of SZ to the extent that they are in fact better defined and measureable. However, even here, caution is important since, as the discussion above with respect to impulsivity made clear, clinically identified symptoms are causally ambiguous and require probing to determine which causal processes are involved in a given case. Thus, links to specific symptoms like hallucinations, delusions, avolition, and anhedonia require theoretical work to establish their mechanistic basis and/or to disentangle different algorithmic processes in a computational model, and to the extent that this can be done, such symptoms can constitute useful research targets. A comparable note of caution applies to more rigorously measured impairments and model-based processes and parameters as well, to the extent that the task impurity problem arises in such cases. Part of the reason for pursuing computational approaches is that they provide tools for resolving such causal ambiguity, as the work of Collins et al. (2014) and Gold et al. (2012) demonstrated.

In sum, the examples of PD and SZ lead to somewhat different conclusions. While PD research demonstrates how research targeting the diagnostic category might effectively proceed, research concerning the diagnostic category of SZ, while of considerable value when suitably understood, points to alternative research strategies focused upon reasonably well-defined clinical symptoms, more rigorously measureable impairments, or other model-based targets.

Conclusion

How well does computational psychiatry fare with respect to the challenges (IC1, IC2, MC1, MC2, CC1, TC1) of extraordinary science? The discussion demonstrates that computational psychiatry has a rich set of representational and methodological resources for meeting the ideological and methodological challenges (IC1, MC1) concerning features of the domain of mental illness. The case study demonstrates that model-based research can be sufficiently productive to (partially) vindicate the substantive assumptions of the research program (IC2) and to provide promising exemplars for research going forward (MC2, TC1). In addition, the case study provides grounds for thinking that computational psychiatry has promise for informing both clinically relevant research and (ultimately) clinical practice (CC1). Finally, although cautionary notes were sounded regarding the use of conventional diagnostic groupings like SZ in research and uncritical reliance on the existing research record based on those groupings, the discussion also demonstrates how such research can be mined for valuable findings and how research not targeting conventional diagnostic categories can be pursued (TC1). Bootstrapping from a foundation of basic research in computational cognitive neuroscience and targeting symptoms, measureable impairments, and model-based mechanisms is one plausible strategy for pursuing research during this transitional period.

Notes

1. See also Wiecki and Frank (2013) and Collins and Frank (2013) for research implicating both processes (viz., top-down biasing influence and direct override) in processes of inhibitory control and hierarchical task set selection, respectively.

2. We note, however, that the model and current state of research is still very incomplete and that there are other related theoretical frameworks that are also useful. Research is needed to further disentangle the sometimes subtle differences between them, and that even within PD there is still some heterogeneity (e.g., degeneration of norepinephrine and 5HT neurons with increased disease progression, different clusters of motor symptoms, etc.).

References

Abi-Dargham, A., R. Gil, J. Krystal, R. M. Baldwin, J. P. Seibil, M. Bowers, C. H. van Dyck, et al. 1998. Increased striatal dopamine transmission in schizophrenia: Confirmation in a second cohort. *American Journal of Psychiatry* 155:761–767.

Artaloytia, J. F., C. Arango, A. Lahti, J. Sanz, A. Pascual, P. Cubero, D. Prieto, and T. Palomo. 2006. Negative signs and symptoms secondary to antipsychotics: A double-blind, randomized trial of a single dose of placebo, haloperidol, and risperidone in healthy volunteers. *American Journal of Psychiatry* 163 (3): 488–493.

Beeler, J. A., M. J. Frank, J. McDaid, E. Alexander, S. Turkson, M. S. Bernandez, D. S. McGehee, and X. Zhuang. 2012. A role for dopamine-mediated learning in the pathophysiology and treatment of Parkinson's disease. *Cell Reports* 2 (6): 1747–1761.

Collins, A., J. K. Brown, J. M. Gold, J. A. Waltz, and M. J. Frank. 2014. Working memory contributions to reinforcement learning impairments in schizophrenia. *Journal of Neuroscience* 34 (41): 13747–13756.

Collins, A., and M. J. Frank. 2012. How much of reinforcement learning is working memory, not reinforcement learning? A behavioral, computational, and neurogenetic analysis. *European Journal of Neuroscience* 35 (7): 1024–1035.

Collins, A., and M. J. Frank. 2013. Cognitive control over learning: Creating, clustering, and generalizing task set structure. *Psychological Review* 120 (1): 190–229.

Collins, A., and M. J. Frank. 2014. Opponent actor learning: Modeling interactive effects of striatal dopamine on reinforcement learning and choice incentive. *Psychological Review* 121 (3): 337–366.

Doll, B., W. Jacobs, A. Sanfey, and M. Frank. 2009. Instructional control of reinforcement learning: A behavioral and neurocomputational investigation. *Brain Research* 1299:74–94.

Eppinger, B., N. W. Schuck, L. E. Nystrom, and J. D. Cohen. 2013. Reduced striatal responses to reward prediction errors in older compared with younger adults. *Journal of Neuroscience* 33 (24): 9905–9912.

Frank, M. 2006. Hold your horses: A dynamic computational role for the subthalamic nucleus in decision making. *Neural Networks: The Official Journal of the International Neural Network Society* 19:1120–1136.

Frank, M. 2008. Schizophrenia: A computational reinforcement learning perspective. *Schizophrenia Bulletin* 34 (6): 1008–1011.

Frank, M. 2011. Computational models of motivated action selection in corticostriatal circuits. *Current Opinion in Neurobiology* 21:381–386.

Frank, M. 2015. Linking levels of computation in model-based cognitive neuroscience. In *An Introduction to Model-Based Cognitive Neuroscience*, ed. B. U. Fortmann and E. Wagenmakers, 163–181. New York: Springer.

Frank, M., and D. Badre. 2015. How cognitive theory guides neuroscience. *Cognition* 135:14–20.

Frank, M. J., and L. Kong. 2008. Learning to avoid in older age. *Psychology and Aging* 23:392–398.

Frank, M., A. Moustafa, H. Haughey, T. Curran, and K. Hutchison. 2007. Genetic triple dissociation reveals multiple roles for dopamine in reinforcement learning. *Proceedings of the National Academy of Sciences of the United States of America* 104 (41): 16311–16316.

Frank, M. J., and R. O'Reilly. 2006. A mechanistic account of striatal dopamine function in human cognition: Psychopharmacological studies with cabergoline and haloperidol. *Behavioral Neuroscience* 120:497–517.

Friston, K., K. Stephan, R. Montague, and R. Dolan. 2014. Computational psychiatry: The brain as phantastic organ. *Lancet. Psychiatry* 1:148–158.

Gold, J. M., G. P. Strauss, J. A. Waltz, B. M. Robinson, J. K. Brown, and M. J. Frank. 2013. Negative symptoms of schizophrenia are associated with abnormal effort-cost computations. *Biological Psychiatry* 74:130–136.

Gold, J. M., J. A. Waltz, T. M. Matveeva, Z. Kasanova, G. P. Strauss, E. S. Herbener, A. Collins, and M. J. Frank. 2012. Negative symptoms and the failure to represent the expected reward value of actions. *Archives of General Psychiatry* 69 (2): 129–138.

Howes, O. D., A. Egerton, V. Allan, P. McGuire, P. Stokes, and S. Kapur. 2009. Mechanisms underlying psychosis and antipsychotic treatment response in schizophrenia: Insights from PET and SPECT imaging. *Current Pharmaceutical Design* 15 (22): 2550–2559.

Huys, Q., M. Moutoussis, and J. Williams. 2011. Are computational models of any use to psychiatry? *Neural Networks* 24:544–551.

Hyman, S. 2010. The diagnosis of mental disorders: The problem of reification. *Annual Review of Clinical Psychology* 6:155–179.

Hyman, S. 2012. Revolution stalled. *Science Translational Medicine* 4 (155): 1–5.

Insel, T. 2013. Director's Blog: Antipsychotics: Taking the long view. Posted on the National Institute of Mental Health website (August 28): http://www.nimh.nih.gov/about/director/2013/antipsychotics-taking-the-long-view.shtml.

Insel, T., B. Cuthbert, M. Garvey, R. Heinssen, D. S. Pine, K. Quinn, C. Sanislow, and P. Wang. 2010. Research Domain Criteria (RDoC): Toward a new classification framework for research on mental disorders. *American Journal of Psychiatry* 167 (7): 748–751.

Kapur, S. 2003. Psychosis as a state of aberrant salience: A framework linking biology, phenomenology, and pharmacology in schizophrenia. *American Journal of Psychiatry* 160 (1): 13–23.

Kendler, K., and K. Schaffner. 2011. The dopamine hypothesis of schizophrenia: An historical and philosophical analysis. *Philosophy, Psychiatry, & Psychology* 18 (1): 41–63.

Kitcher, P. 2011. *Science in a Democratic Society*. Amherst, NY: Prometheus Books.

Kuhn, T. 2012. *The Structure of Scientific Revolutions*. 4th ed. Chicago: University of Chicago Press.

Maia, T., and M. Frank. 2011. From reinforcement learning models to psychiatric and neurological disorders. *Nature Neuroscience* 14 (2): 154–162.

Montague, P. R., R. J. Dolan, K. J. Friston, and P. Dayan. 2012. Computational psychiatry. *Trends in Cognitive Sciences* 16 (1): 1–9.

Moustafa, A., S. J. Sherman, and M. J. Frank. 2008. A dopaminergic basis for working memory, learning, and attentional shifting in Parkinsonism. *Neuropsychologia* 46:3144–3156.

O'Reilly, R., and M. Frank. 2006. Making working memory work: A computational model of learning in the frontal cortex and basal ganglia. *Neural Computation* 18:283–328.

Poland, J. 2014. Deeply rooted sources of error and bias in psychiatric classification. In *Classifying Psychopathology: Mental Kinds and Natural Kinds*, ed. H. Kincaid and J. Sullivan, 29–63. Cambridge, MA: MIT Press.

Poland, J., and B. Von Eckardt. 2013. Mapping the domain of mental illness. In *The Oxford Handbook of Philosophy and Psychiatry*, ed. K. W. M. Fulford, M. Davies, R. G. T. Gipps, G. Graham, J. Z. Sadler, G. Stanghellini, and T. Thornton, 735–752. Oxford: Oxford University Press.

Salamone, J. D., and M. Correa. 2012. The mysterious motivational functions of mesolimbic dopamine. *Neuron* 76 (3): 470–485.

Stephan, K., and C. Mathys. 2014. Computational approaches to psychiatry. *Current Opinion in Neurobiology* 25:85–92.

Strauss, G., M. Frank, J. Waltz, Z. Kasanova, E. Herbener, and J. Gold. 2011a. Deficits in positive reinforcement learning and uncertainty driven exploration are associated with distinct aspects of negative symptoms in schizophrenia. *Biological Psychiatry* 69 (5): 424–431.

Strauss, G., B. Robinson, J. Waltz, M. Frank, Z. Kasanova, E. Herbener, and J. Gold. 2011b. Patients with schizophrenia demonstrate inconsistent preference judgments for affective and nonaffective stimuli. *Schizophrenia Bulletin* 37:1295–1304.

Strauss, G., J. Waltz, and J. Gold. 2014. A review of reward processing and motivational impairment in schizophrenia. *Schizophrenia Bulletin* 40 (Suppl. 2): S107–S116.

Waltz, J. A., M. J. Frank, B. M. Robinson, and J. M. Gold. 2007. Selective reinforcement learning deficits in schizophrenia support predictions from computational models of striatal-cortical dysfunction. *Biological Psychiatry* 62 (9): 756–764.

Waltz, J. A., M. J. Frank, T. V. Wiecki, and J. M. Gold. 2011. Altered probabilistic learning and response biases in schizophrenia: Behavioral evidence and neurocomputational modeling. *Neuropsychology* 25 (1): 86–97.

Waltz, J. A., and J. M. Gold. 2007. Probabilistic reversal learning impairments in schizophrenia: Further evidence of orbitofrontal dysfunction. *Schizophrenia Research* 93:296–303.

Wang, X. J., and J. H. Krystal. 2014. Computational psychiatry. *Neuron* 84:638–654.

Weinberger, D. 1987. Implications of normal brain development for the pathogenesis of schizophrenia. *Archives of General Psychiatry* 44:660–669.

Wiecki, T. V., and M. J. Frank. 2010. Neurocomputational models of motor and cognitive deficits in Parkinson's disease. In *Recent Advances in Parkinson's Disease—Part I: Basic Research, Vol. 183*, ed. A. Bjorklund and M. A. Cenci, 275–297. Progress in Brain Research. Amsterdam: Elsevier.

Wiecki, T., and M. Frank. 2013. A computational model of inhibitory control in frontal cortex and basal ganglia. *Psychological Review* 120:329–355.

Wiecki, T., J. Poland, and M. Frank. 2015. Model-based neuroscience approaches to computational psychiatry: Clustering and classification. *Clinical Psychological Science* 3:378–399.

Wunderink, L., R. Nieboer, D. Wiersma, S. Sytema, and F. Nienhuis. 2013. Recovery in remitted first episode psychosis at 7 years of follow-up of an early dose reduction/discontinuation or maintenance treatment strategy: Long-term follow-up of a 2-year randomized clinical trial. *JAMA Psychiatry* 70 (9): 913–920.

7 Personalized Psychiatry and Scientific Causal Explanations: Two Accounts

Aaron Kostko and John Bickle

Personalized medicine, despite its recent increased attention, is not new (Steele 2009; Offit 2011). Medical practitioners have long sought to include information about the unique aspects of a given patient when offering diagnoses and treatment options. Hippocrates himself is said to have advised that it is more important to know what sort of person has a disease than to know what sort of disease a person has. Attending to unique aspects of a patient has long been recognized as necessary in psychiatry. As McMahon and Insel (2012, 773) point out, "Emphasis on the unique aspects of a patient is, in fact, nothing new for psychiatry. Effective psychiatric care has always been challenging, in part, precisely because it has always been personalized." The reason for the renewed interest in personalized psychiatry is the nature and extent of unique patient information now available. Psychiatrists no longer have to make do with attending only to individual patients' experiences, clinical narratives, and environmental circumstances. To cite just one example: psychiatric pharmacogenomics, which investigates how genes affect responses to specific drugs, now makes it possible to use information about a patient's genome to make more reliable diagnoses or to tailor drugs specifically for individual patients (Mrazek 2010).

Renewed interest in personalized psychiatry has, in turn, renewed attention to another of psychiatry's persistent concerns: its aspirations to scientific legitimacy. These two concerns interrelate. On the one hand, the proper diagnosis and treatment of psychiatric conditions requires that individual patients' experiences, life history, gender, race, socioeconomic status, interpersonal relationships, environmental and biological risk factors, and even self-interpretations and -understandings of one's own conditions predominate clinical assessment. On the other, constructing a scientifically valid and reliable classification of psychiatric conditions and developing more efficacious treatments requires abstracting away from the particular details of individual patients. The scientific legitimacy of psychiatry seems to hinge upon acquiring generalizable results from controlled trials regarding causal mechanisms which generate psychiatric symptoms and treatment responses. Yet, overreliance on generalizable results and preoccupation with causal mechanisms seems incompatible with the aims of personalized psychiatry. It risks ignoring the heterogeneity associated with many psychiatric conditions, leading to potential misdiagnoses and harmful or futile treatments, as well as undervaluing those features specific to individual patients.

Among the many factors contributing to this tension is disagreement over which causal variables should be included in classifying and explaining psychiatric conditions, and whether a single, coherent account of causal explanation can accommodate all relations across these variables. Psychiatry's aim to be more personalized seems to require an account of causal explanation that acknowledges the relevance of the individual variables we mentioned above. James Woodward's (2003, 2008) interventionist account seems to fulfill exactly this aspiration and has already been endorsed (implicitly or explicitly) by several prominent philosophers of psychiatry (Murphy 2006; Campbell 2008; Kendler and Campbell 2009; Kendler 2012, 2014; Graham 2013). The aim of psychiatry to be more scientific, however, may be established more directly if it adopts an account of causal explanation clearly operative within the biomedical sciences. Historically, this aim has tended toward characterizing psychiatry as a branch of clinical medicine, most recently of clinical neuroscience or neurology (Nasrallah 2013; Andersch 2012; Murphy 2006; Insel and Quirion 2005; Martin 2002; Yudofsky and Hales 2002). Silva, Landreth, and Bickle (SLB) (2013) have recently developed an account of causal explanation derived directly from landmark experimental case studies from the cellular and molecular neuroscience of learning and memory. If applicable to the biomedical sciences informing current psychiatry, such an account would support psychiatry's aspired scientific status.

To the extent that Woodward's account accommodates the causal relevance of the variables central to personalized psychiatry, it must also show how these variables can be integrated with those operative within the biomedical sciences. That is, it must show how variables such as individuals' experiences, narratives, and environmental circumstances integrate with hypothesized cellular and molecular mechanisms. Conversely, to the extent that SLB's account accommodates the causal relevance of the variables operative within the biomedical sciences, it must also show how it accommodates the variables central to personalized psychiatry. In this chapter we explore these possibilities by applying each of these accounts to recent research in social neuroscience and environmental epigenetics that bears directly on psychopathology. The first section outlines the two accounts of causal explanation. The next section applies both to two recent examples of basic scientific research in psychiatry. The third section introduces some basic commitments that are constitutive of personalized psychiatry and considers the extent to which both accounts of causal explanation fulfill these commitments. In the end, we suggest that while both accounts realize these commitments, the SLB account better illuminates at least one crucial aspect of actual scientific practice that Woodward's account misses—or at least fails to emphasize.

Two Accounts of Scientific Causal Explanation

The importance of causal-mechanistic details for psychiatric classifications and efficacious treatments seems beyond dispute. This is evidenced by recent attempts to incorporate details from genetics, neuroimaging, cognitive science, and pathophysiology into the *Diagnostic and Statistical Manual of Mental Disorders*, fifth edition (Kupfer and Regier 2011) and by the National Institute of Mental Health's recent launch of the Research Domain Criteria (RDoC) project (Insel et al. 2010). However, despite this recognized relevance, there is no consensus yet as to whether incorporating such details is always necessary or even desirable. Radden (2003), for example, argues instead that a descriptivist classification, which categorizes psychiatric conditions according to their common symptoms, typical course, and prognosis, can be preferable to an etiologically based classification. Descriptivist approaches rely on empirically verifiable hypotheses and remain theoretically neutral with respect to the causes of psychiatric conditions. It is also possible to use probabilistic evidence to provide treatments without knowing the causal mechanisms responsible for the treatment's efficacy; in some cases the treatment itself enables discovery of the causal mechanisms involved. Recent examples include deep brain stimulation (Campaner and Galavotti 2012) and the use of antipsychotic drugs as experimental tools (Tsou 2012).

Despite their potential for developing clinically useful classifications and probabilistically based treatments, descriptivist approaches suffer a major shortcoming: they fail to be *explanatory*. To fully explain the symptoms associated with psychiatric conditions and the efficacy of treatments, an understanding of the relevant causal-mechanistic details is necessary. This is even the case if one hopes to establish a more personalized psychiatry since different causal mechanisms may lead to the same clinically identifiable symptoms or underlie individual variation in treatment response. Of course, which causal-mechanistic details are necessary for establishing a more personalized psychiatry, and which account of causal explanation can best elucidate these details, remains an open question. Woodward's (2003, 2008) interventionist account rests upon the basic idea that two variables are causally related when the value of one "makes a difference" to the value of the other. More specifically, two variables are causally related when an intervention that changes the value of one also changes the value of the other in a regular, stable way. Although there may exist varying degrees of stability between two variables, the general idea is that a stable relationship continues to hold despite changes to other variables within the system, and across a variety of individual and environmental contexts. To illustrate this, consider a hypothesized psychological explanation for clinical depression: negative self-evaluation (M1) causes distressed mood (M2). On Woodward's interventionist account, one can causally explain M2 as the result of M1 to the extent that one can intervene to change an individual's self-evaluation, for example, from positive (or some other value) to negative, in such a way so as to reliably change the individual's mood, for example, from contented (or some other value) to distressed. So long as that relationship between the values of two variables remains invariant despite changes to other variables within the system, and across a variety of individual and environmental contexts—that is, remains "stable"—the interventionist account claims a causal explanation for M2 by M1.

One attractive feature of Woodward's account is that his analysis of an "ideal intervention" captures standard practices of scientific experimental control. Intuitively, the notion is that of an intervention I on X that changes the value of X, and thereby changes the value of Y only by way of the change to X. Thus, intervention I cannot change Y directly; it cannot change some causal intermediary lying between X and Y except by (first) changing X; it cannot be correlated with some other variable C which is a cause of Y; and it must act as a "switch" which controls X, irrespective of any other causes of X. Testing for these possible confounds of an intervention I on X to change Y is part and parcel of the scientific practice of incorporating control conditions into intervention experiments to test causal hypotheses.

Thus, stability for Woodward amounts to a kind of invariance, and invariance requires two crucial features. First, the variables that figure into an invariant generalization must be well-defined. Woodward (2008) characterizes a well-defined variable as follows: "[I]t must be the sort of thing that it makes sense to think of as a target for an intervention and there must be a well-defined, unambiguous answer to the question of what will happen to other variables of interest under this intervention" (142). So for negative self-evaluation to count as a well-defined variable it must be clear what constitutes an intervention onto its value, for only then can the stability of the intervention be judged scientifically. A failure to satisfy either of the conditions that Woodward mentions in the quote above generates the concern that the hypothesized causal variable is not actually the variable upon which one is intervening, or perhaps that one needs to split that variable into more fine-grained species. To return to our hypothetical example above, if negative self-evaluation cannot be well-defined in Woodward's sense, at the very least one might worry that more fine-grained causal variables, for example, negative self-evaluation involving intrusive memories, or negative self-evaluation involving obsessive thoughts, and so on, are the targets of the intervention.

Second, the invariant generalization relating the two variables must exhibit what Woodward refers to as "contrastive focus." He articulates this notion as "the contrast between X's taking some value x and taking some different value x′ that causes the contrast between Y's taking value y and taking some different value y′" (2008, 143). This feature highlights the significance of discovering causal thresholds and the possibility of systems' responding differentially to a particular range of inputs but not to others. Both features are important for disentangling the complex causal processes involved in most psychiatric conditions. For instance, to determine the causal relevance of negative self-evaluation to distressed mood, it will be necessary to establish a certain threshold of self-evaluation that, if exceeded, will bring about a change in mood. It will also be necessary to establish the range or varieties of negative self-evaluation to which a particular individual (or class of individuals) will respond. Failure to establish these features can lead to misleading causal claims and skepticism about the causal relevance of the variable in question. However, to the extent that one can intervene into a well-defined variable so as to reliably bring about a threshold effect or range of effects with respect to another well-defined variable, on Woodward's account it makes no difference if the variables are more coarse-grained or higher level. It also makes no difference if the variables are instantiated in only a single individual.

This applicability of invariance directly to higher-level variables is what makes Woodward's account of scientific causal explanation appealing to personalized psychiatry. His account thereby purports to accommodate both higher-level causal explanations, like our hypothetical example between negative self-evaluation and distressed mood, and interlevel causal explanations, such as an extension of our hypothetical example to negative self-evaluation and hypothesized lower-level mechanisms. This applicability grounds Woodward's (2008) response to Kim's causal exclusion problem for higher-level kinds. According to Woodward, Kim's argument depends upon a mistaken commitment to the existence of fundamental causal explanations. Woodward emphasizes how his interventionist account countenances the causal efficacy of higher-level properties while avoiding the problem of causal exclusion. On Woodward's account two variables are causally related when an (ideal) intervention that changes the value of one well-defined variable changes the value of another in a regular, stable fashion. When applied to our hypothesized causal relation holding between the higher-level variable of negative self-evaluation (M1) and some lower-level neurobiological property, say, P2, the physical realizer of distressed mood (M2), Woodward can claim that M1 causes P2 so long as one can intervene to change an individual's self-evaluation, for example, from positive (or some other value) to negative, in such a way as reliably to change the value of P2.

Woodward's account thus offers a strategy for accommodating the causal relevance of the kinds of higher-level variables central to personalized psychiatry, and for integrating these variables in scientific causal explanations with hypothesized lower-level mechanisms. However, although his account removes any a priori obstacles to establishing the causal relevance of higher-level variables, it leaves as an open empirical question whether there are any actual higher-level causal generalizations or generalizations relating higher-level and lower-level variables that are sufficiently stable to be of practical use within personalized psychiatry. Any such generalizations will need to hold invariantly across changes to other variables within the system, and across a variety of individual and environmental contexts for that individual at least, to inform diagnostic or treatment decisions within psychiatric practice.

In their recent (2013) book Alcino Silva, Anthony Landreth, and John Bickle adopt a purely metascientific perspective on causal explanations in science. Seeking to avoid "external" epistemological and metaphysical assumptions, they instead focus exclusively on describing the practices in landmark examples of causal explanations from recent science. They draw their examples exclusively from the field of *molecular and cellular cognition* (MCC), which studies the cellular and molecular mechanisms of cognitive functions, most successfully those of learning and memory. Their examples include detailed experimental results which, when integrated, have led molecular and cellular neuroscientists to conclude that components of various intraneuronal signaling pathways are a component of the causal mechanisms for cellular long-term potentiation (LTP, a form of activity-dependent synaptic plasticity), and more interestingly specific aspects of learning and memory. They derive a set of experimental conditions directly from these landmark studies that practicing scientists deem sufficient to establish causal mechanistic hypotheses.

SLB's metascientific investigations reveal that three distinct kinds of successful experiments are needed to establish such causal hypotheses with scientific confidence. Each kind is required because each provides a unique type of evidence for the hypothesized causal explanation. *Negative manipulations* decrease the probability or intensity of the hypothesized mechanism (A) and measure the effects on B—more precisely, in MCC experiments, on some behavioral measure widely accepted as indicating (cognitive function) B's occurrence for the purposes of laboratory experimentation. When successful (and properly controlled), negative manipulations establish that hypothesized mechanism A is necessary for B: no (or reduced) A, no (or reduced) B. At present negative manipulations constitute the "bread and butter" of MCC experiments and publications, employing increasingly sophisticated ways both to reduce/eliminate A and measure B. But even the best, most tightly controlled negative manipulations cannot show whether A is a triggering cause of B or a background condition necessary for B to occur. *Positive manipulations* provide evidence for A's being a genuine triggering cause, especially in light of successful negative manipulations. In a positive manipulation experimenters raise the probability or intensity of hypothesized mechanism A and measure for B; when successful, B also increases. Since manipulating background conditions positively above biological baseline rarely produces systematic changes to the target effect, successful positive manipulations typically give good evidence that a hypothesized mechanism, especially one already shown to be causally necessary by negative manipulations, is a genuine triggering cause of B, not merely a necessary background condition. And when positive manipulations mimic the hypothesized cause artificially and generate the effect, they show that the hypothesized cause is sufficient for the effect. Yet, even still, experimenters cannot know whether the successful positive manipulation effects are simply artifacts of the artificial experimental environment (that increased the probability or intensity of A). *Nonintervention experiments*, where occurrences of A and B are measured and correlated in as biologically realistic an environment as making the required measurements will allow, can settle this final question. We can be confident that our positive manipulation experimental results, in light of the negative manipulations, are genuine and nonartifactual if occurrences of A and B are correlated appropriately in nonintervention experiments, where A is not experimentally manipulated.

Two remarks flesh out the above discussion. First, these descriptions of experiment types hold for hypothesized excitatory causal mechanisms for B. For hypothesized inhibitory mechanisms the effects on B of the different manipulations on A are exactly reversed. Second, the term "nonintervention" can confuse. It often takes a lot of "intervening" into the system (especially its nervous system) to make the required measurements to establish these A–B correlations. However, the value of A is not being intervened on—experimentally altered—in these experiments, unlike in the other two kinds. In nonintervention experiments A's co-occurrence with B is simply being tracked. Typically, one needs to manipulate the system experimentally in some way in nonintervention experiments to ensure B's occurrence, to then see if hypothesized mechanism A is correlated properly with B.

On the SLB account, no one kind of these experiments is sufficient to establish a causal hypothesis with full scientific confidence. But when successful and taken together, evidence for a specific causal explanation ($A \rightarrow B$) from all three kinds of experiments provides the first of four critical kinds of *integration of experimental results*, in this case, what SLB refer to as *Convergent 3 Analysis*. Scientists are more confident that a hypothesized causal explanation $A \rightarrow B$ has been justified experimentally when results from all three kinds of experiments testing it have been integrated successfully.[1]

SLB's full account of scientific confidence in causal explanatory practice does not end with the Convergent 3. Other forms of integration of multiple experiments and their results are also crucial toward establishing a causal mechanistic hypothesis relating molecules to cognitive functions. Some of these other forms constitute control experiments done in conjunction with the principal Convergent 3 experiments. *Eliminative Inferences* are control procedures that rule out alternative causal hypotheses. *Consistency Analyses* relate one set of experimental results to others using either identical (*replication analysis*) or altered (*proxy analysis*) experimental protocols (both for manipulating A and measuring B). Experiments and results related by these principles of integration can include those of one or multiple labs. Finally *Mediation Analysis* explores existing gaps lying between the variables of an established causal hypothesis—namely, one for which Convergent 3 evidence has been reported in the published literature and properly controlled by Eliminative Inferences and Consistency Analyses. These gaps are filled by hypothesized mediating causes. Cellular and molecular neuroscientists are never content with even an established causal hypothesis (like CREB activation → late LTP → memory consolidation). They want to know the causes that mediate this established causal connection. This discontent has nothing to do with reductionistic metaphysical scruples, and everything to do with accepted causal explanatory practices in their field of research. Without its integration into a chain of mediating causes, practicing scientists will often remain skeptical of even a molecular mechanism → cognitive function hypothesis for which a full Convergent 3 Analysis has been provided. And eventually each one of those mediating causes must be established experimentally—via Convergent 3 Analysis, Eliminative Inferences, and Consistency Analyses. (For detailed explications and examples drawn directly from landmark MCC publications, see SLB 2013, chapters 3 through 7.)

How does experimental work from higher-level neuroscience—systems, behavioral, cognitive—get integrated into this picture? Answer: in every fashion these components allow. Sometimes as Eliminative Inferences, ruling out specific alternative explanations of the data unveiled by positive and negative manipulation experiments. Sometimes as causal mechanistic hypothesis generators for novel molecular manipulations, a form of Mediation Analysis suggesting cellular and molecular mechanisms that might be good targets for further experimental manipulations. Sometimes for providing better behavioral, or even physiological, measures for specific cognitive functions. Higher-level neuroscience sometimes provides initial causal-mechanistic explanations, as we will see in the next section. Without question higher-level research is critically important for MCC, and not just "heuristically." These data are part of the integrated evidential basis for fully justified causal-mechanistic explanations of cognitive functions by cellular and molecular mechanisms. However, higher-level data and explanations are never judged complete as causal mechanisms in MCC. There are always thought to be mediating causes still to be uncovered, invariably at lower levels of biological organization, which the experimental tools of MCC allow one directly to manipulate and test. With the experimental tools at our current disposal, causal mechanistic explanations currently bottom out in molecular pathways—that is typically the lowest level at which we can intervene directly to generate statistically significant behavioral changes. That, however, is nothing more than a contingent fact about what we can manipulate on the current laboratory bench to affect specific behavioral changes.

Neuroscientists working at higher levels of the field sometimes miss just how prevalent these "ruthlessly reductive" *practices* are in mainstream neuroscience. (Although more often it is philosophical commentators, not scientists, who miss this.) A quote from the previous edition of one of neuroscience's principal textbooks, now almost a decade and a half old, is illuminating:

> This book ... described how neural science is attempting to link molecules to mind—how protein responsible for the activities of individual nerve cells are related to the complexity of neuronal processes. Today it is possible to link the molecular dynamics of individual nerve cells to representations of perceptual and motor acts in the brain and to relate these internal mechanism to observable behavior. (Kandel, Schwartz, and Jessell 2000, 3–4)

This attitude reflects what has been doable experimentally in neuroscience for the past quarter-century, not an allegiance to reductionist metaphysics. MCC has been at the forefront of these experimental efforts.

Two Case Studies

If SLB's (2013) account of scientific causal explanation accurately reflects actual neuroscientific practice in providing evidence for hypothesized causal-mechanistic explanations, then while causal generalizations in neuroscience involving higher-level variables are confirmed by empirical data, cellular and molecular neuroscientists also proceed to Mediation Analysis for further confirming evidence; that is, to search for the lower-level causes that mediate between established higher-level connections. Woodward's (2008) account, on the other hand, sees no fundamental differences between high-level and lower-level causal explanations; interventionism nowhere insists upon anything resembling SLB's Mediation Analysis aimed at lower-level causes as part of the justificational complex for causal hypotheses between higher-level variables (although it does not rule out such endeavors, either). Recent research in social neuroscience and environmental epigenetics intuitively relevant for developing a more personalized psychiatry thus provides interesting case studies toward assessing these differing accounts of scientific causal explanation.

Of particular importance for the themes of this volume is a model of cocaine addiction and anxiety disorder developed by Michael Nader's lab (Nader and Czoty 2005; Morgan et al. 2002; Czoty, McCabe, and Nader 2004), and another of maternal behavior and long-lasting epigenetic effects in offspring developed by Michael Meaney's lab (Weaver et al. 2004). These two models highlight some of the conceptual and methodological tensions that exist between personalized psychiatry and causal-mechanistic science. Both Nader's and Meaney's models attempt to integrate information about the effects of individuals' environmental circumstances on underlying neurobiological and epigenetic mechanisms, a goal toward which personalized psychiatry should strive. More generally, both models illustrate how researchers deal with interlevel causal relations in actual scientific practice—a challenge that proponents of personalized psychiatry encounter regardless of which specific higher- and lower-level variables their clinical practices concern. Whether one is interested in individual patients' experiences, life histories, gender, race, socioeconomic status, interpersonal relationships, environmental and biological risk factors, or interpretations and understandings of their own condition, a fully personalized psychiatry requires an understanding of if and how these variables relate to one another, as well as to lower-level biological causes that few will deny are relevant. The research we will look at in this section provides exemplars toward realizing this goal. A contrast between how Woodward's and SLB's differing accounts of scientific causal-mechanistic explanation illuminate the actual science generating these specific models will thus be crucial toward determining which account offers the better picture of how the science works which potentially informs a personalized psychiatry.

Research in Michael Nader's lab investigates effects of social rank in macaque troop dominance hierarchies on the number and availability of dopamine D_2 receptors in the brain, and on individual monkeys' susceptibility to self-administering cocaine. Previous rodent studies had shown that disruptions to dopaminergic systems alter responses to reward and the reinforcing effects of cocaine. The Nader lab extended this research to nonhuman primates, measuring the impact of individual versus social housing on the number and availability of dopamine D_2 receptors and cocaine self-administration. Morgan et al. (2002) reports that twenty macaque monkeys were individually housed for 1.5 years. Positron emission tomography scans determined the relative distribution of neuronal D_2 dopamine receptors, a class which had previously been implicated in cocaine reinforcement and addiction. All individually housed monkeys, regardless of their eventual place in troop dominance hierarchies following social housing, began the study with statistically similar D_2 receptor distribution volume ratios in their basal ganglia. However, once the transition from individual to social housing (groups of four monkeys) occurred and a stable dominance hierarchy had been established, monkeys that achieved dominant status showed a statistically significant increase in basal ganglia D_2 receptor distribution ratios (compared with their own ratios when housed individually). There were no such increases in monkeys that attained any subordinate status. This receptor increase produces a decreased amount of synaptic dopamine (since more receptors are available for ligand binding). Higher levels of synaptic dopamine, referred to as "dopaminergic hyperactivity," have previously been associated with an increased vulnerability to drug abuse. Consistent with this prior finding, the socially housed dominant monkeys of Nader's lab self-administered cocaine less frequently than the subordinate monkeys, both in terms of the number of intravenous injections self-administered per session and the total amount of cocaine injected. At optimal doses, total cocaine intake per session by individual subordinate monkeys more than doubled that of individual dominants.

While monkeys' social rank had a significant influence on D_2 receptor distribution and cocaine self-administration during initial exposure to the drug, a follow-up study with the same monkeys showed that continued long-term cocaine exposure attenuates this influence. Czoty et al. (2004) found no significant differences, in either D_2 receptor distribution volume ratios in basal ganglia or cocaine self-administration, in all socially housed monkeys who had self-administered cocaine several times a week for 2–5 years, regardless of troop dominance ranking. Continued exposure to cocaine led to increased self-administration by dominant monkeys, suggesting that the drug eventually serves as a reinforcer in all monkeys regardless of social rank. The authors hypothesize that this attenuated effect of social rank indicates a progression of cocaine usage phases. The Morgan et al. (2002) study represents the effects of initial exposure, referred to as the "acquisition" phase. The Czoty et al. (2004) study, on the other hand, tracks the impact of continuous exposure, referred to as the "maintenance" phase. Nader and his colleagues contend that one should not expect that environmental variables influencing cocaine's initial reinforcing effects (acquisition), namely, social rank, need be the same ones influencing the drug's later reinforcing strength (maintenance).

Although these scientists insist that further research is needed to determine the neurobiological states associated with the progression of drug abuse phases, the authors suggest that one implication of their results is clear. Since the changes in D_2 receptor number and distribution in basal ganglia, and susceptibility to self-administer cocaine initially, could not be predicted prior to the emergence of a monkey's status in a group dominance hierarchy, vulnerability to drug abuse acquisition is *more* a consequence of social/environmental factors than of genetic predisposition. Regardless of the relative causal significance of environmental and biological factors, their research clearly establishes the causal relevance of environmental variables. The authors are explicit: "An organism's environment can *produce* profound biological changes that have important behavioral associations" (Morgan et al. 2002, 169). Although neurobiology is necessary to understand changes in D_2 receptor distributions, the Morgan et al. (2002) results seemingly cannot be interpreted correctly without acknowledging the causal relevance of social influences, particularly the monkeys' positions within the group dominance hierarchy at the time of initial cocaine exposure.

Before we apply Woodward's (2008) and SLB's (2013) analyses to this case, it is useful to consider first what a classical reductionist might say. The classical reductionist is likely to resist the Nader lab's interpretation, or at least to reinterpret it in a way that denies that social rank is a genuine cause of D_2 receptor number and distribution in monkeys' basal ganglia. For a genuine causal relationship, the classical reductionist demands a specification of the neuronal mechanisms whereby social rank exerts its influence on behavior, and this would mean that those mechanisms must ultimately connect with the molecular mechanisms that drive D_2 receptor gene expression and protein synthesis in particular neurons. More generally, according to classical reductionism, before one can refer to the environment—or to any cause postulated by higher-level sciences to explain a measured neurobiological or behavioral effect—one must be able to explain how that factor is transduced down to neuronal and molecular mechanisms. For it is only the latter that drive neurotransmitter release into neuromuscular junctions, to elicit muscle contractions (i.e., behavior), and gene expression and protein synthesis that changes receptor numbers and distribution.

This reasoning is exactly what Woodward's interventionist account is intended to avoid. Even if there are relevant causal details regarding gene expression and protein synthesis (which surely there are), these details only add to an already existing causal explanation, rather than replace it. The causal explanation relating the variables of social rank and changed D_2 receptor number and distribution would still hold, if properly established by interventionist procedures, even with the addition of any further causal details. On the interventionist account, so long as social rank is a well-defined variable, and interventions that change the value of that variable bring about changes in D_2 receptor number and distribution in a regular, stable way, then the generalization relating social rank and D_2 receptor number and distribution should be treated as a genuine causal explanation.

If that generalization turns out to admit of numerous exceptions, then it will likely be too unstable to constitute a genuine causal explanation. Classical reductionists would then have good reason to recommend looking down biological levels to find a more stable generalization. However,

Nader's results appear stable enough. In cases of reliably stable higher-level generalizations, satisfying classical reductionist's requirement on a genuine causal-mechanistic explanation seems overly demanding, and in some cases empirically intractable (Harris and Schaffner 1992). Woodward's account minimizes such demands. Although abstracting away from molecular mechanisms and focusing exclusively on social rank may compromise explanatory power, it also provides a greater degree of generality. To the extent that basic scientific research like Nader's ultimately aims at clinical application, this increase in generality may actually provide greater therapeutic utility—for example, by suggesting more tractable variables amenable to clinical manipulation. Of course, whether such increased generality leads to enhanced therapeutic utility is always an open empirical question. If specific molecular mechanisms are discovered that enable researchers to more systematically identify a monkey's position in a dominance hierarchy, and in turn to more reliably intervene so as to change D_2 receptor number and distribution and susceptibility to self-administer cocaine, then, at least in this case, classical reductionism would be vindicated. However, one strength of Woodward's interventionist approach is that it lays the burden of proof on the classical reductionist. Until the reductionist can provide sufficient evidence to show that a lower-level generalization is more stable *and* offers greater therapeutic applicability than one involving higher-level variables, a relatively stable generalization involving higher-level variables should be treated as a genuine causal explanation.

One final note: Nader and colleagues perhaps were too quick to insist on having found a causal explanation of basal ganglia D_2 receptor distribution and increased cocaine self-administration acquisition in terms of group hierarchy ranking (as they claimed in the quotation cited above) when their work is viewed from Woodward's account. For they did not *intervene*, much less ideally (or even approximately ideally) into the social dominance hierarchies. They simply let the hierarchies emerge and measured the hypothesized lower-level effects. More experimental work clearly needs to be done to justify their hypothesized causal explanation from Woodward's perspective. This fact nicely illustrates the logical strength of Woodward's detailed account. Genuine interventions on the hypothesized cause need actually to be done, and not just any old interventions—only ones that approximate the conditions on ideal interventions.

Applying SLB's account likewise illuminates key features and concerns. Notice first that SLB's account separates the two hypothesized causal connections at issue here, social rank → basal ganglia D_2 receptor distribution and social rank → susceptibility to cocaine self-administration in acquisition phase. None of the experiments reported here tests either of the following hypotheses:

- A basal ganglia D_2 receptor distribution → susceptibility to cocaine self-administration in acquisition phase.
- A susceptibility to cocaine self-administration in acquisition phase → basal ganglia D_2 receptor distribution.

One could, of course, hypothesize either for future experimental study.

Second, and more importantly, the Morgan et al. (2002) experiments provide only nonintervention experimental evidence for even these limited hypothesized causal connections. This is for the same reason we noted in applying Woodward's account above: social rank was not experimentally manipulated, either positively or negatively. Thus, taken in their strongest light, on an SLB analysis these experiments only show that social rank in troop dominance hierarchy *is correlated with* both increased basal ganglia D_2 receptor distribution and with increased susceptibility to self-administer cocaine in acquisition phase, in a manner consistent with a genuine causal connection. Recall that on an SLB account, that is the weakest of the types of Convergent 3 experimental evidence required for scientific confidence in a causal hypothesis. It suggests immediate experiments that could be done to bolster scientific confidence. Positive manipulations directly of social rank that show increases in both effects, and negative manipulations that show decreases, under properly controlled conditions (including those of Eliminative Inference and Consistency Analyses) would be the needed next studies. However, where Woodward's account saw the need for genuine experimental interventions that at least approximate the ideal, SLB's account sees the need for various kinds of intervention (manipulation) experiments and their successful integration.

Let's suppose that scientists perform these recommended intervention/manipulation experiment(s), and they are successful. On an SLB account, we would then have full Convergent 3 evidence for the social rank → basal ganglia D_2 receptor distribution and the social rank → increased susceptibility to cocaine self-administration during acquisition phase hypothesized causal explanations. On an SLB analysis, which experiments should be tackled next? One strategy would be to test for a causal connection between these two connections. Do we have connected causal processes, such as social rank → basal ganglia D_2 receptor distribution → increased susceptibility to cocaine self-administration during acquisition phase, or social rank → increased susceptibility to cocaine self-administration during acquisition phase → basal ganglia D_2 receptor distribution? Or are these separate effects themselves unconnected: basal ganglia D_2 receptor distribution ← social rank → increased susceptibility to cocaine self-administration during acquisition phase? Testing each of these causal hypotheses requires Convergent 3 evidence, Eliminative Inferences, and Consistency Analyses, so even if we assume that the experiments hypothesized in the previous paragraph are successful, the scientific work here has only just begun.

There also remains Mediation Analysis. Even with full Convergent 3 evidence for a hypothesized causal connection A → B, cellular and molecular neuroscientists seek mediating mechanisms. In the Nader case, *how* does dominant social rank cause increased D_2 receptor numbers and distribution in primate basal ganglia? *How* do subordinate ranks cause increased susceptibility to cocaine self-administration during the acquisition phase? Even with full Convergent 3 evidence—which, we emphasize again, is *lacking* in the results we surveyed from the Nader lab—cellular and molecular neuroscientists seeking mechanisms of cognitive functions remain less confident in a hypothesized causal connection until experimental evidence for real mediating causes, typically lower level, is found. The SLB account, derived directly from landmark experimental results in these sciences, shares this emphasis with classical reductionism. But *not* for the goal of reductionist metaphysical purity! Rather, as part of an explicit analysis of the typically implicit principles that have driven scientific practice in one central (well-funded and well-published!) field of recent experimental neuroscience. Without question this strategy is tied to the experimental tools available to these scientists and their quarter-century track record of using these tools to find and justify hypothesized lower-level mediating causes.

Clearly, both Woodward's and SLB's accounts of causal explanations avoid difficulties surrounding classical reductionism, especially when applied to a specific case study from the kind of basic science that might inform developments in personalized psychiatry. But before we contrast some specific advantages offered by each approach, let's see how each applies to another, even more influential scientific case study with promise for personalized psychiatry.

Consider a much-cited paper from Michael Meaney's lab on the epigenetic effects of maternal behavior on adult offspring (Weaver et al. 2004). Prior results had shown that rat pups reared by mothers who frequently licked and groomed them (high LG), and used an arched-back style of nursing (ABN), were less fearful and showed a more modest stress response, compared to pups reared by low-LG/ABN mothers, as measured by markers like blood corticosterone levels (a ubiquitous stress hormone) and the amount of time animals spend immobile during a forced swim task. These effects persist into offspring adulthood. Cross-fostering studies had also previously shown that these physiological and behavioral effects were reversible. When offspring from low-LG/ABN mothers were reared by high-LG/ABN mothers, they too became less fearful and showed a more modest stress response. Offspring from high-LG/ABN mothers raised by low-LG/ABN mothers showed exactly the reverse (more fear, increased stress response). These prior findings suggest that variations in maternal behavior serve as a causal mechanism for the nongenomic transmission of persistent individual differences in stress reactivity across life span, extending well beyond the one-week postpartum that rat mothers engage in these behaviors.

One goal of Meaney's research is to determine the mechanisms underlying these long-lasting behavioral effects. They first found that offspring reared by low-LG/ABN mothers had significantly higher levels of methylation of the glucocorticoid receptor (GR) gene in hippocampus neurons, compared to offspring reared by high-LG/ABN mothers. Moreover, they found significantly higher levels of this methylation both in offspring that were born to and reared by low-LG/ABN mothers and those born to high-LG/ABN mothers but cross-fostered to low-LG/ABN mothers, compared to offspring born to and reared by high-LG/ABN mothers and those born to low-LG/ABN but cross-fostered to high-LG/ABN mothers (Weaver et al., 2004).

Leaving aside many of the molecular details, the basic effect here is that increased methylation of the GR gene blocks transcription factors from gaining access to promoter regions, causing decreased gene transcription and ultimately decreased synthesis of GR proteins in hippocampus neurons in the low-LG/ABN offspring. This decrease produces decreased sensitivity to glucocorticoid negative feedback, that is, of feedback which is important for inhibiting the synthesis of corticotropin-releasing factor (CRF, a stress-related hormone) in the hypothalamus–pituitary–adrenal (HPA) axis. Thus, decreased sensitivity to such feedback, due to increased GR gene methylation in the low-LG/ABN-reared offspring, generates higher levels of hypothalamic CRF, leading to the increased stress responses. These epigenetic mechanisms, mediating the maternal behavioral cause through specific gene expression, generate the life-span effects long after the maternal behavior has ceased. Meaney's group acknowledged that further research needed to be done to fully determine how maternal behavior causally interacts with the specifically targeted exon region of the GR gene their research uncovered, but they argue explicitly that their results provide compelling preliminary evidence for "environmental programming of adaptive stress responses across generations" (Weaver et al. 2004, 852).

Meaney's research differs from Nader's in that it seeks initially to provide more of the mechanistic details whereby the hypothesized environmental cause exerts its neurobiological effects. On Woodward's interventionist account, however, the established causal relationship shown to hold between maternal behavior and extent of methylation of the GR gene in offspring hippocampus neurons remains explanatory, even in light of the additional causal details. On Woodward's account, so long as maternal behavior is a well-defined variable, and interventions that change its value bring about changes in methylation of the GR gene in hippocampus neurons in a regular, stable way, then the generalization relating LG/ABN maternal behavior, methylation of the GR gene in hippocampus neurons in offspring, and the measures of decreased stress responses in adult offspring is genuinely causal. Note that Woodward's conditions clearly seem met in the case of Meaney's research. The specific cross-fostering reported in Weaver et al. (2004) at least approximates Woodward-style ideal interventions directly into maternal behavior, and the changes in hippocampus GR gene methylation vary accordingly.

The application of SLB's account to this case is more complicated. For the hypothesized high-LG/ABN maternal behavior → decreased methylation of hippocampus GR gene in offspring connection, Meaney and his colleagues found nonintervention evidence when they simply measured and compared hippocampus GR methylation in offspring from both low-LG/ABN and high-LG/ABN mothers without cross-fostering. However, their cross-fostering studies provide both positive manipulation and negative manipulation evidence, which integrated successfully with each other and with the evidence from the nonintervention study. Rearing offspring of low-LG/ABN mothers by high-LG/ABN mothers is a positive intervention: the hypothesized mechanism, the specific maternal behavior, is increased in these rats. And rearing offspring of high-LG/ABN mothers by low-LG/ABN mothers is a negative intervention. That this positive intervention produced decreases in hippocampus GR gene methylation compared to low-LG/ABN offspring nursed by their low-LG/ABN mothers (the nonmanipulated controls), and the negative manipulation produced the appropriate increases (compared to high-LG/ABN nonmanipulated controls), shows that Meaney and colleagues were able in this single study to provide full and integrated Convergent 3 evidence for the hypothesized causal connection. According to SLB's account, our scientific confidence in this hypothesized causal explanation should increase accordingly.

An SLB account of this study goes further. First, we can hypothesize links between this newly established causal explanation, namely, high-LG/ABN maternal behavior → decreased methylation of hippocampus GR gene (and the related low-LG/ABN counterpart explanation), and other already established causal explanations, such as the following:

- High-LG/ABN maternal behavior → decreased corticosterone levels in adult offspring.
- High-LG/ABN maternal behavior → attenuated stress response in standard behavioral tests.

We can also incorporate the following previously established causal links into our account:

- Decreased methylation of hippocampus GR genes → increased hippocampus sensitivity to glucocorticoid negative feedback → decreased HPA stress response.
- Decreased HPA stress response → decreased bloodstream corticosterone levels and decreased HPA stress response → attenuated stress response in standard behavioral tests.

The result of all these hypothesized connected linkages is a hypothesized *causal pathway*: high-LG/ABN maternal behavior → decreased methylation of hippocampus GR genes → increased sensitivity to glucocorticoid negative feedback → decreased HPA stress response → decreased bloodstream corticosterone levels, and → attenuated stress response in standard behavioral measures, with the last two nodes both connected individually with decreased HPA stress response, but not yet with each other. (We also have the related causal pathway that begins with low-LG/ABN maternal behavior.) Details of the full hypothesized causal pathway become apparent in this graphical representation, and we can fill in at each causal step the full and integrated Convergent 3 experimental evidence that has been obtained and what is still lacking (see Silva, Landreth, and Bickle 2013, chapter 7).

Having established a full and integrated Convergent 3 analysis for the hypothesized high-LG/ABN maternal behavior → decreased methylation of hippocampus GR genes, which investigations did the Meaney lab tackle next? There were numerous candidates. They could have investigated other higher-level variables associated with rat maternal behavior, to spell out further the network of higher-level causes. They could have refined the environmental cause they had confirmed, finding more behavioral distinctions between high- and low-LG/ABN maternal behavior extremes, and tried to link these more specific behavioral variables to more specific measures of hippocampus GR gene methylation. They could have searched for additional higher-level environmental or maternal neural system-wide modulators of this established epigenetic mechanism, perhaps turning to modeling and dynamical systems theory, or to principal component (statistical) analysis, either to abstract away from or seek to isolate, respectively, any number of plausible higher-level modulators. Standard philosophical understanding of social neuroscience practice, of the assumed hierarchical structure and dynamics of environment–system couplings, of the nonlinear interactivity, and of the context sensitivity of the causal variable involved (maternal behavior) would recommend they do one of these or some related higher-level inquiry.

Meaney's lab did nothing of this sort. Instead, and directly in keeping with SLB's metascientific hypothesis about the role and practice of Mediation Analysis in cellular and molecular neuroscience, they turned their attention—and their molecular-biological experimental tools—next to chromatin activity state changes hypothesized to affect DNA methylation. Chromatin gates promoter accessibility to gene transcriptional proteins. Weaver et al. (2004) reports that two measures of active chromatin, histone acetylation and nerve growth factor 1-A (NGF1-A) binding to a specific exon on the GR promoter gene in hippocampal neurons, were significantly increased in adult high-LG/ABN-reared offspring as compared to low-LG/ABN-reared offspring. The results of this nonintervention study suggested that maternal behavior exerts its causal influence on hippocampus GR expression, and subsequent HPA function, through epigenetic alterations regulating NGF1-A binding to that specific exon.

Like typical nonintervention studies on the SLB account, this result immediately suggested additional negative and positive manipulation experiments. To no molecular neuroscientist's surprise, Meaney and colleagues next report the results of one such experiment. In a follow-up SLB-negative manipulation experiment Meaney and colleagues showed that this hypothesized causal mechanism, NGF1-A binding at that specific exon of the hippocampus GR gene, was reversible by use of a histone deacetylase inhibitor in vivo that blocks histone acetylation and subsequent transcription factor binding (Weaver et al. 2004, figures 4 and 5). And this pharmacological reversal had exactly the predicted effects on the behavioral and physiological measures of high-LG/ABN rearing. These are exactly the kinds of lower-level studies that constitute Mediation Analysis on the SLB account of scientific causal-mechanistic explanation.

Despite features of their target phenomenon that so readily prompt philosophers and cognitive scientists—and some systems neuroscientists although their numbers are vastly smaller than their cellular/molecular colleagues—to insist on higher-level investigations, Meaney's lab did instead exactly what SLB's account predicts. They employed the powerful, well-tested, continually successful experimental tools and protocols of molecular biology/neuroscience and found lower-level mediating molecular-genetic mechanisms of their initial epigenetic discovery. This strategy choice was not informed by reductionistic metaphysics but by recognized scientific practices in what has constituted neuroscience's mainstream for more than two decades. Philosophers might wish that more neuroscientists worked at higher levels of biological organization, but most (not all!) neuroscientists realize the promise of working with the experimental tools and strategies that have boosted causal-mechanistic neuroscience to the scientific status it enjoys today, no matter how "dynamic" and "nonlinear" the target phenomenon appears. This strategic choice is central to SLB's account. This account of Mediation Analysis in mainstream neuroscientific practice, plus the emphasis on the integrative nature of evidence for scientific causal explanations, from different kinds of experiments which provide different kinds of evidence, are two features central to SLB's account, which Woodward's account fails to emphasize.

Implications for a Scientific Personalized Psychiatry

The extent to which the Woodward and SLB accounts of scientific causal explanation are compatible with personalized psychiatry depends ultimately on what is required to make psychiatry more personalized. One common and relatively uncontroversial commitment of personalized psychiatry focuses on the ethical or practical dimensions of the psychiatrist–patient relationship and suggests that psychiatrists should strive to be more empathetic when interacting with their patients. Achieving this may require psychiatrists to listen more carefully to patients' narratives, attend more fully to patients' experiences and environmental circumstances, and be more inquisitive about how these conditions are affecting patients' life goals and projects from the perspective of the patient. If personalized psychiatry only entails these minimal extrascientific commitments, then both the Woodward and SLB accounts of scientific causal explanation are fully compatible with personalized psychiatry, primarily because the ability to realize these commitments is independent of and compatible with any particular account of scientific causal explanation.

A stronger personalized psychiatry focuses on the epistemological features of psychiatric practice, and advises psychiatrists to seek out and utilize any potentially relevant information about the unique aspects of individual patients, in order to make more reliable diagnoses of and tailor treatments to individual patients. Such information might include patient experiences, life history, gender, race, socioeconomic status, interpersonal relationships, environmental and biological risk factors, and the patient's own interpretation and understanding of his or her condition. If seeking out and utilizing such information is indeed what personalized psychiatry requires, then Woodward's account would seem to be more compatible with personalized psychiatry than the more reductionistically aligned SLB account. Although the Woodward interventionist interpretation of the two case studies does not show that reductionism, even classical, is necessarily false, it does challenge a priori reasons for ruling out higher-level variables as components of genuine causal explanations. It also provides solid empirical reasons for thinking that such causal explanations exist in actual neuroscience practice, especially in those fields of neuroscience that seem poised to ground a scientific psychiatry. Woodward's account accommodates unabashedly the causal relevance of the sorts of variables that are central to this stronger personalized psychiatry, and provides a strategy for integrating these variables with ones operative within the biomedical sciences. By separating the issue of causal relevance from mechanistic implementation, Woodward's account accommodates the multifactorial nature of causes for psychiatric conditions while remaining consistent with the scientific search for mechanisms. As Kendler (2014, 3) points out, the interventionist approach "can accommodate phenomena occurring at [the] supra-individual level." This result "allows psychiatrists freedom to use whatever family of variables seems appropriate to the characterization of a disorder" (Kendler and Campbell 2009, 883). For this reason, Woodward's account is more compatible with the aims and goals of a stronger personalized psychiatry than is classical reductionism.

With one caveat, SLB's account of scientific causal explanation also seems capable of fulfilling this commitment of a stronger personalized psychiatry. So long as information about the unique aspects of patients can be utilized with some scientific confidence, despite a lack of established mediating causes transduced down to cellular and molecular mechanisms, the SLB account is consistent with this stronger requirement. On SLB's account, Convergent 3 evidence is evidence for a genuine causal relation between any two neuroscientific variables, regardless of their level. Searching for and finding mediating causes, especially lower-level ones concerning the components that compose these higher-level kinds, can still increase scientific confidence that a genuine causal relationship has been established, without *requiring* us to have detailed Mediating Analysis in hand before putting these Convergent 3–established causal explanations to clinical use.

The account therefore recognizes higher-level kinds in the causal links it sees as established by actual neuroscientific research and acknowledges that these kinds can be linked as causes to any kinds of effects, so long as Convergent 3 evidence is either available or under active scientific pursuit. Even here, however, it is important not to underestimate what full Convergent 3 evidence requires; recall from the "Two Case Studies" section above that the Nader results do not provide it for either the hypothesized troop dominance rank → D_2 receptor number and distribution in primate basal ganglia or the troop dominance rank → susceptibility to cocaine self-administration in the acquisition phase connections since no positive or negative manipulation studies were done.

Because of its direct incorporation of more cellular/molecular neuroscientific experimental details into its basic account of scientific causal explanation, SLB's requirements for increased scientific confidence in a causal explanation requires scientific personalized psychiatrists to be more cautious before utilizing certain information about the unique aspects of patients in a clinical context than does Woodward's account. Still, the SLB account seems capable of utilizing this information. However, in another sense these additional requirements of the SLB account might advance the aims of a scientific personalized psychiatry over and above what the Woodward interventionist approach provides.

Consider recent research in psychiatric pharmacogenomics. Scientists have identified structural variations in relevant neurons and genes that carry functional implications for treatment response (Mrazek 2010). The clinical goal of this research is to develop safer and more effective drugs and dosages tailored to individual patients, or at least to specific patient populations. Much of this research has focused on stratifying patient populations with major depressive disorder, schizophrenia, and bipolar disorder based upon biomarkers for altered neural circuitry, for example, cerebrospinal fluid protein expression patterns (Maccarrone et al. 2013), or genes implicated in drug metabolic rates and side effects (Coutts and Urichuk 1999; Binder and Holsboer 2006; Arranz and De Leon 2007). The most significant results involve discovered polymorphisms in cytochrome *P*450 genes, particularly the CYP2D6 and CYP2C19 variants, both of which are implicated in the metabolism of antidepressant and antipsychotic medications for major depressive disorder and schizophrenia. Coutts and Urichuk (1999), for instance, stratified patient populations into poor metabolizers, extensive metabolizers, and ultrarapid metabolizers based upon variations in the CYP2D6 and CYP2C19 polymorphisms. These groupings enabled dosages to be tailored to individual patients to increase efficacy and minimize side effects. Demonstrating the therapeutic utility of these advances still requires clinical information for validation—phenomenological, behavioral, and environmental (Arranz and Kapur 2008). However, the backing by actual science is equally essential to this research and its clinical applicability. The SLB approach seems to capture this second feature. If personalized psychiatry seeks contact with actual biomedical science, it would do itself well to model its approach to basic science on one drawn directly from experimental practices in those very sciences, that is, cellular and molecular biology/neuroscience.

Acknowledgments

Thanks to the volume editors, Şerife Tekin and Jeffrey Poland, for their excellent comments on earlier drafts, which led to numerous improvements.

Note

1. For a related account of causal explanation in cellular and molecular neuroscience, derived from a related set of cases, see Sweatt (2009).

References

Andersch, N. 2012. Time to end the distinction between mental and neurological illnesses. *BMJ (Clinical Research Ed.)* 344:e3454.

Arranz, M. J., and J. De Leon. 2007. Pharmacogenetics and pharmacogenomics of schizophrenia: A review of last decade of research. *Molecular Psychiatry* 12 (8): 707–747.

Arranz, M. J., and S. Kapur. 2008. Pharmacogenetics in psychiatry: Are we ready for widespread clinical use? *Schizophrenia Bulletin* 34 (6): 1130–1144.

Binder, E. B., and F. Holsboer. 2006. Pharmacogenomics and antidepressant drugs. *Annals of Medicine* 38 (2): 82–94.

Campaner, R., and M. C. Galavotti. 2012. Evidence and the assessment of causal relations in the health sciences. *International Studies in the Philosophy of Science* 26 (1): 27–45.

Campbell, J. 2008. Causation in psychiatry. In *Philosophical Issues in Psychiatry: Explanation, Phenomenology, and Nosology*, ed. K. S. Kendler and J. Parnas, 196–215. Baltimore: Johns Hopkins University Press.

Coutts, R. T., and L. J. Urichuk. 1999. Polymorphic cytochromes P450 and drugs used in psychiatry. *Cellular and Molecular Neurobiology* 19 (3): 325–354.

Czoty, P. W., C. McCabe, and M. A. Nader. 2004. Assessment of the relative reinforcing strength of cocaine in socially housed monkeys using a choice procedure. *Journal of Pharmacology and Experimental Therapeutics* 312 (1): 96–102. doi:10.1124/jpet.104.073411.

Graham, G. 2013. *The Disordered Mind: An Introduction to Philosophy of Mind and Mental Illness*. London: Routledge.

Harris, H. W., and K. F. Schaffner. 1992. Molecular genetics, reductionism, and disease concepts in psychiatry. *Journal of Medicine and Philosophy* 17 (2): 127–153.

Insel, T. R., B. Cuthbert, M. Garvey, R. Heinssen, D. S. Pine, K. Quinn, C. Sanislow, and P. Wang. 2010. Research domain criteria (RDoC): Toward a new classification framework for research on mental disorders. *American Journal of Psychiatry* 167 (7): 748–751.

Insel, T. R., and R. Quirion. 2005. Psychiatry as a clinical neuroscience discipline. *Journal of the American Medical Association* 294 (17): 2221–2224.

Kandel, E. R., J. Schwartz, and T. Jessell. 2000. *Principles of Neural Science*. 4th ed. New York: McGraw-Hill.

Kendler, K. S. 2012. The dappled nature of causes of psychiatric illness: Replacing the organic–functional/hardware–software dichotomy with empirically based pluralism. *Molecular Psychiatry* 17 (4): 377–388.

Kendler, K. S. 2014. The structure of psychiatric science. *American Journal of Psychiatry* 17 (9): 931–938.

Kendler, K. S., and J. Campbell. 2009. Interventionist causal models in psychiatry: Repositioning the mind–body problem. *Psychological Medicine* 39 (6): 881–887.

Kupfer, D. J., and D. A. Regier. 2011. Neuroscience, clinical evidence, and the future of psychiatric classification in DSM-5. *American Journal of Psychiatry* 168 (7): 672–674.

Maccarrone, G., C. Ditzen, A. Yassouridis, C. Rewerts, M. Uhr, M. Uhlen, F. Holsboer, and C. W. Turck. 2013. Psychiatric patient stratification using biosignatures based on cerebrospinal fluid protein expression clusters. *Journal of Psychiatric Research* 47 (11): 1572–1580.

Martin, J. B. 2002. The integration of neurology, psychiatry, and neuroscience in the 21st century. *American Journal of Psychiatry* 159 (5): 695–704.

McMahon, F. J., and T. R. Insel. 2012. Pharmacogenomics and personalized medicine in neuropsychiatry. *Neuron* 74 (5): 773–776.

Morgan, D., K. A. Grant, H. D. Gage, R. H. Mach, J. R. Kaplan, O. Prioleau, S. H. Nader, et al. 2002. Social dominance in monkeys: Dopamine D_2 receptors and cocaine self-administration. *Nature Neuroscience* 5 (2): 169–174.

Mrazek, D. 2010. *Psychiatric Pharmacogenomics*. New York: Oxford University Press.

Murphy, D. 2006. *Psychiatry in the Scientific Image*. Cambridge, MA: MIT Press.

Nader, M. A., and P. W. Czoty. 2005. PET imaging of dopamine D2 receptors in monkey models of cocaine abuse: Genetic predisposition versus environmental modulation. *American Journal of Psychiatry* 162 (8): 1473–1482.

Nasrallah, H. A. 2013. Let's tear down the silos and reunify psychiatry and neurology. *Current Psychiatry* 12 (8): 8–9.

Offit, K. 2011. Personalized medicine: New genomics, old lessons. *Human Genetics* 130 (1): 3–14.

Radden, J. 2003. Is this dame melancholy? Equating today's depression and past melancholia. *Philosophy, Psychiatry, & Psychology* 10 (1): 37–52.

Silva, A. J., A. Landreth, and J. Bickle. 2013. *Engineering the Next Revolution in Neuroscience: The New Science of Experiment Planning*. Oxford: Oxford University Press.

Steele, F. R. 2009. Personalized medicine: Something old, something new. *Personalized Medicine* 6 (1): 1–5.

Sweatt, J. D. 2009. *Mechanisms of Memory*. 2nd ed. New York: Academic Press.

Tsou, J. Y. 2012. Intervention, causal reasoning, and the neurobiology of mental disorders: Pharmacological drugs as experimental instruments. *Studies in History and Philosophy of Science. Part C, Studies in History and Philosophy of Biological and Biomedical Sciences* 43 (2): 542–551.

Weaver, I. C. G., N. Cervoni, F. A. Champagne, A. C. D'Alessio, S. Sharma1, J. R. Seckl, S. Dymov, et al. 2004. Epigenetic programming by maternal behavior. *Nature Neuroscience* 7 (8): 847–854.

Woodward, J. 2003. *Making Things Happen: A Theory of Causal Explanation*. Oxford: Oxford University Press.

Woodward, J. 2008. Cause and explanation in psychiatry. In *Philosophical Issues in Psychiatry: Explanation, Phenomenology, and Nosology*, ed. K. S. Kendler and J. Parnas, 132–184. Baltimore: Johns Hopkins University Press.

Yudofsky, S. C., and R. E. Hales. 2002. Neuropsychiatry and the future of psychiatry and neurology. *American Journal of Psychiatry* 159 (8): 1261–1264.

8 The Shift to Mechanistic Explanation and Classification

Kelso Cratsley

Despite widespread recognition that psychiatry would be better served by a classificatory system based on etiology rather than mere description, it goes without saying that much of the necessary work is yet to be done. Most of it will be empirical, but there are also theoretical issues that need to be addressed. In this chapter I take up the increasingly important question of how one particular brand of causal explanation, that of *mechanistic* explanation, fits into larger efforts to build a scientifically sound etiological and nosological framework. The focus here will be on the broad theoretical outlines of several key issues. I will not rehearse the details of the various critical exchanges stirred by publication of the *Diagnostic and Statistical Manual of Mental Disorders*, fifth edition (DSM-5; American Psychiatric Association 2013), initiation of the Research Domain Criteria (RDoC; Insel et al. 2010; Insel 2013), and ongoing work on the *International Classification of Diseases*, eleventh revision (World Health Organization 2012; First et al. 2015). I primarily focus on mechanistic explanation, and address several challenges it faces in the context of psychiatric research, but many of these issues also have implications for classification.

Mechanistic explanation is committed to the identification of the components that make up the workings of the mind, characterized at complementary levels of explanation. This is standard fare in the allied cognitive sciences, and there has been a noticeable shift toward including psychiatry in this alliance, with the implication that it should also be in the business of elucidating mechanisms (Murphy 2006; Kendler 2008). This has included calls for the identification of dysfunctional mechanisms in the service of research frameworks that may eventually provide the basis for classification, such as the RDoC (Insel et al. 2010; Cuthbert and Insel 2013; Cuthbert 2014a; Insel 2014). Perhaps unsurprisingly, though, there are a number of issues that arise when mechanistic assumptions are brought to bear on psychiatric conditions.

In what follows, I pay particular attention to the challenge of explaining conditions that do not appear to have stable surface features or involve discrete underlying dysfunction.[1] Standard cognitive mechanisms are commonly thought to be relatively enduring structures with regular operations, the result of genetic and developmental effects. But if psychopathology is conceptualized as the product of the breakdown of specific, otherwise stable mechanisms, then a number of psychiatric symptoms appear to belie this notion, given their causal heterogeneity, substantial variability, and diversity of presentation. For example, the symptoms associated with psychotic disorders have been hypothesized to be the result of a staggering array of causal factors and tend to vary in timing and severity. Needless to say, this complicates efforts to identify impaired underlying structures. But as I will explain, there are ways in which a mechanistic framework can accommodate these features—at least for the most part. Briefly put, a relatively broad construal of mechanism allows for something less than the flawless execution of internal operations, appeals to the influence of contextual factors, and attends to organizational relations both within the mechanism and across the wider cognitive system. Such points of emphasis can help clarify how the mechanistic approach can be constructively applied to the study of psychopathology.

Here is how I proceed. I begin by setting out some of the basics of mechanistic explanation, highlighting several key features of this approach, including the explanatory significance of causal regularity, levels of explanation, and network analysis. Following this, the remaining discussion is structured as a series of potential challenges to the application of mechanism to psychiatric research, most of which I suggest are relatively manageable. The first has to do with the fact that multifactorial models of psychopathology increasingly appeal to social and environmental influences, which raises issues for reductive explanation given that causal factors "cross levels." I next consider a set of closely related difficulties encountered when attempting to identify and decompose the dysfunctional mechanisms at work in psychiatric conditions, including the transient nature of many symptoms, the complex organization of underlying systems, and the fact that many disorders are the product of a nonstandard developmental course. I conclude by considering several remaining issues that need to be addressed going forward.

Mechanistic Explanation and Psychiatry

Part of the appeal of mechanistic explanation is that it helps move theorizing away from an interest in discovering general laws toward a focus on the actual explanatory practices of scientists. The literature on mechanism is filled with examples of its application in scientific research, especially in cognitive neuroscience (Craver 2007; Bechtel 2008; Craver and Darden 2013), as well as several discussions of its potential application in psychiatry (Kendler 2008; Tabery, 2009; Kendler, Zachar and Craver, 2011). What I want to do first is fairly modest, underscoring aspects of this kind of causal explanation that are particularly relevant to the study of psychopathology. In doing so, I endorse a relatively broad, noncontroversial brand of mechanism, drawing largely from the work of Craver, Bechtel, and colleagues. Of course, tensions exist within this program, sometimes referred to as the "new mechanism" approach, as well as between it and alternative accounts (reviewed in Andersen 2014; Craver & Tabery, 2016). The endorsement is appropriate in the present context, however, because this is exactly the notion of mechanism operative—indeed, explicitly referenced—in the relevant psychiatric literature (Kendler 2008; Cuthbert and Kozak 2013; Cuthbert 2014a). The focus here, then, is not on evaluating the program itself but merely its application to psychopathology.

Mechanism

In its roughest form, mechanistic explanation follows from the strategies of "functional analysis" (Cummins 1975) and "functional decomposition" (Bechtel and Richardson 1993/2010) in seeking to identify the causal processes responsible for various phenomena. Within cognitive science, this usually involves the idea that explanations of mental capacities should appeal to underlying information-processing systems that can be broken down into simpler and simpler components. The details of this approach are the subject of ongoing debate and refinement, but a highly influential and widely shared assumption is that cognitive processes can be decomposed into hierarchically structured, functionally specifiable mechanisms (Machamer, Darden, and Craver 2000; Craver 2007; Bechtel 2008; Craver and Darden 2013). This is first and foremost a heuristic strategy, regarding the shape that successful explanations often take, but it also frequently implies an *ontic* conception of what is actually out in the world. So understood, mechanisms are causal entities and activities with several key features, including the phenomena they produce, the components out of which they are built, the interactions of these components, and their spatial and temporal organization. The discovery of mechanisms and the full characterization of these features is a gradual process, including intermediary steps of sketches and schemas, driven by an ever-expanding range of methodologies that include various observational techniques and experimental interventions.

An important part of this process is the tracking of causal regularity. Mechanisms are commonly thought to reliably produce phenomena (Machamer et al. 2000; Craver 2007). Indeed, it is the recurrence of certain phenomena that opens up the possibility that an underlying mechanism is responsible. Such causal patterns lead the search for mechanisms; they help pick out mechanisms from the often random, chaotic context in which they are embedded (Andersen 2012a, 2014). This is an element of the "new mechanism" approach that separates it from other traditions which deploy mechanism as a complete explanation of the world and all causal relations within it. On the latter view, absent a regularity assumption, phenomena such as accidents of history or circumstance can be reasonably construed as mechanistic. But the "new" approach has the advantage of using the criterion of recurrence—or repeatability in response to intervention—to individuate mechanisms from other causal forces. An important implication of this is that not all causation will be the work of mechanisms. Singular or highly irregular causal connections may fall outside the mechanistic purview. This comes with the caveat that the working notion of regularity must be relatively broad. Many mechanisms do not operate at anything close to deterministic standards, or even "always for the most part" (as in Machamer et al. 2000). But there are good reasons to think that a broadened conception of regularity can still describe phenomena that do not exhibit fully predictable patterns, such as neurotransmitter release by presynaptic neurons (Andersen 2012a).[2]

Another basic feature of this style of explanation is its commitment to multiple levels of explanation. This is obviously closely connected to the general presumption in cognitive science of mutually constrained levels. For instance, Craver's (2007) well-known example of the mechanism responsible for spatial memory in mice includes several distinct levels: (1) the animal navigating through a maze, (2) the hippocampus generating a spatial map, (3) neurons inducing long-term potentiation, and (4) the activation of NMDA (*N*-methyl-D-aspartate) receptors. For Craver, this mechanism sketch, while admittedly incomplete and open to the addition of further detail (and levels), captures the hierarchical—from higher to lower—components that produce a mouse's capacity for spatial memory. As such, it appeals to the phenomenon in question (e.g., psychological capacity), computations performed by neural systems, cellular-electrophysiological activity, and molecular activity. On each of these levels there are components that "do different things" within the broader mechanism (Bechtel 2008). Thus, mechanistic explanation implicates any number of separate working parts that collectively give rise to a phenomenon.[3]

Notice that this approach represents a departure from the standard account of levels of explanation in cognitive science. Following Marr's highly influential work, explanations of any particular aspect of the mind are usually expected to include accounts of (I) the goal or task of the computational system, (II) the algorithm or set of operations required to carry out this task, and (III) the physical structures responsible (Marr 1982/2010).[4] Each of these three levels captures important explanatory properties, distinctly characterized. Levels in this sense represent different perspectives on a single entity or phenomenon, varied ways of understanding the same cognitive process. This is primarily an epistemic framework, but it also implies a constitutive relation of *realization*. The properties tracked by higher levels are realized or implemented by those on the lower levels (for recent commentary on Marr's levels, see the articles in Peebles and Cooper, 2015).

In contrast, levels for Craver, Bechtel, and colleagues are constitutive in the sense of part–whole relations. The different 'levels of mechanism' represent the components—entities and activities—that contribute to the phenomenon in question. They are best understood as levels of organization or composition; in this way they are decidedly non-Marrian (Craver 2007; Bechtel 2008). There is an explicit commitment to *non*realization across levels, and thus nonreduction more generally, with each level explanatorily autonomous and no single, fundamental level of analysis. This strategy is, of course, reductive in a way, in that it seeks to break down or decompose phenomena into mechanistic components. Call this "weak" reduction (Godfrey-Smith 2014). Mechanistic reduction is ultimately metaphysically neutral when it comes to stronger forms of reduction. As in the example from Craver, mechanisms are typically thought to be physical entities of some sort, thus precluding certain metaphysical possibilities. But beyond that there is nothing, in principle, barring mechanisms from a variety of possible implementational relations. Again, there is certainly a diversity of applications of the concept of mechanism, all of which carry different metaphysical implications. But for Craver and Bechtel, mechanistic levels are most importantly *organizational*.

The reasons for neutrality are another matter. Space does not allow for a full discussion of the larger debates surrounding, for example, level reduction versus the autonomy of the psychological. For Craver and Bechtel, mechanistic decomposition is necessarily multilevel because of several closely related considerations. Craver (2007) places an emphasis on the causal relevance of entities and activities at each different level. An explanation of the spatial memory mechanism would be incomplete without reference to the components at each level because all the components play a significant role in the collective production of the capacity (the components at all levels are "causally relevant" to the functioning of the overall mechanism). For Bechtel (2008), stress is placed on the epistemic importance of an interlevel perspective. Without an understanding of the organization of components across levels, the mechanistic picture will be incomplete; studying the entities and activities at each level in isolation is relatively uninformative.[5] In addition, the *environment* in which the organism is embedded is explanatorily important. In the example of spatial memory, the nature of the experimental intervention—in this case what type of maze the mouse is run through—is vital information. A full explanation needs to appeal to external, contextual factors alongside mechanisms internal to the organism.[6]

Within the organism, mechanisms capture both the functional and neural properties of cognitive processes, thus arguably bridging the divide between psychology and neuroscience (Bechtel, 2008; Piccinini and Craver 2011). This is significant because the extent to which these two abstract away from each other, explanatorily if not fundamentally, has implications for broader projects in cognitive modeling. Most pressingly, recent work has made it clear that cognitive functions are underpinned by widely distributed neural circuits (e.g., Sporns 2010). This means that in many cases there is not a strict one-to-one relation between function and neural region or pattern of activity. Rather, there appear to be numerous long-range networks that overlap in their functional responsibilities, with specific connections activated for specific functions (Anderson 2014). What such nonisomorphy requires from mechanistic explanation is further attention to networked interactions.

From the start, the "new mechanism" approach has been both critical of strict localization claims and interested in mechanistic renderings of the feedback loops and cyclical processing that are essential to a systems neuroscience approach (Bechtel and Richardson 1993/2010; Bechtel 2008). The mechanism framework is flexible enough to accommodate such phenomena, especially if start-up and termination conditions are not required of the relevant activities (compare Bechtel 2008 to Machamer et al. 2000). These kinds of issues are subject to ongoing debate. For example, advocates of situated or dynamical approaches have been critical of mechanistic assumptions (Chemero 2009) while mechanists have maintained that the two approaches are complementary (Kaplan and Bechtel 2011). It is certainly true that specifying the details of complex interactions often lags behind the modeling of the more basic features of a mechanism. The same goes for the overall organization of the mechanism and the broader system of which it is part. In particular, there are significant challenges to identifying the components of highly integrated systems, where individual parts are dependent on activities throughout the mechanism. I will return to this issue below when I discuss several potential obstacles to decomposing impaired mechanisms.

Psychopathology

The study of pathology has played a central role in the history of the cognitive sciences. This includes well-known research on incapacities in domains such as vision, language, and memory, advanced by way of studying the "natural" interventions of accidental damage to the brain (Shallice 1988; Bechtel and Richardson 1993/2010; Bechtel 2008). This has largely been the work of cognitive neuropsychology, with its emphasis on understanding standard cognition by way of lesion studies. Such research follows the rough logic that an association between a relatively discrete lesion and an anomalous behavioral profile in one particular capacity is suggestive of the physical location of a specialized cognitive mechanism, sometimes inferred from *double dissociations* (Shallice 1988; Davies 2010). More recently, this approach has been extended to the study of conditions traditionally defined as psychiatric by work in cognitive neuropsychiatry (David 1993; Frith 2008). And currently, with a broader set of explanatory resources, including epidemiology, neuroimaging, and statistical modeling, much of the wider field of psychiatry is increasingly committed to the search for impaired mechanisms. As noted at the outset, this includes programs such as the RDoC that promote the search for hierarchically structured mechanisms as the basis for a fundamental science of brain and behavior.

Given the recency of the shift toward this style of explanation in psychiatry, it is relatively unsurprising that it is not yet clear how this is supposed to work. One of the appeals of mechanistic explanation in this context is that it provides a framework with which we can identify the broken parts of a system. The starting assumption is usually that the signs and symptoms of a disorder represent a form of cognitive incapacity, or set of incapacities, that is the manifestation of impairments to underlying mechanisms. This is a gross simplification, and of course it involves several problematic notions, not least of which is the presumption that we can establish what should qualify as mental disorder (and incapacity). It should also be noted that nothing precludes the possibility of normally functioning mechanisms playing a proximal causal role in disorder. The influence of cognitive neuropsychology still looms large, but just as the notion of strictly localized lesions has proven increasingly unhelpful in psychiatry, the assumption that relevant mechanisms are broken or disenabled may be unnecessary for any given etiological account. This does not resolve the related worry, though, that we do not yet have a complete model of *normal* cognitive functioning from which to work. This underscores the importance of basic scientific research as a necessary foundation for the identification of both standard and impaired mechanisms, an issue that will come up again below in relation to the RDoC.[7]

If we set these questions to one side for the moment and proceed with the rough and ready assumption of impairment to standard mechanisms, this leads to a range of explanatory options. Broadly speaking, (A) there can be a problem with the activities or internal operations of the mechanism itself, (B) an otherwise normally operating mechanism can receive deviant input from the environment or other mechanisms that leads to problematic output, or (C) there may be a disconnection between mechanisms (all of these options include the possibility of cascading effects across multiple mechanisms).[8] As described elsewhere (Murphy and Stich 2000; Cratsley and Samuels 2013), similar forms of mechanistic impairment can be found in a number of influential theories of psychiatric disorder. These kinds of irregular arrangements become more complicated in the context of mechanistic *networks*, where there may be multiple circuits implicated in any one particular disorder or, alternatively, singular impairment implicated in multiple disorders.

This is only meant to signal the kinds of details that mechanistic theories of psychopathology will ultimately require. And of course the types of entities and activities at each level of the mechanism in question will impact the resulting explanation. Once again, this style of explanation usually carries with it a commitment to multiple levels of explanation, and the psychiatric literature increasingly includes multilevel theories. A frequently referenced example is research suggesting that major depression can be traced to several different factors, including genetic predisposition, such as an atypical variant of the serotonin transporter gene (5-HTTLPR), personality traits, such as neuroticism, along with a history of childhood abuse or substance abuse and more recurrent forms of social stress such as social humiliation (e.g., Kendler, Gardner, and Prescott 2006). Data of this kind obviously suggest a wide range of causal factors, all of which are required in order to model the diversity of pathological trajectories. This increasingly looks like the right approach more generally given the multifactorial nature of many psychiatric disorders. Theory building therefore needs to appeal to findings from several disciplines and their attendant methodologies, with explanations that traffic in distinct kinds of entities and activities.

Cross-Level Challenges

In recognizing the causal multiplicity of psychopathology, several interesting things follow. These have been commented on by Murphy (2008, 2010a, 2013), covering a range of closely related concerns, but at least two central strands can be drawn out. The first is that multifactorial models must grant a central place to social and environmental factors—for example, stress and poverty become important parts of the causal story. This does not bode well, however, for the conventional view within cognitive science that reductive explanation should only target mechanisms within a relatively closed physical structure. And in attempting to explain disorders by way of the interaction between multiple factors that are effectively on different levels, psychiatry appears to part ways with cognitive science even more substantially. As I have already described, the traditional Marrian conception of levels denotes varied perspectives on a *single* aspect of the mind, whereas explanations in psychiatry are concerned with explaining the aberrant interactions of disparate phenomena. If levels represent relationships governed by realization, then this leaves no room for causation that effectively crosses levels. Second, if causal perturbations can arise on any given level, then not only should we pursue them wherever we can find them (following Schaffner, 2008), but perhaps we should also proceed without a prior commitment to the filling out of *all* the standard levels of explanation. Thus, there do seem to be tensions between the emerging empirical picture in psychiatry and the conventions of cognitive science. But these are often more apparent than deeply problematic. Building on my previous description of mechanistic explanation, several points of emphasis can help provide some resolution.

Contextual Factors and Reduction

For a start, mechanistic explanation need not exclusively feature causal factors internal to the organism. That is simply to say that it can, and should, appeal to social and environmental influences. As I previously described, understanding the external context in which mechanisms are embedded is crucial to the success of this style of explanation (Bechtel 2008). The discovery and decomposition of cognitive mechanisms is consistent with research on all sorts of relevant phenomena external to the organism, including causal factors less amenable to decomposition into physical mechanisms.[9] In the study of psychopathology this will involve appealing to social and environmental stressors alongside dysfunctions internal to the individual. Research programs focusing on contextual factors, such as in psychiatric epidemiology, are therefore essential. An example of this is recent work on psychotic disorders, which is increasingly driven by population-level data on various risk factors, including childhood trauma, urbanicity, and migration (Murray, Di Forti, and Howes 2010; van Os, Kenis and Rutten, 2010;). Research has also started to take up the challenge of explaining how the contextual factors correlated with aberrant mental states impact neural mechanisms, such as in the study of the effects of childhood socioeconomic disadvantage on the brain (Holz, Laucht, and Meyer-Lindenberg 2015).

The causal role of contextual factors, though, may also have implications for reduction more generally. As Murphy (2008, 2013) has pointed out, the causal influence of effects such as exposure to environmental pathogens or social humiliation will be difficult to reduce to a more fundamental level of explanation. And so even if we are content to model contextual factors alongside mechanisms as part of an integrated explanatory approach, the prospects for strong reduction do not look good. Now, there is a question as to whether environmental influences are simply background features rather than partially determining factors of pathology. If they are the former, then reduction can arguably go through (Mitchell 2008b). Forms of pathology with clear genetic origins, for example, may be susceptible to environmental effects to some degree while their explanation can still safely operate on just one level. But disorders traditionally defined as psychiatric generally do not fit this picture, given their polygenetic origins and the fact that environmental factors play a substantial role. Therefore, it is probably right that no one level of explanation will be fundamental.[10] The point to emphasize here is that proponents of mechanistic explanation share a similar nonfundamentalism, due to the interplay between contextual factors and mechanisms as well as the organizational hierarchy of levels within any one mechanism (Craver 2007).

This relates to the issue of non-Marrian levels in psychiatric etiology. One way of diagnosing this problem is to blame the occasional conflation in the literature of causal and constitutive claims—or, more precisely, a lack of clarity when discussing causal trajectories versus reductionist commitments. These two kinds of explanatory projects are separable. The need for multifactorial theories that include genetic, developmental, and social factors requires contributions from many disciplines, with the goal of a causally integrated account. This is particularly helpful when modeling disorders that involve processes that occur gradually over long periods of time. It may be that just these kinds of considerations are reflected in the methodological pluralism that appears to predominate in current psychiatric research (Kendler 2014). Such an approach can be maintained without any fundamental or metaphysical commitment to how the various factors relate, and thus it is distinct from matters of strong reduction. But when a particular mental state is investigated in order to understand its fundamental nature, not necessarily synchronically but as a kind of snapshot or distillation, then the more pressing questions concern the "mapping relations" between brain and behavior (as in the RDoC, e.g., Cuthbert and Insel 2013). This latter approach more closely resembles the traditional understanding of levels of explanation and therefore raises reductive questions. We should be careful, then, to distinguish between causal claims and those that engage questions of leveled constitution.

As I have already mentioned, levels of explanation, and the relations between levels, can be variously described. Again, an interest in the mapping relations between phenomena described in either neural or behavioral terms inevitably runs up against the question of strong reduction. Murphy is right to observe that this makes more implementational conceptions of levels potentially unfit for psychiatry (given multiple causal factors that cross levels diachronically). But this neglects the weaker form of reduction pursued by mechanistic explanation. This way of understanding levels, as organizational hierarchies, foregrounds the contributions that components on separate levels make to the overall phenomenon. Entities and activities at each level are causally relevant to the action of the whole mechanism, and the mechanisms interact with other mechanisms and the environment in ways that drive the behavior of the organism. One of the potential appeals of the mechanistic approach is that it aims to provide a causal story without overly strong metaphysical commitments.[11]

Requisite Levels

The second, related worry is that the multifactorial nature of psychiatric disorders may require an abandonment of any prior commitment to levels of explanation. Murphy (2010a, 2013) has suggested something like this, going beyond the inability of Marrian levels to handle cross-level effects to the point of criticizing the standard expectation of mutually constrained levels as an epistemic hindrance. The argument for this view touches on a number of issues, following the more provocative proposal developed by Campbell (2008, 2009, 2013) that the commitment to complementary levels of explanation is driven by the misguided desire to find causal relations penetrable to reason. These suggestions warrant a more extensive discussion than can be provided here, but the main concern appears to be that the nonfundamentalism necessitated by multiple causal factors implies that the assignment of levels should be secondary to the discovery of causal relations, no matter what form they take. To proceed any differently only burdens the process with unnecessary constraints. For example, if depression is caused by social stressors, then we should not be too troubled by incomplete lower-level, neuroscientific explanations. On the other hand, if dopamine dysfunction is in fact the cause of psychotic disorder, then perhaps this is a satisfactory etiology without complete higher-level, psychological detail. Nonfundamentalism is taken seriously and causal relations should be taken wherever they are found.

This is another challenge to the Marrian view, and, interestingly enough, it might also apply to the levels that comprise mechanisms. Mechanistic or organizational levels are interdependent as part of a larger causal structure, but if a component is identified that is especially causally relevant, then perhaps components on other levels should take an explanatory backseat. Because of this possibility, the proposal is fairly intriguing. That said, there are good reasons to resist it. It is true that one possible response to nonfundamentalism is to sanction a certain amount of selectivity when choosing which cause on what level is the most explanatorily salient. But another option is to take it as a good indication that attention must be paid to *all* of the standard levels, per the convention. We certainly do not want to add to the already challenging task of explaining complex phenomena, which seems to be one of Murphy's chief concerns (and Campbell's, for that matter). But the inadequacy of a candidate explanation pitched at a specific level, such as a purely genetic theory of depression, is not reason enough to reject a multilevel approach. If we are trying to avoid the unwarranted prioritization of either higher or lower levels, then one rather sensible way of ensuring such nonfundamentalism is simply to continue to require explanation on all levels.

Another approach is to take each case on its own merits. This strategy grants the permissibility of selective levels. As it happens, this is also the strategy initially proposed by Marr, whose original framework was less prescriptive than it is now often taken to be. On his account, not only are levels described as loosely related, but their application should also be appropriate to the phenomena in question. This leaves open the possibility that "some phenomena may be explained at only one or two of them" (Marr 1982/2010, 25). The example of visual afterimages—for example, after staring at a lightbulb—makes his point, as they are readily explained by way of physical implementation alone. Other phenomena demand explanations on multiple levels. Here Marr mentions the Necker cube illusion, where both neural systems (a bistable network) and psychological effects (two different visual interpretations) are important pieces of the explanatory story. The nature of the phenomenon in question guides the choice of necessary levels. Leveled explanations are thus driven by empirical considerations, but the choice of levels is also partially pragmatic, dependent upon disciplinary and program-specific considerations (which also applies to levels of mechanism, as in Craver 2007; Craver and Darden 2013).

When this strategy is applied to the complex mental states studied by psychiatry, it is quite likely that multiple levels are necessary. The levels might not be strictly Marrian or implementational, given the need to capture contextual effects, but this is where levels of mechanism are useful. Again, epistemically, the point is that both top-down and bottom-up perspectives are necessary for understanding the mechanisms subserving cognitive capacities (Bechtel 2008). Certain phenomena will escape explanation unless we have a grasp of the overall organizational relation of its components. In something like depression, a full explanatory picture may involve causal contributors described on levels roughly corresponding to genetic liability, limbic and prefrontal structure and activity, cognitive competence and deficits, personality, thinking style and reasoning biases, occurrent thoughts and felt experience, as well as developmental effects and other contextual factors such as poverty or social humiliation. For example, a mechanism sketch of depression might include levels comprised of (i) the person impacted by stressful life events, (ii) the amygdala and cingulate responsible for chemical responses to environmental stressors, (iii) the serotonin transporter involved in synapse transmission, and (iv) the 5-HTTLPR gene mediating protein synthesis (Tabery, 2009).

In terms of causation, the mechanism sketch is filled out by levels that correspond to the causally relevant components of the mechanism (Craver 2007). This suggests that only those components that are doing causal work are included. By these terms, levels are not an empirically unhelpful commitment. The search for causal relations drives the explanatory project, and those causal components deemed significant are included in the mechanism's levels. So it is not entirely clear how or why this would slow down or impede the explanatory project. We attempt to identify causal relations as part of a larger effort to develop a complete mechanistic understanding. This may mean that two separate steps are involved, with causal connections first established, by way of experimental and natural interventions, followed by mechanism elaboration (Kendler and Campbell 2009). But this does not undermine the overall usefulness of mechanistic levels. For his part, Murphy (2010a) confirms that levels are unobjectionable just as long as they simply represent assorted causal variables. The mechanistic approach is more substantial than this, but a relatively broad, flexible understanding of mechanism allows for something similar.[12]

Decompositional Challenges

Up to this point, the challenges discussed have largely had to do with reconciling contextual factors with a multilevel mechanistic framework. There are other potential obstacles to explanation and classification in mechanistic terms, however. It is common in the literature to point out that psychiatric conditions not only derive from multiple causal factors but also result in highly heterogeneous symptoms and often exhibit unstable courses of illness.[13] This marks them out from the kinds of phenomena that are the standard targets of cognitive science, such as the relatively constant psychological capacities of vision, memory, attention, and so forth. In contrast to the study of cognition proper, the tools of cognitive science may not be suited for explaining the distinctive features of psychopathology. While there is something to this charge, it falls short of a damning critique. Methodological adjustments may need to be made to accommodate the idiosyncrasies of mental disorder, especially with the increased focus on networked models, but a wholesale overhaul will not be required. The heterogeneity of symptoms, for instance, need not forestall mechanistic theorizing due to the fact that scientific explanation often proceeds by way of targeted idealizations—exemplars or prototypes—of the relevant phenomena, and psychiatry is no exception (Murphy 2006, 2010a,b; Schaffner 2012, 2013).[14]

In this section I address three other aspects of psychiatric symptomatology that represent potential challenges to mechanistic decomposition, building on issues discussed elsewhere (Murphy 2010b; Cratsley and Samuels 2013). All of these raise questions about the difficulties involved in moving inward into the organism, tracing phenomenal and behavioral features all the way down to core mechanisms—in other words, decomposing or weakly reducing apparent incapacities into mechanisms and their components. The first is the already mentioned issue of temporal instability, or the fact that many psychiatric symptoms tend to wax and wane over time. Next, there is the presumed complexity of the mechanisms underpinning mental capacities, as the highly integrated nature of many systems represents a potential roadblock to the individuation of components. Lastly, there is the question of developmental effects, products of the interplay between contextual factors and internal mechanisms that may lead to the creation of thoroughly atypical internal structures. For most of these issues there are explanations available that can help smooth the way for empirical investigation.

Temporal Instability

The questions surrounding temporal instability are particularly relevant to the symptoms associated with depression and psychotic disorders (this is especially true of the mood-related symptoms in both disorders; see Broome et al. 2015). In these conditions the tendency for atypical states to come and go over time does not fit well with the mechanistic expectation of stable underlying processes that have somehow gone awry. But explanatory options are on offer. Most notable is the idea of partial impairment, which has been discussed primarily in the context of the positive symptoms of psychosis (Coltheart 2010). The suggestion is that the implicated mechanisms do not suffer complete breakdown; rather, the operative dysfunction may only be partial. The mechanism in question can be compromised to a degree at which it is intermittently operable, at times failing to function but at other times sputtering back to life. Or it may be compromised in highly selective ways, only impacting one component within the larger mechanism, allowing other components to compensate. If a mechanism is on the blink in these ways, versions of option A from above, then its aberrant outputs may only lead to occasional incapacity and fluctuations in the presence and/or severity of symptoms.

In addition, harking back to the earlier discussion of the fundamentals of this style of explanation, the notion of regularity at work need not be overly strict or deterministic. There are good reasons to think that a criterion of regularity is essential to mechanism, but in order to fit many of the activities of the brain it needs to be relatively forgiving. Indeed, standard mechanisms *fail* to fulfill their functional duties with some degree of regularity. But a broadened conception of regularity can be retained (again, see Andersen 2012a). For the purposes of this discussion, the key point is that the degree of irregularity exhibited by otherwise normally functioning mechanisms may help explain the instability of symptoms. The relevant mechanisms may not actually be impaired or broken, they just exhibit a lower degree of regularity. Alternatively, if they are in fact impaired, then it may be the case that they still work with some degree of regularity.

These possibilities are consistent with the larger point that relatively normal processes may be involved in the disruption of standard capacities and production of aberrant mental states. This can also include mechanisms that receive bad input from other sources, as in option B from above. Poorly functioning mechanisms can produce cascading effects across connected systems simply by passing on bad information. If the input is erratic, then the eventual products of the recipient systems will be as well. Notice that this grants additional importance to the role of contextual factors external to any given mechanism and the organism as a whole. Most importantly, social and environmental input of an atypical variety can throw off otherwise normal mechanisms (as well as those that are impaired to some degree). Fluctuations of input of this type are probably enough to lead to the temporal instability of symptoms in many cases. For example, psychotic symptoms can fluctuate on a daily or hourly basis, presumably because of affective responses to social factors and interactions (reviewed in Myin-Germeys and van Os 2007); recently this moment-to-moment instability has been linked to hypofunction in the ventromedial prefrontal cortex (Hernaus et al. 2015).[15] In conjunction with research of this type, empirical attention should also be turned to *compensatory* factors represented by general cognitive resources such as executive function and personality. It would seem likely that in many cases there is an ongoing competition between impaired and protective processes that creates symptomatic fluctuation.

Complex Systems

Aside from the fact that psychiatric symptoms are often a moving target of sorts, there are additional difficulties involved in the identification and decomposition of the relevant mechanisms. Most notably, many forms of psychopathology do not avail themselves of the clear behavioral and neural profiles that would allow for the discovery of specific mechanisms. Despite impressive advances in experimental interventions and imaging technology, the empirical state of play remains one in which decisive dissociations between incapacities—tracked by performance on various measures and differential patterns of neural activity—are exceedingly rare. This is plausibly due to their inherently confounded nature. The most notorious example is psychotic disorder, where symptoms have been correlated with any number of cognitive and neural irregularities, including what many take to be global cognitive impairment (Schaefer et al. 2013; Barch and Sheffield 2014). The point should not be overstated, as relatively specific impairments have been identified, particularly in neural structure and activity, and this important research continues apace (Haller et al. 2014). But the broader methodological point is that the patterns of impairment and sparing that warrant inferences about the presence of specific neurobiological and cognitive mechanisms, like those found in classic double dissociations, are largely absent from psychotic disorders as well as other psychiatric conditions.

None of this is news to those working on etiological models, since in one way or another the challenge of specifying dysfunctional mechanisms continues to drive the development of increasingly sophisticated research methods. Something similar applies to efforts to uncover the mechanisms that underpin standard cognition. But again, without adequate models of normal functioning we do not have solid ground on which to build models of impairment. There remains the possibility of directly modeling the impairment involved in certain disorders, but there are not many precedents for this approach, and it is not entirely clear how to structure this kind of theory building without *some* reference to standard cognition (more on this below). An increasingly convincing explanation of the ongoing difficulties with decomposing both standard and irregular cognition is that the mechanisms comprising the mind are highly codependent and thus difficult to individuate. Breaking down a system into mechanisms and components can run up against limits when it is to a large extent integrated, with the overall organization of the system more significant than the contribution of any individual part.

Human cognition appears to be just such a system, as most capacities require contributions from a combination of processing systems, and thus identifying and decomposing specific mechanisms and their components can be especially challenging. Proponents of mechanism acknowledge this limitation, with a high degree of functional integration resulting in minimally decomposable or even nondecomposable systems (Bechtel and Richardson 1993/2010). The decomposition of *impaired* mechanisms will run up against these same explanatory limitations, as a number of commentators have noted (Kendler 2008; Mitchell 2008a; Schaffner 2008; Murphy 2010b). There may be some instances of highly selective impairment, but the more integrated the system, then the less discrete the pattern of breakdown. If this is right, at least about the mechanisms involved in many forms of psychopathology, then the rarity of isolable defects or separately modifiable systems is exactly what one might expect (in contrast to canonical findings from neuropsychology). Clearly, then, this stands as one of the biggest potential challenges for modeling disorder in mechanistic terms.

It need not undercut the general utility of mechanistic assumptions, however, as there will be implicated processes that are decomposable to a significant degree. This is consistent with the optimistic assessment that areas of local decomposability can be targeted first as part of the gradual process of explanation (Kendler 2008). Such optimism is buoyed by examples of the successful explanation of highly complex processes, such as fermentation or the citric acid cycle (Bechtel 2008). Regardless of the degree of complexity, the phenomena in question are the result of the interactions between components. And so at least the basic challenge is fairly straightforward: specify the interactions and wider organizational relations. That said, investigative efforts may find it hugely difficult, or perhaps even impossible, to trace the workings of a system along each and every one of its multiple connections (Bechtel and Richardson 1993/2010). Therefore, the possibility of nondecomposability signals the potential for limit cases.[16]

A forward-looking perspective can embrace the emerging picture of dense, widely distributed networks, conceptualized as specific circuits and activations that represent dedicated mechanisms of a sort. This holds much promise although the empirical details are yet to be fully worked out. There are good examples of current research programs committed to the identification and decomposition of mechanisms in terms of relatively specific network disruption. Recent work on prediction-error processes and the positive symptoms of psychosis follows this line (Corlett et al. 2010), as well as work on schizophrenia more generally (Narr and Leaver 2015). And there is similar work on other forms of disorder (Rubinov and Bullmore 2013). But once again, it is important to note that research of this kind will necessarily involve a contrastive premise. Inferences about impairment rely upon a reciprocal relationship with assumptions about standard cognition. There is nothing inherently flawed with this approach, but it is worrisome in cases where both sides of the equation are not yet on solid empirical ground. Unfortunately, this predicament is still the rule rather than the exception for the study of most of the higher functions of the mind.

To mention one prominent example, the processes collectively known as working memory have been implicated in many forms of psychopathology, including depression (Kircanski, Joormann, and Gotlib 2012) and psychosis (Barch and Sheffield 2014). They have also been cited as a phenomenon understood—or "reliably characterized"—in sufficient detail to use as one of the domains of functioning or constructs within the RDoC (Cuthbert 2014a, 31).[17] But this is probably a bit hasty. The empirical status of important aspects of working memory remains unresolved (Diamond 2013; D'Esposito and Pastle 2015). In fairness to the RDoC program, it recognizes that its constructs are provisional and thus may be fractionated following additional investigation, just as it acknowledges the possibility of substantial relations between constructs (Sanislow et al. 2010; Cuthbert and Insel

2013). What makes the recent research on working memory so interesting, though, is that it has revealed it to be dependent on a widely distributed network running between prefrontal and parietal areas (and other regions) that supports *generalized* functions above and beyond the maintenance and manipulation of active representations (see the meta-analysis by Rottschy et al. 2012). The still-emerging complexity of the processes involved in standard working memory, then, may go some way toward explaining the ongoing difficulties in characterizing the nature of the impairments to this capacity that plague various forms of psychopathology.[18]

Developmental Effects

Finally, another challenge follows closely from these concerns that has to do with the decomposition of disorders thought to be the product of non-standard development. This deserves a fuller treatment, especially as many psychiatric conditions look to be the product of atypical development, including psychotic disorders (Murray et al. 2010), depression (Whittle et al. 2014), and personality disorder (De Fruyt and De Clercq 2014). Here I will only gesture toward the general problem, originally presented in the context of cognitive neuropsychology and debates over nativism versus constructivism. It is based on the observation that dissociative evidence rarely, if ever, reveals clean patterns of impairment and preserved capacity. More often than not, the impairment is only partial and what might appear to be a preserved capacity is often compromised in subtle ways. With reference to just this kind of data from research on developmental disorders such as Williams syndrome, it has been proposed that atypical development does not result in cognitive and neural systems where broken mechanisms reside alongside "residually normal" mechanisms (Karmiloff-Smith 1992; D'Souza and Karmiloff-Smith 2011).[19] Rather, given the highly interconnected nature of neurobiological mechanisms, aberrant developmental trajectories create knock-on effects for each and every mechanism, resulting in thoroughly atypical minds and brains. If this is the case, then it precludes the possibility of drawing sound inferences about specific mechanisms by contrasting capacity and incapacity.

This critique has been responded to in several ways, with much of the disagreement hinging on the interpretation of empirical evidence. For example, it has been argued that the extant data are more supportive of partially impaired mechanisms than comprehensively atypical mechanisms (Machery 2011). This is based on the entirely sensible notion that even messy or "impure" dissociations can factor into constructive abductive inference (Davies 2010). In addition, it may be that developmental trajectories are robust or buffered enough to largely withstand aberrant developmental effects, thus preserving a sufficient degree of "normality" to allow for contrastive inference (for a version of this argument, see Machery 2011). This latter claim is difficult to evaluate. Some instances of disorder afford identification of fairly specific deficits. And where this is not available, it may be that inferences across cases, in a piecemeal fashion, can still help in theory construction about specific capacities and incapacities and their underpinnings. On the other hand, there are examples of developmental delay and global impairment that would seem to require the direct modeling of impairment, such as severe cases of autism, general intellectual disability, and perhaps the extensive cognitive deficits present in some instances of schizophrenia. In other words, such a broad swath of the cognitive economy has been affected that contrastive inferences may be uninformative. At the very least, we should be especially careful about the evidential status of contrastive inference in the context of nonstandard developmental trajectories.

Provisional Conclusions and Implications

The shift to mechanistic explanation within psychiatry is a welcome development, especially as it provides theoretical tools for etiological accounts that can eventually help form the basis of a new classificatory system. Psychiatric conditions present several explanatory challenges to mechanistic-style explanation, but as I have described, most of them can be managed in one way or another. What is required is a relatively broad notion of mechanism as well as the incorporation of contextual factors in theory building. In concluding, I would like to briefly draw attention to several implications of the shift toward mechanistic explanation and classification.

The first is the question of demarcating mechanistic and diagnostic thresholds. While the RDoC program purposefully avoids thresholds, it does hold out hope for the delineation of tipping points or cut points where the functional variation in any given domain slides into the pathological (Cuthbert and Insel 2013; Cuthbert 2014a). The idea seems to be that the sheer severity of symptomatology is not always indicative of dysfunction and thus that there may be "nonlinear" causal action that creates breaking points. To be sure, identifying mechanistic thresholds will be no easy task. In terms of symptomatology, the dimensional measures supported by the RDoC and included in the supplemental section of the DSM-5 rely upon scores of degrees of severity. Now, as others have helpfully emphasized, establishing thresholds along a gradient of symptomatology can be grounded upon *nonarbitrary* distinctions, such as in hypertension and obesity, where certain scores are reliable, probabilistic markers of poor outcomes (Haslam 2014).[20] The question of functional thresholds in underlying mechanisms is a separate concern.[21]

The rough idea would seem to be that research should target the internal operations and external interactions of mechanisms that, when disrupted, can create breaking points in the ensuing phenomena. There are interesting precedents in other fields, such as in systems ecology, where shifts from one relatively stable equilibrium to another can be readily observed and investigated mechanistically (Horan et al. 2011). In research on psychotic disorders, the search for nonlinear thresholds is consistent with the proposal that the transition to psychosis is not simply the product of the overall "load" of symptoms; rather, it is the result of a distinctive coalescence of multiple causal factors, including developmental and environmental effects and the persistence of emotional and cognitive dysfunction (Kaymaz and van Os 2010). Research on psychotic thresholds will likely benefit from particular attention to the specific mechanics and causal interactions at the *onset* of illness, where it has been proposed, for example, that dopamine dysregulation is the final step in a nonstandard developmental trajectory (Murray et al. 2010).

There is clearly work to be done, and much of it should proceed with respect to complementary disciplinary contributions. As previously discussed, it will be helpful to distinguish between causal accounts and those that claim a stake on fundamentally metaphysical grounds. The causal multiplicity that is increasingly central to theories of psychopathology demands pragmatic reconciliation between studies of diverse factors using a wide range of methodologies (even if the resulting attempts at integration are messy and piecemeal—Craver and Tabery, 2016). Research programs with etiological ambitions mostly respect this interdisciplinary requirement. This includes the RDoC, which, despite appropriate concerns that its focus on "brain disorders" risks overly favoring lower levels of explanation (Lilienfeld 2014; Poland 2014), recommends—at least on paper—an *integrated* framework (Cuthbert and Insel 2013; Cuthbert 2014a). Its proponents have even gone so far as to defend themselves against charges of "eliminative reductionism" (Cuthbert and Kozak 2013; Cuthbert 2014b). Of course there is a difference between a repudiation of eliminativism and a principled commitment to explanatory pluralism and nonfundamentalism. Even mainstream nonreductive physicalism can in practice veer toward a prioritization of neuroscientific explanation. Research programs need to take care to grant equal weight to contextual factors such as social, environmental, and developmental effects, something the RDoC has also been criticized for neglecting (Wakefield 2014).

There have been few attempts at setting out models of what multifactorial, cross-level explanation should look like in the service of classification (e.g., Schaffner 2012). An essential piece of this work going forward will involve filling in the necessary theoretical and empirical detail. The example of working memory is instructive. It demonstrates how increased detail can lead to the decomposition of processes into increasingly specific mechanisms. It also highlights how challenging decomposition can be when it comes to the mechanisms involved in *higher* cognition. Certain capacities appear to be served by wide-ranging networks, while relatively circumscribed neural regions appear to be involved in multiple functions. Even a cursory familiarity with the literature, for instance, makes it clear just how much we have asked the dorsolateral prefrontal cortex to do, both in standard cognition and psychopathology.

We need to continue to push forward, with classification in mind. These efforts should be guided by network analysis in mechanistic terms. Such an approach has already formed the basis of promising classificatory proposals, such as that of Buckholtz and Meyer-Lindenberg (2012). This particular proposal aspires to the identification of relatively precise dysfunctional circuits that are responsible for specific cognitive deficits and symptoms. Like the RDoC, it has run into legitimate criticism on the grounds that it underplays the role of contextual factors (Poland and Von Eckardt 2013). There are other diagnostic proposals that place both contextual and diachronic factors at the core of the framework (van Os et al. 2013). Therefore, with the necessary adjustments, these kinds of approaches can provide the basis for a classificatory system based on contextually embedded, highly networked cognitive mechanisms.

Acknowledgments

I would like to thank the editors, Serife Tekin and Jeff Poland, for helpful comments on an earlier version of this chapter.

Notes

1. This is distinct from concerns about the "instability" of the constructs used in research on both standard and nonstandard cognition, given inconsistent operationalization and mixed methodology within and across scientific disciplines (Sullivan 2014).

2. It has been argued that fairly minimal—though still explanatorily useful—requirements for regularity can be set by several parameters, including organizational location (or component connections within a mechanism), strength of connection between operating stages, and patterns of failure (Andersen 2012a). Sporadically operating mechanisms, such as the action potentials that drive the release of neurotransmitters by vesicles in presynaptic neurons, can still be described along these parameters, albeit at the more irregular boundaries.

3. On this view, the assignment of a component to a specific level is governed by whether it can be considered part of another, higher component. If so, then it belongs to a lower level within the mechanism (Craver 2007). Thus two components of roughly the same physical type may be found on different levels if they are making different contributions to the mechanism (Bechtel 2008). On the other hand, there are ways in which one might try to distinguish, for example, neurons from molecules based upon a criterion like size or frequency of interaction. For discussion of potential level demarcations, see Craver (2007, 2015), Bechtel (2008), Young (2012) and Craver and Tabery (2016).

4. Marr's computational, algorithmic, and implementational levels are closely related to a number of other proposals, such as Pylyshyn's (1984) semantic, syntactic, and physical levels.

5. Interestingly enough, the most common argument against level reduction, that of multiple realization, is challenged by Bechtel (2008). He emphasizes the ways in which mechanistic systems, including dense networks, are constrained by the range of actual realizations available. For a helpful recent discussion of multiple realization, see Piccinini and Maley (2014).

6. The boundaries of a mechanism, both in relation to other mechanisms and the outside world, are set by consideration of what is causally relevant to the phenomenon in question. But this is dependent upon prior assumptions about the phenomenon itself (Craver 2007; Craver and Tabery 2016). Craver recognizes the difficulty in establishing the boundaries of any given mechanism, then, while also recognizing that cognitive mechanisms rely upon resources outside the skull. This position is distinct, however, from the view that cognition is dependent upon—or actually constituted by—external structures, that is, "extended cognition." That said, proponents of mechanism could do more to emphasize the role of contextual factors. For example, Craver has been criticized in the past for neglecting *external* sources of representational content (Von Eckardt and Poland 2004). Interestingly enough, it has recently been suggested that Marr's computational level should be read as incorporating the role of environmental factors (Bechtel and Shagrir 2015).

7. A couple of points are worth making. First, when it comes to the question of what defines mental disorder, there obviously are no easy answers. But the mechanistic approach certainly does not have a monopoly on this problem. Second, it is

also important to emphasize that the mechanistic approach's lack of an assumption of broken components is consistent with the idea that not all mental disorders are brain disorders. This point is not new and has recently been made in relation to the RDoC (Poland 2014; Wakefield 2014). Simply put, while physicalism entails that all mental states are brain states, and thus that all disordered mental states are brain states of some sort, it need not follow that such brain states are disordered.

8. This does not exhaust all of the possible forms of breakdown. In addition to those listed, it is also possible for a functional system to be thrown off by a change in the order of operations between components, a shift of the functional responsibilities of an individual component, or the addition of a new functional component (Von Eckardt Klein 1977). Similar points have been made in relation to the difficulties involved in predicting mechanistic response under intervention (Andersen 2012b). There are cases where medical treatment proceeds on the basis of a relatively complete mechanistic picture of normal functioning but is ultimately ineffective (e.g., lavage and debridement as treatment for knee osteoarthritis). This raises the possibility that the causal structure of the impaired mechanism is significantly different from the healthy version of the mechanism because of changes wrought by disease. A truly complete mechanistic picture, then, must detail the variety of ways in which a mechanism can be impaired, including those which may depart from what would be predicted based upon what is known about the *un*impaired version of the mechanism.

9. There is a sense in which social and environmental factors are causal "mechanisms." This may be true if the implication is simply that they have causal force. As noted, though, the version of mechanistic explanation endorsed here distinguishes between mechanistic causation and causation more generally, based upon a regularity assumption (Andersen 2012a, 2014). On the other hand, causal forces in the environment that can be decomposed into biological mechanisms are likely to meet this standard. It's also worth noting that mechanists appear to be increasingly open to the idea of "social mechanisms" (Craver and Tabery 2016).

10. The story does not end here, as there are many versions of reductionism, some of which may be able to handle the possibility of substantial contextual effects (Brigandt and Love 2015). For example, a "wide" reductionism can appeal to *horizontal* relations at lower levels, such as those between an organism's cells and the microbes in its immediate environment (as briefly discussed, for example, in Barker 2013).

11. It is important to note that Craver and Bechtel are wary of claims of causation *between* the levels of a mechanism. Their concern is that interlevel causation would imply certain metaphysical oddities related to self-causation, such as the lack of a distinction between cause and effect, the possibility that causes do not temporally precede effect, and the possibility that causes and effects do not come into direct contact (Craver and Bechtel 2007, Craver, 2015). To square these traditional assumptions with the compositional, part–whole relations of mechanistic levels requires

that causation be understood as mechanistically mediated—that is, *intra*level. For a recent discussion and defense of this position, see Romero (2015).

12. There are a number of related issues that require more extensive discussion, particularly regarding Campbell's (2008, 2009, 2013) view. His critique of levels and mechanisms has several targets, including the overly reductive prioritization of neurobiological explanation and theories that hold causation to be exclusively mechanistic. However, as I have tried to show, more recent treatments of mechanism are both nonreductive and inclusive of nonmechanistic causation. On the other hand, Campbell also appears to make more of a modal claim about the poor prospects for detailing higher cognition and its breakdown in functional terms (i.e., *can* we tell a story on the computational level?). This is an interesting skeptical line to take; somewhat similar worries are discussed in the next section on decompositional challenges.

13. See Poland (2014) for a comprehensive list of the distinctive features of psychiatric conditions that make them especially challenging explananda.

14. Notice that I am bracketing the question of whether psychiatric conditions are natural kinds. From a mechanistic perspective, natural kinds are phenomena with shared properties explained by way of similar mechanisms (Craver and Tabery 2016). But, as I've indicated, there is a good case to be made that scientific explanation can proceed simply on the basis of targeted exemplars. In addition, it's important to recognize the degree of pragmatism required of natural kinship claims. In the case of psychiatric conditions, given their causal heterogeneity, the search for natural kinds will inevitably appeal to significant practical considerations, including the explanatory target, level of detail, and broader aims of any particular research program (Craver 2009; Kendler et al. 2011; Zachar 2014). For a helpful taxonomy of natural kinship claims in psychiatry, see Haslam (2014).

15. This is part of a broader interest in the role of stress in many forms of psychopathology—for example, see the recent special section edited by Harkness, Hayden, and Lopez-Duran (2015).

16. In the context of psychopathology, some instances of delusion may represent just such a limit case, given the likely involvement of impairments to higher cognition. See the discussion of related issues in Murphy (2006).

17. According the language of the RDoC, several "domains" of functioning are broken down into more specific "dimensions," represented by provisional "constructs." For example, the domain of "cognitive systems" includes the following dimensions/constructs: attention, perception, working memory, declarative memory, language behavior, and cognitive control (Cuthbert and Insel 2013; Cuthbert 2014a). These are the *rows* of the RDoC's matrix, and as such are meant to capture various behavioral and neural capacities, measured by the "units of analysis" listed in the *columns* of the matrix: genes, molecules, cells, circuits, physiology,

behavior, and self-reports. In relation to levels of explanation, the columns will play an important role in integrating the findings from various disciplines and methodologies, while Craver's (2007) "levels of mechanism" have more immediate relevance to the processes that underlie the constructs listed in the matrix's rows.

18. Something similar is afoot in research on theory of mind capacities (Schaafsma et al. 2015), with potential implications for the RDoC's construct of "perception/understanding of others."

19. Williams syndrome, a disorder associated with impairments to visuospatial cognition but preserved social cognition and facial recognition, is often contrasted with disorders such as prosopagnosia, which involves impaired facial recognition but preserved visuospatial cognition. Any apparent double dissociation, though, is complicated by what appear to be subtle impairments in social cognition and facial recognition in Williams syndrome. These kinds of findings are taken by Karmiloff-Smith to suggest that developmental disorders do not selectively impair and preserve neural systems.

20. This is not to minimize the difficulties involved in establishing symptomatic thresholds. Beyond the empirical challenges, such efforts can also be heavily influenced by nonscientific factors, such as the vested interests of industry (Greene 2007), similar to more general concerns about industry influence on classification (Cosgrove and Krimsky 2012).

21. Beyond the question of thresholds, the functional variation, or 'dimensionality,' posited by the RDoC could be taken as a further challenge to the mechanistic approach. If capacities operate on a spectrum, then we need an account of how mechanisms with regular interfaces and activities produce such a diverse range of outputs. And in terms of pathology, a gradient of symptom severity caused by the cumulative effects of multiple causal factors may seem at odds with the positing of impairment to specific, otherwise stable mechanisms. But there are means by which an appeal to mechanisms can facilitate explanation. Again, there are various ways in which mechanisms within an organism can function and fail to function—including irregularities in internal operations, problems with networked relations, and sensitivity to contextual factors—all of which can lead to output of graded quality. There are also ways to reconcile mechanistic regularity with population-wide phenotypic variation, including susceptibility to mental disorder (Tabery, 2009). These considerations are consistent with the broader motivations for dimensional *classification*, such as the multiplicity of causes and symptoms within traditional diagnostic categories, shared symptoms and causal factors across categories, and the overall prevalence of comorbidity.

References

American Psychiatric Association. 2013. *Diagnostic and Statistical Manual of Mental Disorders*. 5th ed. Arlington, VA: American Psychiatric Association.

Andersen, H. 2012a. The case for regularity in mechanistic causal explanation. *Synthese* 189:415–432.

Andersen, H. 2012b. Mechanisms: What are they evidence for in evidence-based medicine? *Journal of Evaluation in Clinical Practice* 18:992–999.

Andersen, H. 2014. A field guide to mechanisms: Part I & II. *Philosophy Compass* 9 (4): 274–293.

Anderson, M. L. 2014. *After Phrenology: Neural Reuse and the Interactive Brain*. Cambridge, MA: MIT Press.

Barch, D. M., and J. M. Sheffield. 2014. Cognitive impairments in psychotic disorders: Common mechanisms and measurement. *World Psychiatry: Official Journal of the World Psychiatric Association (WPA)* 13:224–232.

Barker, M. J. 2013. Biological explanations, realism, ontology, and categories (Reviewing J. Dupré, *Processes of Life: Essays in the Philosophy of Biology*). *Studies in History and Philosophy of Biological and Biomedical Sciences* 44:617–622.

Bechtel, W. 2008. *Mental Mechanisms: Philosophical Perspectives on Cognitive Neuroscience*. New York: Routledge.

Bechtel, W., and R. C. Richardson. 2010. *Discovering Complexity: Decomposition and Localization as Strategies in Scientific Research*. Cambridge, MA: MIT Press. (Originally published by Princeton University Press in 1993.)

Bechtel, W., and O. Shagrir. 2015. The non-redundant contributions of Marr's three levels of analysis for explaining information-processing mechanisms. *Topics in Cognitive Science* 7 (2): 312–322.

Brigandt, I., and A. Love. 2015. Reductionism in biology. In *The Stanford Encyclopedia of Philosophy*. Fall 2015 ed., ed. E. N. Zalta. http://plato.stanford.edu/archives/fall2015/entries/reduction-biology/.

Broome, M. R., K. E. A. Saunders, P. J. Harrison, and S. Marwaha. 2015. Mood instability: Significance, definition and measurement. *British Journal of Psychiatry* 207:283–285.

Buckholtz, J. W., and A. Meyer-Lindenberg. 2012. Psychopathology and the human connectome: Toward a transdiagnostic model of risk for mental illness. *Neuron* 74:990–1004.

Campbell, J. 2008. Causation in psychiatry. In *Philosophical Issues in Psychiatry: Explanation, Phenomenology and Nosology*, ed. K. S. Kendler and J. Parnas, 196–215. Baltimore: Johns Hopkins University Press.

Campbell, J. 2009. What does rationality have to do with psychological causation? Propositional attitudes as mechanisms and as control variables. In *Psychiatry as Cognitive Neuroscience: Philosophical Perspectives*, ed. L. Bortolotti and M. Broome, 137–149. Oxford: Oxford University Press.

Campbell, J. (2013). Causation and mechanisms in psychiatry. In *The Oxford Handbook of Philosophy and Psychiatry*, ed. K. W. M. Fulford, M. Davies, R. G. T. Gipps, G. Graham, J. Z. Sadler, G. Stanghellini, and T. Thornton, 935–949. Oxford: Oxford University Press.

Chemero, A. 2009. *Radical Embodied Cognitive Science*. Cambridge, MA: MIT Press.

Coltheart, M. 2010. The neuropsychology of delusions. *Annals of the New York Academy of Sciences* 1191:16–26.

Corlett, P. R., J. R. Taylor, X.-J. Wang, P. C. Fletcher, and J. H. Krystal. 2010. Toward a neurobiology of delusions. *Progress in Neurobiology* 92:345–369.

Cosgrove, L., and S. Krimsky. 2012. A comparison of DSM-IV and DSM-5 panel members' financial associations with industry: A pernicious problem persists. *PLoS Medicine* 9 (3). doi:10.1371/journal.pmed.1001190.

Cratsley, K., and R. Samuels. 2013. Cognitive science and explanations of psychopathology. In *The Oxford Handbook of Philosophy and Psychiatry*, ed. K. W. M. Fulford, M. Davies, R. G. T. Gipps, G. Graham, J. Z. Sadler, G. Stanghellini, and T. Thornton, 413–433. Oxford: Oxford University Press.

Craver, C. 2007. *Explaining the Brain: Mechanisms and the Mosaic Unity of Neuroscience*. Oxford: Oxford University Press.

Craver, C. 2009. Mechanisms and natural kinds. *Philosophical Psychology* 22:575–594.

Craver, C. 2015. Levels. In *Open MIND*, ed. T. Metzinger and J. M. Windt. doi:10.15502/9783958570498.

Craver, C., and W. Bechtel. 2007. Top-down causation without top-down causes. *Biology & Philosophy* 22:547–563.

Craver, C., and L. Darden. 2013. *In Search of Mechanisms: Discoveries across the Life Sciences*. Chicago: University of Chicago Press.

Craver, C., and J. Tabery. 2016. Mechanisms in science. In *The Stanford Encyclopedia of Philosophy*. Spring 2016 ed., ed. N. Zalta. http://plato.stanford.edu/archives/spr2016/entries/science-mechanisms/.

Cummins, R. 1975. Functional analysis. *Journal of Philosophy* 72:741–764.

Cuthbert, R. 2014a. The RDoC framework: Facilitating transition from ICD/DSM to dimensional approaches that integrate neuroscience and psychopathology. *World Psychiatry: Official Journal of the World Psychiatric Association (WPA)* 13 (1): 28–35.

Cuthbert, R. 2014b. Response to Lilienfeld. *Behaviour Research and Therapy* 62:140–142.

Cuthbert, B. N., and T. R. Insel. 2013. Toward the future of psychiatric diagnosis: The seven pillars of RDoC. *BMC Medicine* 11 (126). doi:10.1186/1741-7015-11-126.

Cuthbert, B. N., and M. J. Kozak. 2013. Constructing constructs for psychopathology: The NIMH Research Domain Criteria. *Journal of Abnormal Psychology* 122 (3): 928–937.

David, A. S. 1993. Cognitive neuropsychiatry? *Psychological Medicine* 23:1–5.

Davies, M. 2010. Double dissociations. *Mind & Language* 25 (5): 500–540.

De Fruyt, F., and B. De Clercq. 2014. Antecedents of personality disorder in childhood and adolescence: Toward an integrative developmental disorder. *Annual Review of Clinical Psychology* 10:449–476.

D'Esposito, M. D., and B. R. Pastle. 2015. The cognitive neuroscience of working memory. *Annual Review of Psychology* 66:115–142.

Diamond, A. 2013. Executive functions. *Annual Review of Psychology* 64:135–168.

D'Souza, D., and A. Karmiloff-Smith. 2011. When modularization fails to occur: A developmental perspective. *Cognitive Neuropsychology* 28 (3&4): 276–287.

First, M. B., G. M. Reed, S. E. Hyman, and S. Saxena. 2015. The development of the ICD-11 clinical descriptions and diagnostic guidelines for mental and behavioural disorders. *World Psychiatry: Official Journal of the World Psychiatric Association (WPA)* 14 (1): 82–90.

Frith, C. 2008. In praise of cognitive neuropsychiatry. *Cognitive Neuropsychiatry* 13 (1): 1–7.

Godfrey-Smith, P. 2014. *Philosophy of Biology*. Princeton, NJ: Princeton University Press.

Greene, J. A. 2007. *Prescribing by Numbers: Drugs and the Definition of Disease*. Baltimore: Johns Hopkins University Press.

Haller, C. S., J. L. Padmanabhan, P. Lizano, J. Torous, and M. Keshavan. 2014. Recent advances in understanding schizophrenia. *F1000prime Reports* 6 (57). doi: 10.12703/P6-57.

Harkness, K. L., E. P. Hayden, and N. L. Lopez-Duran, ed. 2015. Special section: Stress sensitivity in psychopathology: Mechanisms and consequences. *Journal of Abnormal Psychology* 124 (1): 1–231.

Haslam, N. 2014. Natural kinds in psychiatry: Conceptually implausible, empirically questionable, and stigmatizing. In *Classifying Psychopathology: Mental Kinds and Natural Kinds*, ed. H. Kincaid and J. A. Sullivan, 11–28. Cambridge, MA: MIT Press.

Hernaus, D., D. Collip, J. Lataster, W. Viechtbauer, E. Myin, J. Ceccarini, K. Van Laere, J. van Os, and I. Myin-Germeys. 2015. Psychotic reactivity to daily life stress and the dopamine system: A study combining experience sampling and [^{18}F]fallypride positron emission tomography. *Journal of Abnormal Psychology* 124 (1): 27–37.

Holz, N. E., M. Laucht, and A. Meyer-Lindenberg. 2015. Recent advances in understanding the neurobiology of childhood socioeconomic disadvantage. *Current Opinion in Psychiatry* 28:365–370.

Horan, R. D., E. P. Fenichel, K. L. S. Drury, and D. M. Lodge. 2011. Managing ecological thresholds in coupled environmental–human systems. *Proceedings of the National Academy of Sciences of the United States of America* 108 (18): 7333–7338.

Insel, T. 2013. Director's Blog. Transforming diagnosis. http://www.nimh.nih.gov/about/director/2013/transforming-diagnosis.shtml.

Insel, T. 2014. The Research Domain Criteria (RDoC): Precision medicine for psychiatry. *American Journal of Psychiatry* 171 (4): 395–397.

Insel, T., B. Cuthbert, M. Garvey, R. Heinssen, D. S. Pine, K. Quinn, C. Sanislow, and P. Wang. 2010. Research Domain Criteria (RDoC): Toward a new classification framework for research on mental disorders. *American Journal of Psychiatry* 167:748–751.

Kaplan, D. M., and W. Bechtel. 2011. Dynamical models: An alternative or complement to mechanistic explanations? *Topics in Cognitive Science* 3:438–444.

Karmiloff-Smith, A. 1992. *Beyond Modularity: A Developmental Perspective on Cognitive Science*. Cambridge, MA: MIT Press.

Kaymaz, N., and J. van Os. 2010. Extended psychosis phenotype—yes: Single continuum—unlikely. *Psychological Medicine* 40:1963–1966.

Kendler, K. S. 2008. Explanatory models for psychiatric illness. *American Journal of Psychiatry* 165:695–702.

Kendler, K. S. 2014. The structure of psychiatric science. *American Journal of Psychiatry* 171:931–938.

Kendler, K., and J. Campbell. 2009. Interventionist causal models in psychiatry: Repositioning the mind–body problem. *Psychological Medicine* 39:881–887.

Kendler, K. S., C. O. Gardner, and C. A. Prescott. 2006. Towards a comprehensive developmental model for depression in men. *American Journal of Psychiatry* 163:115–124.

Kendler, K. S., P. Zachar, and C. Craver. 2011. What kinds of things are psychiatric disorders? *Psychological Medicine* 41:1143–1150.

Kircanski, K., J. Joormann, and I. H. Gotlib. 2012. Cognitive aspects of depression. *Wiley Interdisciplinary Reviews: Cognitive Science* 3:301–313.

Lilienfeld, S. O. 2014. The Research Domain Criteria (RDoC): An analysis of methodological and conceptual challenges. *Behaviour Research and Therapy* 62:129–139.

Machamer, P., L. Darden, and C. F. Craver. 2000. Thinking about mechanisms. *Philosophy of Science* 67 (1): 1–25.

Machery, E. 2011. Developmental disorders and cognitive architecture. In *Maladapting Minds: Philosophy, Psychiatry, and Evolutionary Theory*, ed. P. Adriaens and A. De Block, 91–116. Oxford: Oxford University Press.

Marr, D. 2010. *Vision: A Computational Investigation into the Human Representation and Processing of Visual Information.* Cambridge, MA: MIT Press. (Originally published by Freeman in 1982.)

Mitchell, S. D. 2008a. Explaining complex behavior. In *Philosophical Issues in Psychiatry: Explanation, Phenomenology and Nosology*, ed. K. S. Kendler and J. Parnas, 19–38. Baltimore: Johns Hopkins University Press.

Mitchell, S. D. 2008b. Comment: Taming causal complexity. In *Philosophical Issues in Psychiatry: Explanation, Phenomenology and Nosology*, ed. K. S. Kendler and J. Parnas, 125–131. Baltimore: Johns Hopkins University Press.

Murphy, D. 2006. *Psychiatry in the Scientific Image*. Cambridge, MA: MIT Press.

Murphy, D. 2008. Levels of explanation in psychiatry. In *Philosophical Issues in Psychiatry: Explanation, Phenomenology and Nosology*, ed. K. S. Kendler and J. Parnas, 99–125. Baltimore: Johns Hopkins University Press.

Murphy, D. 2010a. Explanation in psychiatry. *Philosophy Compass* 5/7:602–610.

Murphy, D. 2010b. Complex mental disorders: Representation, stability and explanation. *European Journal of Analytic Philosophy* 6 (1): 28–42.

Murphy, D. 2013. The medical model and the philosophy of science. In *The Oxford Handbook of Philosophy and Psychiatry*, ed. K. W. M. Fulford, M. Davies, R. G. T. Gipps, G. Graham, J. Z. Sadler, G. Stanghellini, and T. Thornton, 966–986. Oxford: Oxford University Press.

Murphy, D., and S. Stich. 2000. Darwin in the madhouse: Evolutionary psychology and the classification of mental disorders. In *Evolution and the Human Mind: Modularity, Language and Meta-Cognition*, ed. P. Carruthers and A. Chamberlain, 62–92. Cambridge: Cambridge University Press.

Murray, R. M., P. Di Forti, and O. Howes. 2010. Integrating the epidemiology and pathogenesis of schizophrenia: From the street to the striatum. In *Advances in Schizophrenia Research 2009*, ed. W. F. Gattaz and G. Busatto, 357–366. New York: Springer.

Myin-Germeys, I., and J. van Os. 2007. Stress-reactivity in psychosis: Evidence for an affective pathway to psychosis. *Clinical Psychology Review* 27:409–424.

Narr, K. L., and A. M. Leaver. 2015. Connectome and schizophrenia. *Current Opinion in Psychiatry* 28:229–235.

Peebles, D., and R. P. Cooper. 2015. Special section: Thirty years after Marr's vision: Levels of analysis in cognitive science. *Topics in Cognitive Science* 7 (2): 187–335.

Piccinini, G., and C. Craver. 2011. Integrating psychology and neuroscience: Functional analyses as mechanism sketches. *Synthese* 183:283–311.

Piccinini, G., and C. J. Maley. 2014. The metaphysics of mind and the multiple sources of multiple realizability. In *New Waves in Philosophy of Mind*, ed. M. Sprevak and J. Kallestrup, 125–152. New York: Palgrave Macmillan.

Poland, J. 2014. Deeply rooted sources of error and bias in psychiatric classification. In *Classifying Psychopathology: Mental Kinds and Natural kinds*, ed. H. Kincaid and J. A. Sullivan, 29–63. Cambridge, MA: MIT Press.

Poland, J., and B. Von Eckardt. 2013. Mapping the domain of mental illness. In *The Oxford Handbook of Philosophy and Psychiatry*, ed. K. W. M. Fulford, M. Davies, R. G. T. Gipps, G. Graham, J. Z. Sadler, G. Stanghellini, and T. Thornton, 735–752. Oxford: Oxford University Press.

Pylyshyn, Z. 1984. *Computation and Cognition*. Cambridge, MA: MIT Press.

Romero, F. 2015. Why there isn't inter-level causation in mechanisms. *Synthese* 192 (11): 3731–3755.

Rottschy, C., R. Langner, I. Dogan, K. Reetz, A. R. Laird, J. B. Schulz, P. T. Fox, and S. B. Eickhoff. 2012. Modeling neural correlates of working memory: A coordinate-based meta-analysis. *NeuroImage* 60:830–846.

Rubinov, M., and E. Bullmore. 2013. Fledgling pathoconnectomics of psychiatric disorders. *Trends in Cognitive Sciences* 17 (12): 641–647.

Sanislow, C. A., D. S. Pine, K. J. Quinn, M. J. Kozak, R. K. Heinssen, P. S. Wang, and B. N. Cuthbert. 2010. Developing constructs for psychopathology research: Research Domain Criteria. *Journal of Abnormal Psychology* 119:631–639.

Schaafsma, S. M., D. W. Pfaff, R. P. Spunt, and R. Adolphs. 2015. Deconstructing and reconstructing theory of mind. *Trends in Cognitive Sciences* 19 (2): 65–72.

Schaefer, J., E. Giangrande, D. R. Weinberger, and D. Dickinson. 2013. The global cognitive impairment in schizophrenia: Consistent over decades and around the world. *Schizophrenia Research* 150:42–50.

Schaffner, K. F. 2008. Etiological models in psychiatry: Reductive and nonreductive approaches. In *Philosophical Issues in Psychiatry: Explanation, Phenomenology and Nosology*, ed. K. S. Kendler and J. Parnas, 48–90. Baltimore: Johns Hopkins University Press.

Schaffner, K. F. 2012. A philosophical overview of the problems of validity for psychiatric disorders. In *Philosophical Issues in Psychiatry II: Nosology*, ed. K. S. Kendler and J. Parnas, 169–189. Oxford: Oxford University Press.

Schaffner, K. F. 2013. Reduction and reductionism in psychiatry. In *The Oxford Handbook of Philosophy and Psychiatry*, ed. K. W. M. Fulford, M. Davies, R. G. T. Gipps, G. Graham, J. Z. Sadler, G. Stanghellini, and T. Thornton, 1003–1022. Oxford: Oxford University Press.

Shallice, T. 1988. *From Neuropsychology to Mental Structure*. Cambridge: Cambridge University Press.

Sporns, O. 2010. *Networks of the Brain*. Cambridge, MA: MIT Press.

Sullivan, J. 2014. Stabilizing mental disorders: Prospects and problems. In *Classifying Psychopathology: Mental Kinds and Natural Kinds*, ed. H. Kincaid and J. A. Sullivan, 257–281. Cambridge, MA: MIT Press.

Tabery, J. 2009. Difference mechanisms: Explaining variation with mechanisms. *Biology & Philosophy* 24:645–664.

van Os, J., G. Kenis, and B. P. F. Rutten. 2010. The environment and schizophrenia. *Nature* 468:203–212.

van Os, J., P. Delespaul, J. Wigman, I. Myin-Germeys, and M. Wichers. 2013. Beyond DSM and ICD: Introducing "precision diagnosis" for psychiatry using momentary assessment technology. *World Psychiatry; Official Journal of the World Psychiatric Association (WPA)* 12 (2): 113–117.

Von Eckardt, B., and J. S. Poland. 2004. Mechanism and explanation in cognitive neuroscience. *Philosophy of Science* 71:972–984.

Von Eckardt Klein, B. 1977. Inferring functional localization from neurological evidence. In *Explorations in the Biology of Language*, ed. W. Walker, 27–66. Montgomery, VT: Bradford Books.

Wakefield, J. 2014. Wittgenstein's nightmare: Why the RDoC grid needs a conceptual dimension. *World Psychiatry; Official Journal of the World Psychiatric Association (WPA)* 13 (1): 38–40.

Whittle, S., R. Lichter, M. Dennison, N. Vijayakumar, O. Schwartz, M. L. Byrne, J. G. Simmons, et al. 2014. Structural brain development and depression onset during adolescence: A prospective longitudinal study. *American Journal of Psychiatry* 171:564–571.

World Health Organization. 2012. *International Classification of Diseases-11 Beta Draft*. http://apps.who.int/classifications/icd11/browse/l-m/en.

Young, A. 2012. Levels of analysis. *Wiley Interdisciplinary Reviews: Cognitive Science* 3:315–325.

Zachar, P. 2014. Beyond natural kinds: Toward a "relevant" "scientific" taxonomy in psychiatry. In *Classifying Psychopathology: Mental Kinds and Natural Kinds*, ed. H. Kincaid and J. A. Sullivan, 75–104. Cambridge, MA: MIT Press.

9 Classification, Rating Scales, and Promoting User-Led Research

Rachel Cooper

Those who talk of a "crisis" in psychiatric research tend to worry that research based on categories drawn from the American Psychiatric Association's *Diagnostic and Statistical Manual of Mental Disorders* (DSM) has proved less successful than some researchers hoped, and that a new and more "science-based" classification may be required. This chapter focuses on an orthogonal crisis; many patients and mental health professionals have lost faith in psychiatric research. Over the past decade, concerns that much psychiatric research serves the interests of funders (mainly the pharmaceutical industry) rather than the interests of patients have become mainstream. Some worry that research tends to be directed at treatments that are potentially profitable rather than those that might best benefit patients. Some worry that data from drug trials is no longer trustworthy—various researchers have been found to have engaged in the manipulation of results. Such concerns are not unique to psychiatry but extend to many areas of science. One way in which such concerns can be ameliorated is via the development of more amateur/citizen/user-led research. I argue that promoting research conducted outside of traditional academic settings promises a range of benefits—both to the amateur researchers themselves and to others who want truths to be discovered. Having argued that it would be a good idea to have more user-produced research, I shall discuss how research by users might be facilitated or hindered by changes to the informational infrastructure of science. In particular, I discuss how different styles of classification, and rating scale, can facilitate the work of some research communities and set back the work of others. I finish by considering how changes to classification and rating scales in psychopathology might facilitate user-led research.

A Crisis in Current Research

Over the past decade, concerns that much psychiatric research serves the interests of industry rather than the interests of patients have become mainstream. These concerns are too well-known to require discussing in detail here, but I shall present a brief overview for any readers not familiar with the issues.

Much research in mental health is now funded by pharmaceutical companies. It is in the nature of such companies that they invest funding in research that they hope might yield profitable results; they fund drug trials rather than studies into the importance of social interventions, and research into the effects of patentable chemicals rather than old ones. A consequence is that a great many issues that may be of interest to patients (and, of course, other people) are underresearched. For example, a 2009 study found that patients would like more research into alternative treatments (nutrition, creativity, etc.), consumer surveys, and medication side effects (e.g., Del Vecchio and Blyler 2009). None of these issues are commercial priorities.

A further problem caused by the prevalence of pharmaceutical funding is that trust in results reported from company-sponsored studies has been eroded. Around 60% of drug trials are industry funded (Perlis et al. 2005). Trials funded by pharmaceutical companies are more likely to find "positive" results—a phenomenon known as "sponsor bias." Perlis et al. (2005) examined a sample of clinical trials and found that those that reported conflict of interest were 4.9 times more likely to record positive results for the drug under study. Though the explanation of sponsor bias is contested, it at least raises the possibility that many reported results are unreliable.

Furthermore, scandal after scandal has emerged, further destroying public confidence. In one well-known case, industry researchers had data that suggested that SSRIs (a family of antidepressant drugs including Prozac) plausibly induced suicidal thought in some patients, but they massaged their published findings to disguise this link (Healy 2006). As another example, consider the work of Joseph Biederman, who has played a key role in promoting the idea that children can suffer from bipolar disorder. Biederman is very influential; in 2007 he was ranked the second most cited psychiatrist worldwide, with 217 papers cited a total of 6,030 times over the past ten years (In-cites 2007). He worked at the Johnson & Johnson Center for Pediatric Psychopathology at Massachusetts General Hospital.[1] Johnson & Johnson funded some of Biederman's work, and they also manufacture Risperdal, one of the drugs that is used in the treatment of children diagnosed with bipolar disorder. Such a setup is not unusual; it has become common for work that is in the interests of a pharmaceutical company to be funded by that company. However, reports in *The New York Times* also discuss evidence unearthed during a congressional investigation which suggests that Biederman transgressed current norms. He is said to have told Johnson & Johnson that clinical trials he had yet to perform would show good results for their drug, and to have failed to disclose to his university the full extent of his payments (Harris 2008, 2009). The Biederman case is interesting because it is hard to judge whether the wrongdoings of which Biederman stands accused are evidence of deep corruption, or minor technicalities. Predicting the results of a trial that has yet to be conducted sounds bad in a newspaper article, but in reality most scientists can predict with fair accuracy the likely results of their studies. Still, such cases are enough to raise doubts about the credibility of research. It is important to bear in mind that for the credibility of academic research to be undermined it is not necessary for widespread corruption to be proved; as soon as it becomes a realistic possibility that research might be manipulated, trust is damaged.

Such concerns have become well-known. In recent years, article after article, and book after book, has chronicled the ways in which psychiatric research, and medical research more broadly, has become corrupted. The titles alone sketch the argument: Marcia Angell (2005) *The Truth about the Drug Companies: How They Deceive Us and What to Do about It*; Daniel Carlat (2010) *Unhinged: The Trouble with Psychiatry—A Doctor's Revelations about a Profession in Crisis*; David Healy (2012) *Pharmageddon*.

Angell sums up the situation:

> [I]t would be naive to conclude that bias is only a matter of a few isolated instances. It permeates the entire system. Physicians can no longer rely on the medical literature for valid and reliable information. This is the conclusion I reluctantly reached toward the end of my 2 decades as an editor of the *New England Journal of Medicine*, and it has been reinforced in subsequent years. Clinicians just do not know anymore how safe and effective prescription drugs really are, but these products are probably nowhere near as good as the published literature indicates. (Angell 2008, 1070–1071)

I suggest that the crisis of credibility that affects psychiatry should be understood as part of a wider problem. Much university research across a broad range of areas is now industry sponsored. There are good reasons to think that this quite generally leads to research on questions that are profitable (which may not be the same as those questions that are interesting or useful) and to findings potentially being distorted to fit with industry interest (for a review of the issues focused on biomedical research, see Krimsky 2004; for a more general discussion, see Washburn 2008). Concerns similar to those that now plague psychiatry have been raised in a wide variety of areas, including, but not limited to, research on the human health impact of industrial and agricultural chemicals (Hardell et al. 2007), the nutritional value of foods (Lesser et al. 2007), genetically modified crops (Myhr and Traavik 2003), the effects of tobacco (Bero 2005), criminology (with the rise of private prisons in the United States) (Geis, Mobley, and Shichor 1999), and even research on the effectiveness of punitive legal payments (Freudenburg 2005). There is a general crisis of trust in scientific research. The crisis that currently faces psychiatry should be situated within this broader picture.

The Potential for Amateur Science/Citizen Science/User-Led Research

Current concerns that much scientific research may have been co-opted by industry stem from the fact that researchers have become dependent on business money. Since the professionalization of science in the nineteenth century, research has come to be dominated by salaried researchers—who either work for universities or in industry research facilities (Golinski 1998, chapter 2; Morrell 1990). However, there are good reasons to think that quite generally, and specifically in the case of mental health research, it would be a good thing for this trend to be partially reversed. Numerous terms are employed to refer to research performed by lay people who are not university-employed academics—"amateur science," "citizen science," "user-led science." I will use "amateur research" to refer to any type of research conducted by unpaid volunteers working outside of a traditional research-conducting institution (university, industry laboratory). When talking specifically about such research as conducted in the mental health field, I will sometimes switch to talk of "user-led" research, as this term has become so established. I will argue that it would be a good thing for more research to be undertaken by amateurs. I think that amateur-produced research can not only play a role in restoring trust in areas where trust has been lost, but is also a good idea because (as I shall argue) having a more diverse research community has general epistemic advantages.

The term "amateur" sometimes takes on derogatory connotations—the amateur researcher is sometimes distinguished from the "real," "professional," "reliable" researcher. Here, by "amateur," I mean simply "not employed to do the research." In this sense "amateur" researchers may be just as knowledgeable, skilled, and reliable as university employees (they may even be university employees conducting their own research projects in their spare time). I am principally interested here in considering the possible benefits of research that is conducted independently of institutional backing. In the mental health context this might be undertaken by individuals or groups of patients seeking to find things out on their own initiative.

In mental health research, "user-led" research now also takes place within universities—some employ salaried user researchers on projects. Such initiatives are valuable for various reasons (some of which I discuss in Cooper 2007, chapter 8; 2014a, chapter 3), but they are not the sorts of research that primarily interest me here. Here, I focus on the potential of research conducted by independent researchers who are not being paid to undertake the research.

Some associate "user-led" research with claims that I wish to distance myself from. In *Postpsychiatry*, Patrick Bracken and Philip Thomas (2005) link user-led research with a postmodernist account of truth. Although I haven't time to argue it here, I think their approach mistaken and I do not think that user-led research and postmodernism need be linked. I hope for user-led research that seeks truths in exactly the same sort of sense as traditional researchers should but that might find out truths that traditional researchers have overlooked or hidden.

Another strand of thought that I wish to distance myself from links user-led research with the use of certain methodologies, typically qualitative, often narrative based (Campbell 2009). I think that qualitative studies have their place, but I also think that quantitative methods are appropriate for addressing many legitimate questions and might be employed by users. In particular, quantitative studies are required to guide rational decision making regarding treatment choices (Cooper 2014b). To take an example, suppose one is trying to decide whether to agree to electroconvulsive therapy (ECT) treatment. Qualitative studies suggest that some people who have ECT find it very helpful, while others suffer a range of side effects, such as memory loss. While this is good to know, in order to judge whether undergoing ECT treatment is a risk that is worth taking, statistics from which one can gauge the odds of being helped or harmed are required. Of course, quantitative methods generally require researchers to possess some statistical know-how, and many have supposed them to be beyond the competence of amateurs. I suspect that the supposed incompetence of amateurs is overstated and that there are amateurs who are capable of employing sophisticated statistical methodologies (consider that various projects requiring technical expertise have been successfully undertaken by unpaid workers in other areas—such as the software developed by the Open Source movement).

In short, I think that all truth-seekers (whether traditional researchers or amateur researchers) seek truths in the same sense and can employ the same methods. The difference between traditional researchers and amateur researchers in the sense that interests me is merely that traditional researchers are paid to conduct research whereas amateur researchers are not.[2] I shall argue that amateur science is now possible and timely for a number of interconnected reasons.

Until very recently, researchers working in universities, and in other traditional research settings, such as industrial laboratories, have enjoyed tremendous advantages over amateurs. Typically, professional researchers, but not amateurs, had access to education, journals and books, computing power, critical discussion with peers, and so on. This is now all changing.

The rise of university-level education means that many more people than in earlier times have been trained in research methodologies. I do not believe that competent researchers will necessarily have PhDs, but still, having a PhD is good evidence that an individual is capable of conducting high-level research. It is worth noting that most people with PhDs are not currently employed as researchers. Most people with PhDs are either retired or never gained a research position.[3] Thus many individuals who have been trained to conduct research are "at large" in the public. The Internet has also made self-education easier than ever before; freely available online lecture courses mean that anyone with access to the Internet can find out fairly much whatever they want.

The means of conducting research are also increasingly accessible. In the past only those with access to academic libraries had access to journals; now very many research papers are freely available online. Computer software for statistical analyses can be run on home computers; specialist equipment can often be purchased from online retailers. Maintaining contact with others who are able to critique and support research efforts is also crucial for most researchers, and the Internet makes it easier for amateurs to become integrated in communities of researchers.

Not only is amateur research now possible, but it promises various benefits, both to the amateur researchers themselves and to the wider society. Most obviously, much amateur-produced research is politically motivated. Knowledge is power, and those who conduct research are in a position to find out what they want to know to make their lives better and to spot when those in authority are seeking to mislead them. For example, Gwen

Ottinger (2010) discusses the role of amateur research in enabling residents in the Diamond subdivision in Norco, Louisiana, to successfully lobby for greater protection from air pollutants released from a nearby Shell chemical plant. Residents had long suspected that air pollutants from the plant were damaging their health. Still, although the air sometimes smelled bad, residents' concerns were dismissed by regulators who monitored long-term average pollutant levels and found them to be within "acceptable" ranges. The tide turned when residents became able to monitor short-term spikes in pollutants themselves using a simple air-sampling technology known as "buckets." Originally developed during the mid-1990s, "buckets" provide a cheap and easy means of monitoring "grab-samples" of air. They are now distributed through nonprofit environmental organizations such as the Louisiana Bucket Brigade. Residents can use buckets to monitor air quality at a point in time—for example, on occasions when they smell something and suspect pollutants have been released. While the reliability of bucket data is contested, they can be used to produce quantitative data that regulators take seriously enough to prompt further investigation. This example nicely illustrates multiple points: citizens sometimes need to conduct their own research; a little technical know-how can go a long way (developing buckets required engineering expertise, using them does not); and networks of activists are capable of supporting amateurs to obtain data that is fairly reliable (the Louisiana Bucket Brigade will supply buckets and provides training).

Knowledge is sometimes urgently required to enable action, but research that is of no immediate use is also worth doing. Knowledge gained may turn out to be of use at some future point. Knowledge that will always be useless is also often worth gaining; many people obtain pleasure from knowing things and finding things out (for a description of the pleasures that motivate naturalists, see, e.g., Ellis 2011). Generally, knowledge is a good thing,[4] and amateur-produced research can lead to truths being discovered that would not otherwise be known for a variety of reasons.

Most obviously, some research questions will never be addressed by traditional researchers because the funding will never be made available. Some research is so labor-intensive that it would be prohibitively expensive if researchers were paid. Consider, for example, Galaxy Zoo (http://www.galaxyzoo.org/), a project started in 2007 by researchers at the University of Oxford. Images of galaxies are best classified by the human eye, but the volume of data to be processed is huge. Galaxy Zoo makes use of volunteer research labor. Those clicking on a website classify images of galaxies as "round," "spiral," and so on. In the first year 50 million classifications were received. Although not an amateur-initiated project, Galaxy Zoo helps illustrate the potential of amateur research labor.

Some research questions could be investigated fairly cheaply but will never be studied by paid researchers because they are of no interest to funders. In mental health, patients groups regularly call for research into topics that are not considered priorities by industry or grant givers. In many cases these questions might be addressed by groups of patients, who could conduct their own studies looking, for example, at the effects of lifestyle changes on symptoms (caffeine, exercise, etc.). When it comes to drug trials, company-sponsored studies generally examine whether a drug reduces average symptoms in a pool of patients over some shortish period of time. Questions connected to drug use that are of importance to patients, but of no commercial interest, tend not to be investigated. For example, even if a drug produces benefits in most of those who take it, for any individual the question of whether the medication produces benefits in his or her particular case remains. Patients might also want themselves to investigate the effects of long-term use and any side effects. Some of the most successful user-initiated research projects to date have involved groups of patients conducting their own surveys of unwanted drug reactions. For example, Mind, the UK mental health charity, published reports in 1996 and 2001 which helped highlight concerns about links between SSRI use and feelings of violence and suicide (Cobb 1996; Cobb, Darton, and Juttla 2001). After the Mind reports, these concerns were taken up by mainstream researchers.

Even when money is not an issue, amateurs can often gain access to places, things, and people that university researchers cannot. Some phenomena are very rare. Projects that depend on relocating previously tagged fish rely on fishermen, not marine biologists, to find the fish (Smith and Scharf 2010). Schoolchildren can find rare ladybirds missed by professional scientists (Losey, Perlman, and Hoebeke 2007). Sometimes data will be hidden from professional researchers but not from amateurs. For example, patients and care assistants are much more likely than visiting social scientists to see evidence of physical abuse in institutional settings. As another sort of example, patients clearly have better access to their own subjective experiences than do traditional researchers. Work on the phenomenology of mental disorder might be well done by patients. More subtle effects also occur. What observers notice and how they interpret what they see depend on their interests and assumptions. For example, Donna Haraway (1989) shows how male and female primatologists have tended to see the social role of female chimps differently. Male scientists saw female chimps as passive bit players in a social drama controlled by males. Female scientists noticed behavior that had previously been missed; in their telling, female chimps make active decisions regarding their mates and play a role in negotiating social hierarchies. Researchers coming from different backgrounds are likely to discover different truths.

To sum up, work by amateur researchers is now possible and promises to enable the discovery of truths that would otherwise remain unknown. Amateurs can find things out that professional researchers cannot in a range of circumstances; professional researchers may lack the funding or incentive to investigate a question, professionals may be deliberately hiding information, and professionals may lack access to the phenomena to be investigated.

Worries: Can Amateur Research Be Trusted?

Some will consider the discussion so far naive. I have argued that amateur-produced research both is possible and can be a good thing, but so far I have not talked about two serious reasons for doubt. First, much amateur-produced research would be of poor quality. Second, patient groups can be co-opted to the interests of industry in exactly the same way as can university researchers. Some patient groups have already become the focus of conflict-of-interest allegations (see Rose 2013). In light of such accusations, why suppose that research conducted by user groups is any more credible than that conducted by university researchers? How can the reliability of user-generated research be guaranteed?

Note first that the old idea that all and only papers published in peer-reviewed journals can be trusted is in any case dying, and new methods that enable work to be assessed postpublication are quite generally required. Concerns that large chunks of medical research have become so corrupted by industry as to be unreliable have already been discussed. There are also widespread concerns about the misleading conclusions that can be drawn from reviewing a literature that privileges the publishing of positive results and tends to underreport negative findings (Nosek, Spies, and Motyl 2012). In many fields, attempts to replicate published findings are rare, but those studies that have been done suggest that replicating reported findings can often be impossible (Prinz, Schlange, and Asadullah 2011; Begley and Ellis 2012). Regardless of whether more research comes to be done by amateurs, new systems for evaluating research reports need to be developed. Here, I can only offer a few pointers on how readers might decide whether a report is reliable. First, and most obviously, those trying to figure out which research findings to trust will need to read reports critically, whether those reports are from traditional or amateur researchers. Systems of postpublication peer review might be developed to enable communities of readers to critique published reports. I have argued in this chapter that the possibility that researchers might be bought is a real concern. To a certain extent such possibilities can be investigated. It is generally possible to find out how research has been funded and to find out whether the funders might have an interest in particular results being found. Meta-analyses can be used to compare results obtained from a variety of differently funded studies and can sometimes uncover evidence of funder bias (or, more hopefully, its absence). Some researchers have a past history of having been involved in problematic research activities. These can normally be uncovered via web searches. Sometimes researchers may be personally known to readers, and this might give readers reason to consider a report trustworthy (or not).

To move away from such generalities, when amateur researchers report results there are three possibilities:

1. The amateur research is the only research that addresses some issue.
2. The amateur research finds the same results as have been reported by traditional researchers.
3. The amateur research finds different results than have been reported by traditional researchers.

In the first case, when amateur research is the only research that addresses some issue, it must be taken on its own merits. In the second case, when amateur and professional researchers report the same results, this does not guarantee that such results are correct. It might be that both groups are making the same methodological mistake or are both biased in the same way. Still, agreement in results gives some reason to consider them reliable. Agreement is especially convincing in cases where we can suppose that the distinct research groups are likely to have very different interests and biases (as would generally be the case if an industry-sponsored study and a user-led project reported similar results).

What, though, of the third case, when the results reported by traditional and amateur researchers conflict? To take an example, studies on the effects of ECT conducted by traditional researchers and patient groups have found conflicting results (Rose et al. 2003). Studies by traditional researchers suggest that most of those who receive ECT find it helpful. Studies by user groups find far less patient satisfaction. When different groups of researchers report different results, then there must be some explanation for the discrepancy. In their paper, Rose et al. investigate possible methodological reasons for the different results: Studies by traditional researchers tended to ask patients for their views fairly soon after treatment, the interviewer was often a mental health professional, and fixed option questionnaires were often used. In contrast, studies by user groups often elicited patient views long after treatment, no mental health professionals were involved in the studies, and an open response format was more often employed. Selection effects might also explain the different results; some studies by patient groups might have disproportionately collected data from patients who had experienced problems post-ECT. Here we have an example where critical engagement between different groups of researcher can facilitate progress in discovering truths. Questionable assumptions can be challenged, and methodologies can be improved (e.g., the possibility of selection bias has prompted user groups to initiate prospective studies of experiences of ECT, and traditional researchers are now exploring whether ECT may have long-term side effects not captured by short-term studies). As a result, and over time, a clearer picture with respect to the effects of ECT should be achieved. In such a situation, conflict between different groups of researcher is useful as it prompts a more thorough critique of assumptions and methodology than might otherwise be the case. Through such conflict more reliable research findings can be obtained (as discussed further by Helen Longino 1990 and in Cooper 2007, chapter 8). The fact that researchers from different backgrounds and with different interests look at problems differently, and can spot and correct different types of problems in scientific research, provides a further reason why it is a good thing to have more research conducted by amateurs.

What's This Got to Do with Rating Scales and Classification?

I have argued that user-led research is both possible and a good idea. I will now go on to consider how different types of rating scales and classification can help or hinder amateur research. I focus on classifications and ratings scales, but the discussion here can be read as a case study that explores a more general phenomenon. Researchers rely on "the infrastructure of science"—by which I mean the social, conceptual, and material systems that enable scientists to do research (systems of accessing journals, of peer review, rating scales, classification systems, methods of statistical analysis, etc.). Quite generally, such systems can be set up to make life more or less difficult for amateurs. Here, I focus on classifications (and, later, ratings scales). The first stage of my argument depends on showing that multiple distinct classifications can be "natural" or "valid." There is more than one "scientifically legitimate" classification. The second stage of the argument depends on showing that any given classification can help, or hinder, research by a particular research community. This means that one of the factors to be considered when constructing a classification is which research communities will be best able to use it.

First, for the argument that multiple classifications will be equally legitimate: John Dupré, a philosopher of biology, argues for a position he calls promiscuous realism (Dupré 1981, 1993). Although Dupré originally developed his position when thinking about classification in biology, it can also be considered applicable to other areas, including mental disorders. Dupré notes that different subdisciplines in biology classify organisms in different ways: Evolutionary theorists find it best to classify on the basis of evolutionary descent. Ecologists prefer classifications that focus on current behavior. Microbiologists struggle to trace evolutionary lineage or find out much about the behavior of the organisms they study; they classify on the basis of DNA. Which of these classifications is right? In Dupré's account all of these classifications are legitimate. Each focuses on (some of) the real similarities and differences between organisms.

At a more abstract level, Dupré suggests that the world is complicated enough to enable very many potentially fruitful classifications. We can imagine the properties of some domain mapped out in a multidimensional property space, as in cluster analysis. In such a space, entities that are very similar will be found close together while those that share fewer properties will be far apart. If we were to map biological organisms, some clusters would correspond to traditional biological species. However, other clusters could also be picked out. Depending on the level of resolution, we may see one cluster or a grouping of smaller clusters. We could focus in on particular dimensions and just classify with regard to particular properties; for example, we might classify mushrooms on the basis of DNA, or depending on whether or not they are edible. Dupré's account is realist—the ways in which entities cluster depend on the properties that they possess, but it is promiscuous as the world is such that many distinctions could be drawn and so decisions have to be made as to which distinctions are of importance (which, of course, varies with context and interest).

Dupré notes how different classifications can facilitate work on different types of research questions. Classifications based on evolutionary lineage are best for research into questions connected to evolutionary theory, classifications based on current behavior are best for ecology, and so on. Here, I want to go beyond Dupré's point and consider how different types of classifications also facilitate research by different types of researchers. The natural historical sciences offer good case studies for thinking through the tensions that can emerge between professionals and amateurs over classification. There is a strong tradition of amateur involvement in natural history, and these are paradigmatic examples of classification-based sciences.

Amateurs tend to be excluded from laboratory-based sciences; access to most labs is restricted, and these sciences tend to use expensive or dangerous equipment. In contrast, the natural world cannot be locked up and is easy to see; plants, bugs, and birds are all around us. Many people enjoy some amateur spotting, and some individuals develop great skill in specimen identification. Some types of organism are such that they can only be distinguished by those who have spent hours and hours developing their perceptual skills. Brambles and mosses, for example, are particularly tough groups. Those individuals who can distinguish different types of organism have undeniable abilities but historically have often not been the sorts of people that science has traditionally been comfortable granting epistemic authority. In the nineteenth century, for example, some of the most skilled English naturalists were to be found in the "botany societies" of Lancashire, where working-class men met in pubs to identify and study plant specimens (Secord 1994a,b). Today, it remains the case that the skills of amateur naturalists command recognition; lorry drivers present conference posters on mushrooms (Meyer 2010), and published papers are often written by amateurs (Hopkins and Freckleton 2002).

However, although the natural historical sciences have a long tradition of amateur research, there have been ongoing tensions between professionals and amateurs over classification (Hopkins and Freckleton 2002). At base the disputes are over whether classification should be based on technologically advanced methods (favoring university-based researchers) or on skilled human perception (putting university researchers and amateurs on a level playing field). John Dean (1979) documents the rifts in plant taxonomy that arose from the 1920s between traditionalists, who split species on the basis of morphological differences, and experimental taxonomists, who employed a range of techniques, such as hybridization studies (which examine whether plants can produce offspring) and the microscopic examination of chromosomes. The different approaches better fit the needs of distinct research communities. Those who are interested in mapping intraspecific genetic variation find a classification that uses experimental techniques and seeks to track patterns of interbreeding most useful. Those who conduct research that requires identifying species in the field tend to prefer classifying on the basis of morphological differences. Often the two approaches will classify organisms similarly, but sometimes the species recognized differ depending on the techniques considered legitimate.

Gilia inconspicua looks to be five sibling species of small blue flower if one uses microscopic examination of the chromosomes, but one species if one relies on morphological characteristics. Conversely, *Gilia tenuiflora-latiflora* is made up of several morphologically distinct groups (of slightly different-looking small blue flowers), but these groups can be shown to be capable of interbreeding. The traditional taxonomist focuses on morphology and sees *Gilia inconspicua* as one species, and *Gilia tenuiflora-latiflora* as a complex made up of several distinct species. The experimental taxonomist takes the opposite stance and sees *Gilia inconspicua* as a complex of five species, and *Gilia tenuiflora-latiflora* as a single species. Different ways of classifying best fit different research questions (generally, morphology is more important for questions of ecology and various conservation projects; genetics is more important for research into evolutionary theory). Different ways of classifying also promote the interests of different research communities; realistically, amateurs can only make use of morphologically based classifications.

In recent years, these long-standing tensions between technology-heavy classification and traditional classification have been reinvigorated as many types of natural history have faced a crisis. Over the course of the twentieth century, university-based taxonomy lost ground to more fashionable sciences, and as a result there are fewer and fewer professionals who have the skills required to identify specimens (see, e.g., Löbl and Leschen 2005, Hopkins and Freckleton 2002). For a striking illustration of the demise of professional taxonomy, consider the difficulties faced by a project seeking beetle specialists to catalog species living in Europe: "[O]nly four skilled British coleopterists [beetle specialists] could be found … three of them retired" (Löbl and Leschen 2005, 287). At the same time as university-based expertise in taxonomy has declined, concerns about mapping and managing biodiversity mean that demand for species identification and monitoring remains strong. The skills shortage has led to two types of response. On the one hand, some seek to cultivate amateur knowledge. Various research projects now depend on the identification skills of amateurs (Ellis and Waterton 2004; Bell et al. 2008). The other response has been to seek a technological solution; some hope to replace skilled human perception with DNA bar coding (Ellis, Waterton, and Wynne 2010).

The use of DNA sequencing in the classification of biological organisms sharply illustrates the divergent interests of professional and amateur researchers. Only professional researchers have access to DNA technology. Any move to require DNA sequencing data privileges such researchers and would make contributing to taxonomic research impossible for amateurs.

Some researchers object to the increased use of DNA sequencing on such grounds:

> Most current taxonomy is pursued using low-cost technology. Mandatory introduction of DNA sequences into taxonomy seems to us a retrograde step. In most instances, a quick survey of morphology will serve the same purpose and, although morphology has its problems, DNA has as many pitfalls. A sufficiently different sequence might warrant the description of a new species, as will a sufficiently different morphology. An expensive and centralized DNA-based taxonomy would only add to the North–South divide in taxonomy, and might exclude the many taxonomists who have limited access to sequencing. (Seberg et al. 2003, 64)

We can generalize the point; some classifications can only be used by those with access to particular types of technology—such classifications act to exclude those who lack access to the technology from research communities. Quite generally, the classification systems that might best support research by university-based professionals may be distinct from those that would best enable research by amateurs.

What Sorts of Classifications and Rating Scales Might User-Led Research in Mental Health Need?

Not all user-led research into issues related to mental health will make use of classifications or ratings of psychopathology. User-led research into drug side effects, for example, relies on asking people who are taking a particular drug to note their experiences. For such projects, there is no need for people to be classified according to their diagnosis or symptoms. Similarly, projects that examine the lived experience of care do not need to classify patients by condition or symptomatology (such projects might instead use ratings from scales such as the Community Oriented Programs Environment Scale; Moos 1974).

Other possible projects, however, would rely on there being classifications of psychopathology that can be used by users. Currently, most users will have been given one (or more) diagnoses by mental health professionals and can compare their experiences with others who have been similarly diagnosed. People usually know their DSM diagnoses, and the DSM is sufficiently intelligible to lay readers for users to have a fairly good idea of whether the diagnosis they have been given seems reasonable or might have changed. Online tests that can confirm the plausibility of any given diagnosis are also available for many disorders.

In mental health research, classifications and rating scales are closely connected. Many symptoms can only be reliably measured by the use of rating scales, and users will need access to rating scales in order to address many possible questions. To take a simple example, consider someone who wants to find out whether a drug they have been prescribed seems to be helping them. They might well want to chart the severity of their symptoms in order to see. Similarly, if user researchers are to be able to conduct their own studies to look at whether, say, exercise helps with mood, they may need to use scales to measure mood.

Some rating scales can equally easily be used by user researchers or traditional researchers. These will often refer to measures that are easily observable. To take an example, consider the "clutter scale" (http://www.hoardingconnectioncc.org/Scale.cfm), which can be used to assess the severity of clutter as it occurs in hoarding. The scale consists of a set of photos of different rooms in the house (bedroom, kitchen, lounge) showing differing amounts of clutter. To use the scale, one looks at the rooms to be assessed and picks the image on the scale that most closely matches it. One's judgment can easily be checked by asking a friend to also make a rating. This is an example of a scale that is easy to use and also freely available online. Because users can make use of it themselves, they are empowered to conduct their own research and are also able to make sense of the research findings that use the scale that are published by professional researchers.

Other scales that can be used by users do not rely on ratings of things that are readily publically observable but ask about subjective experiences. For example, the Internal State Scale (Bauer et al. 1991) asks patients to score statements such as "I feel sped up inside," "My thoughts are going faster," "I feel energized," and so on. Over the last few decades a great many rating scales have been developed that could be used by patients to rate their own symptoms (e.g., Altman et al. 1997; Connor et al. 2000; Marks and Mathews 1979; Zung 1965). For the most part, these scales have been developed with the aim of saving clinician time; the idea has been that patients should rate their own symptoms in the waiting room and then pass on the results to their clinician. However, many of these scales would be suitable for use in user research—if they were made publically available (some, such as the Beck Depression Inventory, are currently sold on a commercial basis and may be inaccessible to users).

One strand of user-led research holds that monitoring changes in symptomatology may not be the best way to conduct research that meets the needs of users (Del Vecchio and Blyler 2009). Rather than focusing on symptom reduction, some users will be more interested in examining the factors that promote quality of life or "recovery." Measures of quality of life/recovery, and of symptomatology, can come apart for a variety reasons. Consider that some drug treatments are effective in reducing symptoms but have side effects. Those taking such drugs may find that their symptoms are reduced but their quality of life also goes down. As another example, some "symptoms" may not cause patients any problems. For example, some people hear voices that do not bother them. In such cases a reduction in symptoms may bring no benefits to the patient. In response to such concerns, various scales that seek to measure recovery have been developed (Campbell-Orde et al. 2005). Insofar as some users are more interested in measuring recovery than symptom reduction, such scales might be useful for user-led research.

Even where a classification or rating scale is not going to be employed by users in their own research, I suggest that one desirable feature for a classification or rating scale is for it to be "transparent" in the sense that nonexperts are able to understand it (or fairly easily find out how to understand it). Transparency is a virtue in that it makes it possible for lay people to make intelligent use of classifications and ratings and to challenge them. Not all will be in favor of increasing transparency. The professional interests of elite groups are often promoted by using classifications and ratings scales that are obscure to outsiders. Conducting research in terms that no one else can understand can bring professional advantages in that it can make researchers appear clever, and it also insulates a research community from possible criticism. I think that transparency is desirable because it enables broad debate about science, but it must be noted that is not the only desideratum for a classification system. The system must also seek to be, for example, valid, reliable, and scientifically fruitful. In some cases, it might not be possible to achieve all these aims together, and sometimes transparency might need to be sacrificed in the pursuit of other goods. All things being equal, however, a system that can be understood by many rather than few is to be preferred.

The DSM is a relatively transparent classification system. Most of the terms it uses can be understood by nonexperts, and clear rules for diagnosis are given. Owen Whooley (2010) links what he regards as psychiatry's ambivalent regard for the DSM to this transparency. Compared to the obscure mystique of psychoanalytic diagnosis, recent versions of the DSM have rendered psychiatric diagnosis transparent to nonexperts. This helped to defend psychiatry from the 1970s antipsychiatrists; the DSM-III helped make it clear why some people and not others might justifiably be considered mentally disordered. At the same time, however, the transparency of the DSM has rendered psychiatry vulnerable to detailed critique from bureaucrats and lay people. Administrators can look in the DSM and see that a patient should not retain a diagnosis of adjustment disorder for a long period of time; a patient can see that a brief psychotic episode is differentiated from schizophrenia chiefly on the basis of the duration of symptoms.

However, although the DSM and many of the rating scales currently used in psychiatric research are fairly transparent, mental health research is currently at a crucial juncture. The RDoC project poses both risks and opportunities when it comes to transparency. On the one hand RDoC moves psychiatry further in the direction of high-tech, lab-based science. As such, the ratings employed by projects that make use of the RDoC framework are likely to be less accessible to lay people than are current projects that depend on DSM categories. On the other hand, the RDoC framework includes a multiplicity of classifications, and, by implication, suggests that further classifications might also be legitimate. Against such a background, it is timely to push for the development and maintenance of classifications and rating scales that might facilitate research by user researchers.

In this chapter I have argued that the crisis of trust that currently faces psychiatric research should be seen as part of a broader problem. Across many areas of science, research has become commercialized. This has led to research that is conducted into areas that are potentially profitable rather than in the public interest, and to concerns that published research findings are being manipulated. At the same time the prospects for amateur research are better than ever before. The rise of university-level education means that many members of the public have been trained in research methodologies, and the Internet makes it possible for amateurs to be embedded in support networks that will enable them to conduct research. For a variety of reasons, amateur researchers can discover truths that traditional researchers have either hidden or overlooked. As such, making it possible for more amateurs to conduct research can be expected to increase the total sum of useful human knowledge to the benefit of all, and to decrease the risk that biased findings rest unchallenged. All researchers rely on the "infrastructure of science" (systems of accessing journals, rating scales, classifications, statistical methods, etc.) in conducting their research. For amateurs to be able to conduct research, the systems that make research possible need to be open to use by amateurs. As a case study, I consider in some detail how classification systems and ratings scales might best support research by users. I suggest that there is a need for classifications and rating scales that rely on data that can either be easily observed by anyone (e.g., the clutter scale) or on symptoms that can be reliably self-reported by users.

As psychiatric research moves into the RDoC era, there is a risk that greater interest in research into basic neuroscience will lead to less research into other areas, such as the phenomenology of mental illness, sociocultural contexts, individual agency, and so on. However, it is worth noting that in this chapter I have presented a picture of research in which distinct research projects need not compete in a zero-sum game. First, Dupré's promiscuous realism offers a picture of classification where multiple classifications can be employed in investigating different questions. Second, greater use of amateur research would mean that different research projects need not compete for a limited amount of funding or researcher time. In this picture, the world is rich enough and the talents of amateurs are potentially great enough for a wide variety of different research projects to legitimately be pursued.

Acknowledgments

This work was funded by a mid-career fellowship from the British Academy (Evaluating the Diagnostic and Statistical Manual of Mental Disorders, MD120060) and I am grateful for their support. A version of this chapter was presented at a workshop held at Lancaster University and sponsored by the Royal Institute of Philosophy, "Patient Knowledge and Involvement in Healthcare," May 2014, and I have benefitted from the comments of those present. I also thank Jeff Poland and Şerife Tekin, who gave me many helpful comments on an earlier draft.

Notes

1. Biederman's affiliation is given in a paper he co-authored (Faraone et al. 2003). This paper also lists Biederman as a recipient of a grant from Johnson & Johnson.

2. Research by graduate students and retired professors can be hard to categorize. Frequently these researchers are not paid. Sometimes they are "part of the system," for example, in the case of a PhD student who toes the line in the hope of securing an academic position. Sometimes they can act more independently than salaried academics.

3. As an indication in 2009 in the United States only 14% of those graduating with PhDs in biology and the life sciences had an academic position within five years (Vastag 2012).

4. Though there are some research questions that are best left unstudied—for example, research that aims to develop methods of torture.

References

Altman, E. G., D. Hedeker, J. L. Peterson, and J. M. Davis. 1997. The Altman self-rating mania scale. *Biological Psychiatry* 42 (10): 948–955.

Angell, M. 2005. *The Truth about the Drug Companies: How They Deceive Us and What to Do About It.* New York: Random House.

Angell, M. 2008. Industry-sponsored clinical research: A broken system. *Journal of the American Medical Association* 300 (9): 1069–1071. doi:10.1001/jama.300.9.1069.

Bauer, M., P. Crits-Christoph, W. Ball, E. Dewees, T. McAllister, P. Alahi, J. Cacciola, and P. Whybrow. 1991. Independent assessment of manic and depressive symptoms by self-rating: Scale characteristics and implications for the study of mania. *Archives of General Psychiatry* 48 (9): 807–812.

Begley, C., and L. Ellis. 2012. Drug development: Raise standards for preclinical cancer research. *Nature* 483 (7391): 531–533.

Bell, S., M. Marzano, J. Cent, H. Kobierska, D. Podjed, D. Vandzinskaite, H. Reinert, A. Armaitience, M. Grodzińska-Jurczak, and R. Muršič. 2008. What counts? Volunteers and their organisations in the recording and monitoring of biodiversity. *Biodiversity and Conservation* 17 (14): 3443–3454.

Bero, L. 2005. Tobacco industry manipulation of research. *Public Health Reports* 120 (2): 200–208.

Bracken, P., and P. Thomas. 2005. *Postpsychiatry: Mental Health in a Postmodern World.* Oxford: Oxford University Press.

Campbell, J. 2009. We are the evidence: An examination of service user research involvement as voice. In *Handbook of Service User Involvement in Mental Health Research*, ed. J. Wallcraft, B. Schrank, and M. Amering, 113–138. Oxford: Wiley-Blackwell.

Campbell-Orde, T., J. Chamerlin, J. Carpenter, and H. S. Leff. 2005. *Measuring the Promise: A Compendium of Recovery Measures. Vol. II.* Cambridge, MA: Evaluation Center. http://www.power2u.org/downloads/pn-55.pdf.

Carlat, D. 2010. *Unhinged: The Trouble with Psychiatry—A Doctor's Revelations about a Profession in Crisis.* New York: Free Press.

Cobb, A. 1996. *Mind's Yellow Card Scheme Reporting the Adverse Effects of Psychiatric Drugs. First Report. May 1996.* London: Mind.

Cobb, A., K. Darton, and K. Juttla. 2001. *Mind's Yellow Card for Reporting Drug Side Effects: A Report of Users' Experiences.* London: Mind.

Connor, K. M., J. R. Davidson, L. E. Churchill, A. Sherwood, E. Foa, and R. H. Weisler. 2000. Psychometric properties of the Social Phobia Inventory (SPIN) new self-rating scale. *British Journal of Psychiatry* 176 (4): 379–386.

Cooper, R. 2007. *Psychiatry and Philosophy of Science*. Stocksfield, UK: Acumen.

Cooper, R. 2014a. *Diagnosing the Diagnostic and Statistical Manual of Mental Disorders*. London: Karnac Books.

Cooper, R. 2014b. On deciding to have a lobotomy: Either lobotomies were justified or decisions under risk should not always seek to maximise expected utility. *Medicine, Health Care, and Philosophy* 17 (1): 143–154.

Dean, J. 1979. Controversy over classification: A case study from the history of botany. In *Natural Order: Historical Studies of Scientific Culture*, ed. B. Barnes and S. Shapin, 211–230. Beverly Hills, CA: Sage.

Del Vecchio, P., and C. Blyler. 2009. Identifying critical outcomes and setting priorities for mental health services research. In *Handbook of Service User Involvement in Mental Health Research*, ed. J. Wallcraft, B. Schrank, and M. Amering, 99–112. Oxford: Wiley-Blackwell.

Dupré, J. 1981. Natural kinds and biological taxa. *Philosophical Review* XC:66–90.

Dupré, J. 1993. *The Disorder of Things*. Cambridge, MA: Harvard University Press.

Ellis, R. 2011. Jizz and the joy of pattern recognition: Virtuosity, discipline and the agency of insight in UK naturalists' arts of seeing. *Social Studies of Science* 41 (6): 769–790.

Ellis, R., and C. Waterton. 2004. Environmental citizenship in the making: The participation of volunteer naturalists in UK biological recording and biodiversity policy. *Science & Public Policy* 31 (2): 95–105.

Ellis, R., C. Waterton, and B. Wynne. 2010. Taxonomy, biodiversity and their publics in twenty-first-century DNA barcoding. *Public Understanding of Science (Bristol, England)* 19 (4): 497–512.

Faraone, S. V., J. Sergeant, C. Gillberg, and J. Biederman. 2003. The worldwide prevalence of ADHD: Is it an American condition? *World Psychiatry; Official Journal of the World Psychiatric Association (WPA)* 2 (2): 104–113.

Freudenburg, W. 2005. Seeding science, courting conclusions: Re-examining the intersection of science, corporate cash, and the law. *Sociological Forum* 20 (1): 3–33.

Geis, G., A. Mobley, and D. Shichor. 1999. Private prisons, criminological research, and conflict of interest: A case study. *Crime and Delinquency* 45 (3): 372–388.

Golinski, J. 1998. *Making Natural Knowledge: Constructivism and the History of Science*. Chicago: University of Chicago Press.

Haraway, D. J. 1989. *Primate Visions: Gender, Race, and Nature in the World of Modern Science*. London: Routledge.

Hardell, L., M. J. Walker, B. Walhjalt, L. S. Friedman, and E. D. Richter. 2007. Secret ties to industry and conflicting interests in cancer research. *American Journal of Industrial Medicine* 50 (3): 227–233.

Harris, G. 2008. Research center tied to drug company. *The New York Times*. November 25, p. A22, New York Edition.

Harris, G. 2009. Drug maker told studies would aid it, papers say. *The New York Times*. March 19, p. A16, New York Edition.

Healy, D. 2006. Did regulators fail over selective serotonin reuptake inhibitors? *British Medical Journal* 333:92–95.

Healy, D. 2012. *Pharmageddon*. Berkeley: University of California Press.

Hopkins, G., and R. Freckleton. 2002. Declines in the numbers of amateur and professional taxonomists: Implications for conservation. *Animal Conservation* 5 (3): 245–249.

In-cites. 2007. The most-cited researchers in psychiatry/ psychology. Last accessed November 21, 2014. http://in-cites.com/top/2007/second07-psy.html.

Krimsky, S. 2004. *Science in the Private Interest: Has the Lure of Profits Corrupted Biomedical Research?* Lanham, MD: Rowman & Littlefield.

Lesser, L., C. Ebbeling, M. Goozner, D. Wypij, and D. Ludwig. 2007. Relationship between funding source and conclusion among nutrition-related scientific articles. *PLoS Medicine* 4 (1): e5.

Löbl, I., and A. Leschen. 2005. Demography of coleopterists and their thoughts on DNA barcoding and the phylocode, with commentary. *Coleopterists Bulletin* 59 (3): 284–292.

Longino, H. E. 1990. *Science as Social Knowledge: Values and Objectivity in Scientific Inquiry*. Princeton, NJ: Princeton University Press.

Losey, J. E., J. E. Perlman, and E. R. Hoebeke. 2007. Citizen scientist rediscovers rare nine-spotted lady beetle, *Coccinella novemnotata,* in eastern North America. *Journal of Insect Conservation* 11 (4): 415–417.

Marks, I. M., and A. M. Mathews. 1979. Brief standard self-rating for phobic patients. *Behaviour Research and Therapy* 17 (3): 263–267.

Meyer, M. 2010. Caring for weak ties—the Natural History Museum as a place of encounter between amateur and professional science. *Sociological Research Online* 15 (2): 9.

Moos, R. H. 1974. *Community Oriented Programs Environment Scale*. Palo Alto, CA: Consulting Psychologists Press.

Morrell, J. B. 1990. Professionalisation. In *Companion to the History of Modern Science*, ed. R. Olby, G. Cantor, J. Christie, and M. Hidge, 980–989. London: Routledge.

Myhr, A. I., and T. Traavik. 2003. Genetically modified (GM) crops: Precautionary science and conflicts of interests. *Journal of Agricultural & Environmental Ethics* 16 (3): 227–247.

Nosek, B., J. Spies, and M. Motyl. 2012. Scientific utopia. II. Restructuring incentives and practices to promote truth over publishability. *Perspectives on Psychological Science* 7 (6): 615–631.

Ottinger, G. 2010. Buckets of resistance: Standards and the effectiveness of citizen science. *Science, Technology & Human Values* 35 (2): 244–270.

Perlis, R., C. Perlis, Y. Wu, C. Hwang, M. Joseph, and A. Nierenberg. 2005. Industry sponsorship and financial conflict of interest in the reporting of clinical trials in psychiatry. *American Journal of Psychiatry* 162 (10): 1957–1960.

Prinz, F., T. Schlange, and K. Asadullah. 2011. Believe it or not: How much can we rely on published data on potential drug targets? *Nature Reviews. Drug Discovery* 10 (9): 712.

Rose, D., P. Fleischmann, T. Wykes, M. Leese, and J. Bindman. 2003. Patients' perspectives on electroconvulsive therapy: Systematic review. *British Medical Journal* 326 (7403): 1363.

Rose, S. L. 2013. Patient advocacy organizations: Institutional conflicts of interest, trust, and trustworthiness. *Journal of Law, Medicine & Ethics* 41 (3): 680–687.

Seberg, O., C. J. Humphries, S. Knapp, D. W. Stevenson, G. Petersen, N. Scharff, and N. Andersen. 2003. Shortcuts in systematics? A commentary on DNA-based taxonomy. *Trends in Ecology & Evolution* 18 (2): 63–65.

Secord, A. 1994a. Corresponding interests: Artisans and gentlemen in nineteenth-century natural history. *British Journal for the History of Science* 27 (4): 383–408.

Secord, A. 1994b. Science in the pub: Artisan botanists in early nineteenth-century Lancashire. *History of Science* 32 (97): 269–315.

Smith, W., and F. Scharf. 2010. Demographic characteristics of southern flounder, *Paralichthys lethostigma*, harvested by an estuarine gillnet fishery. *Fisheries Management and Ecology* 17 (6): 532–543.

Vastag, B. 2012. U.S. pushes for more scientists, but the jobs aren't there. *The Washington Post*. July 7, 2012. Last accessed November 27 2014. http://www

.washingtonpost.com/national/health-science/us-pushes-for-more-scientists-but-the-jobs-arent-there/2012/07/07/gJQAZJpQUW_story.html.

Washburn, J. 2008. *University, Inc.: The Corporate Corruption of Higher Education*. New York: Basic Books.

Whooley, O. 2010. Diagnostic ambivalence: Psychiatric workarounds and the *Diagnostic and Statistical Manual of Mental Disorders*. *Sociology of Health & Illness* 32 (3): 452–469.

Zung, W. W. 1965. A self-rating depression scale. *Archives of General Psychiatry* 12 (1): 63–70.

10 Six Myths about Schizophrenia: A Paradigm Well Beyond Its Use-By Date?

Richard P. Bentall

In 2007, the *British Medical Journal*, one of the world's leading outlets for medical research, published an editorial by Jeffrey A. Lieberman and Michael B. First (2007), entitled "Renaming Schizophrenia: Diagnosis and Treatment Are More Important than Semantics." The editorial was a response to a suggestion by some critics of psychiatry that the concept of schizophrenia lacked scientific or clinical validity and that the term should therefore be replaced with something else.

The authors of the editorial can fairly be called leaders of American psychiatry. Lieberman is Lawrence E. Kolb Professor and chairman of psychiatry at the Columbia University College of Physicians and Surgeons and director of the New York State Psychiatric Institute. First is a professor of psychiatry in the same institution and has been heavily involved in the development of internationally accepted diagnostic criteria for schizophrenia and other psychiatric conditions. In their editorial, they say,

> The charge that schizophrenia does not define a specific illness is clearly unwarranted. ... For more than 100 years schizophrenia has been an integral part of our nosology and has facilitated research and treatment of people affected by this disease. People qualify for the diagnosis if their clinical signs and symptoms conform to the operational diagnostic criteria that define schizophrenia. Many studies have shown that these diagnostic criteria can be applied reliably and accurately by trained mental health professionals. Although a diagnosis of schizophrenia depends on the presence of a pattern of symptoms (such as delusions, hallucinations, disorganised speech, disorganised or catatonic behaviour, and negative symptoms such as lack of motivation), evidence shows that these are manifestations of brain pathology. Schizophrenia is not caused by disturbed psychological development or bad parenting. Compared with normal controls, people with schizophrenia have abnormalities in brain structure and function seen on neuroimaging and electrophysiological tests. In addition, the evidence that vulnerability to schizophrenia is at least partly genetic is indisputable.

These claims are a defense of the familiar, biomedical conception of schizophrenia, which perhaps should surprise no one given the status of the authors within the mainstream of American psychiatry. However, a careful examination of the available research literature reveals that the widely accepted assumptions about the nature of schizophrenia cataloged in this article are at best questionable and, in many cases, refuted by empirical data. It is striking, therefore, that leaders in the field can make bold statements such as these when the scientific research evidence points to starkly different conclusions. In this chapter it is not my intention to question the motives of these authors; surely they are honorable, and Lieberman and First were stating assumptions about schizophrenia that were so sincerely held that they were mistaken as fact. Rather, I want to argue that the endurance of the schizophrenia concept in the face of mounting evidence of its inadequacy is a testament to the power that scientific paradigms hold over the minds of researchers, and of the failure of the normal process of empirical refutation that ensues.

Schizophrenia as a Paradigm

The concept of schizophrenia can be traced back to the late years of the nineteenth century and, in particular, the work of Emil Kraepelin (1899/1990), who set out to develop a system of classifying psychiatric disorders that would serve both the researcher and the clinician.

Kraepelin believed that disorders could, in principle, be classified in three ways, but that each method would lead to the same result:

> Judging from our experience in internal medicine it is a fair assumption that similar disease processes will produce identical symptom pictures, identical pathological anatomy and an identical aetiology. If, therefore, we possessed a comprehensive knowledge of any of these three fields—pathological anatomy, symptomatology, or aetiology—we would at once have a uniform and standard classification of mental diseases. A similar comprehensive knowledge of either of the other two fields would give us not just as uniform and standard classifications, but *all of these classifications would exactly coincide*. (Kraepelin 1907, italics mine)

In Kraepelin's time, very little was known about the pathological anatomy or etiology of psychiatric disorders, but within this framework, classifying disorders according to how symptoms aggregate or follow a common course should provide a kind of Rosetta stone by which the language of madness can be decoded. The researcher simply has to group together people with the same diagnosis (defined according to signs, symptoms, and course) and compare them with suitable controls; whether the researchers are interested in genes, brains, or indeed psychological functions, those who have the diagnosis should have something in common (indicative, hopefully of an etiological process) which is absent in the controls, and meaningful science should follow.

As is well known, by studying the signs, symptoms, and outcomes of a large number of patients (by 1896 he had collected over 1,000 case studies, which he considered hardly enough for his purposes) Kraepelin came to identify two major classes of severe psychiatric disorder which continue to preoccupy psychiatric researchers today (Bentall 2003). First he identified a group of patients whose illness typically developed in early adulthood, whose symptoms included hallucinations and delusions against a background of pronounced cognitive impairment, and who progressively deteriorated over time; the term he gave for this condition was *dementia praecox* (literally, senility of the young). Second, he identified another group of patients whose outcomes were generally better and who suffered from pronounced mood difficulties (typically depression but in some cases mania); these patients were said to suffer from *manic depression* (the historian of psychiatry David Healy [2011] has suggested that this latter diagnosis—which, in Kraepelin's account, encompassed what we know as unipolar depression as well as bipolar disorder—emerged as a foil to the dementia praecox concept; in order to establish the validity of a form of mental illness which had a very poor outcome, it was necessary to identify an equally severe type of psychiatric disorder with a good prognosis).

Both of these concepts have been passed down to the present time in a process that might be compared to the telephone game, in which they have gone through a series of transformations as they have been passed from one expert to the next. It was the Swiss psychiatrist Eugen Bleuler (1911/1950) who reformulated dementia praecox as *schizophrenia* (or actually "the group of schizophrenias"), rejecting the idea that the condition was necessarily praecox (always appearing in the young) or indeed a dementia (although full recovery rarely if ever occurred, some degree of restitution could be expected). For Bleuler, who was partly influenced by Freud, it was not the cognitive deterioration identified by Kraepelin that was the core of the disorder but the more subtle processes of inappropriate affect, loosening of the associations, emotional ambivalence, and autism (by which he meant a retreat into a preferred world of fantasy). However, Bleuler's view that what we now call positive symptoms were secondary to these psychological processes was largely forgotten after the German psychiatrist Kurt Schneider (1959), in an attempt to develop a pragmatic approach to diagnosis, proposed a list of eleven first-rank symptoms, which were all types of hallucinations or delusion. Despite Schneider's explicit denial that these symptoms were necessarily the most important for understanding the disorder—they were merely easy to spot—his account presaged the focus on positive symptoms enshrined in modern diagnostic manuals such as the American Psychiatric Association's *Diagnostic and Statistical Manual of Mental Disorders* (DSM). Small wonder that (in contrast to Lieberman and First's claim that "[f]or more than 100 years schizophrenia has been an integral part of our nosology and has facilitated research and treatment of people affected by this disease") some commentators have questioned whether, when describing the disorder, Kraepelin, Bleuler, and Schneider were talking about the same thing (Boyle 1990).

Enthusiasm for the Kraepelinian system waned during the middle years of the twentieth century, under the influence of Adolf Meyer (1951), who thought that patients should be treated as individuals and that psychiatric problems were always a reaction to some kind of adverse life experience (Meyer famously quipped that "[w]e should classify plants, not people"). However, the system was revived again in the later decades of the last century by a group of American psychiatrists who explicitly described themselves as neo-Kraepelinians. The neo-Kraepelinians wished to return psychiatry to its medical roots; it is no accident that, when photographed, many of the leading advocates of this approach were often wearing white coats (as does Jeffrey Lieberman on his Wikipedia page).

One of the neo-Kraepelinians, Samuel Guze (1989), suggested that "there is no such thing as a psychiatry that is too biological." Another, Gerald Klerman (1978), authored what amounted to a manifesto for the movement, which explicitly listed nine assumptions about mental illness, including that a clear line could be drawn between mental illness and normal behavior and that there are a discrete and discoverable number of psychiatric disorders.

Perhaps the neo-Kraepelinians' greatest achievement, other than diverting psychiatric research funding so that it focused almost exclusively on biological measurements, was to author the influential third edition of the American Psychiatric Association's (1980) DSM in which methods for diagnosing different psychiatric disorders were laid out using operational criteria. Although revised several times since (the latest version, DSM-5, was published in 2013), the essential structure of the manual remains little changed from the 1980 version. Lieberman, in particular, has been a staunch defender of the manual against a wide range of critics and, in a recent blog, famously described DSM-5 as an "up-to-the-minute diagnostic GPS" (Lieberman 2013).

Building on his studies in the history of science, and in particular of the struggles by Galileo and others to establish the heliocentric model of the universe, the philosopher Thomas Kuhn (1970) noted that scientific progress often proceeds in leaps or "scientific revolutions," interspersed by periods of "normal science" in which a paradigm or conceptual framework is widely accepted without question. (For instance, the notion that space is best described by Euclidian geometry was universally accepted by physicists until Einstein's theory of general relativity suggested that space could be curved.) During the periods of "extraordinary science" in which revolutions occur, vigorous attempts are made to defend the existing paradigm, the rules of research are often relaxed in an attempt to resolve anomalies, and philosophical issues are brought to the fore, until, after intense debate, a strong alternative paradigm at last emerges. This account, which regards science as in part a sociological phenomenon, contrasts markedly with the more traditional Popperian conception in which scientists readily abandon their theories in the face of empirical refutation (Popper 1963); according to Kuhn, it is only after the accumulation of overwhelming evidence that is inconsistent with the paradigm that a new framework will be accepted. The paradigm, in this model, is not simply a way of looking at the world: it is a tacit set of assumptions about the nature of reality through which scientific information is filtered. For the researcher lost in the paradigm, its walls are the walls of the world itself and it is only in the face of extraordinary evidence that it is possible to see beyond them.

In the case of the concept of schizophrenia, and the Kraepelinian approach to psychiatric diagnosis in general, evidence challenging the tacit set of assumptions underlying conventional psychiatric theory now exists in abundance. And yet, despite increasing disquiet in the psychiatric community about the limited achievements of research based on categorical diagnoses (as most notably reflected in the National Institute of Mental Health's new Research Domain Criteria strategy, which suggests that researchers should instead focus on core transdiagnostic mechanisms such as inhibition and negative cognition; see Insel et al. 2010), it seems that leading psychiatric researchers throughout the world are reluctant to abandon it. This gap between evidence and continuing belief in the paradigm can be seen when we examine some of the claims and assumptions about schizophrenia evident in Lieberman and First's editorial.

Myth 1: Schizophrenia Is a Reliable Concept

In their editorial, Lieberman and First assert that "[m]any studies have shown that these diagnostic criteria [for schizophrenia] can be applied reliably and accurately by trained mental health professionals."

The authors of DSM-III realized that psychiatric diagnoses needed to meet two tests of their usefulness: reliability and validity. The first refers to the extent to which clinicians can agree on the application of the diagnostic criteria, for example, on who does or does not have schizophrenia. The second concerns whether the diagnoses are scientifically valid, which is to say whether they are usefully associated with other meaningful scientific (etiology, biomarkers) or clinical constructs (e.g., the course and outcome of the disorder or response to treatment). Note that there is no single index of validity, and different researchers may emphasize different tests. Clearly, therefore, this second criterion is much more difficult to establish, but, for the moment, it is important to note that there is nonetheless an asymmetrical relationship between reliability and validity. As recognized by the authors of DSM-III, whereas a diagnosis might be reliable without being valid (which would be the case, e.g., if I defined "Bentall's disease" in terms of such easy to measure and yet completely unconnected "symptoms" as being more than six feet tall, having red hair, and having more than two Pink Floyd albums in one's album collection), "assuredly an unreliable diagnosis cannot be valid" (Spitzer and Fliess 1974). If we cannot agree on who has schizophrenia and who does not, then there is no way of researching whether schizophrenia has a specific cause or responds to a specific treatment.

The standard way of assessing reliability is by arranging for independent clinicians to diagnose a population of patients and then examining the extent to which they agree. Robert Spitzer, the editor of DSM-III, and his statistician colleague Joseph Fliess, were aware that, in a study of this kind, the number of diagnoses employed and the characteristics of the population studied would heavily affect the extent to which clinicians agreed about diagnoses by chance (e.g., if there are only two diagnoses, chance agreement would be at 50%). To account for this difficulty they introduced a standard metric, known as the kappa statistic, for estimating the extent to which diagnostic agreement is better than chance. Kappa can be calculated for any population and any number of diagnostic choices and varies between 0 (chance agreement) and 1 (complete agreement). Although there is clearly no magic point above which agreement is adequate, Spitzer and Fliess reported that, at that time, only three diagnoses (mental deficiency, organic brain syndrome, and alcoholism) had a "satisfactory" kappa value of 0.7 or above.

From DSM-III onward the authors of the diagnostic manual conducted field trials to determine whether their proposed criteria were reliable. After the publication of DSM-III, Gerald Klerman (1986) claimed that the reliability problem had "in principle been solved" and Spitzer and his colleagues claimed that the reliability of the manual was "extremely good" (Hyler, Williams, and Spitzer 1982). Critics of the field trials noted that they were often unrealistic, in the sense that the diagnosticians received special training, used structured interview schedules when interviewing patients, and often spent much more time over their diagnoses than would be typical in routine practice. Nonetheless, they often failed to achieve reliabilities that exceeded the (admittedly arbitrary) 0.7 criterion (Kutchins and Kirk 1997).

What about DSM-5? Just before the publication of this "up-to-the-minute diagnostic GPS," the results of the field trials appeared in a series of papers in the *American Journal of Psychiatry* (Regier et al. 2013). Only one diagnosis (major neurocognitive disorder) exceeded the 0.7 threshold regarded as "satisfactory" by Spitzer and Fliess. Bipolar I disorder scored 0.56, schizophrenia 0.46, and major depressive disorder 0.28. Mixed anxiety-depressive disorder, a proposed diagnosis that was included in the field trials, was dropped after it scored a derisory –0.04. Far from advancing the goals of psychiatric research and clinical consistency, this latest version of the manual therefore appears to be a step backward. However, this was perhaps not obvious to many observers because the DSM-5 researchers now declared that any kappa values above 0.4 indicated "good agreement" (Freedman et al. 2013), a clear demonstration of how the rules of research may be relaxed in a last-ditch effort to defend a paradigm.

Myth 2: There Is a Clear Dividing Line between Schizophrenia and Healthy Functioning

When Gerald Klerman (1978) drew up his manifesto for the neo-Kraepelinian movement, he argued that "[t]here is a boundary between the normal and the sick." While this issue is not raised in the Lieberman and First editorial in the *British Medical Journal*, it is clearly important in the way that biological psychiatrists think about schizophrenia and has been the subject of intense debate in recent times (David 2010; Lawrie et al. 2010; Linscott and van Os 2010).

Before proceeding to consider this issue further, it is important to acknowledge that the idea of a continuum between schizophrenia and normal functioning is not *logically* fatal to a biomedical account; many physical ailments exist on continua with normal functioning. This is true, for example, for hypertension; although there is no clear cutoff point at which blood pressure become problematic, high levels of hypertension are regarded as causes for medical concern for good reason—they are associated with life-threatening medical emergencies (heart attack and stroke). Nonetheless, a continuum view of schizophrenia would require a more nuanced approach to treating severe mental illness than conventional psychiatric classification would allow. In particular, we would have to allow some debate about how best to help—or even whether to offer help at all—in the case of individuals who lie close to an arbitrary boundary, and perhaps admit that whether or not we should intervene should depend on factors other than conventional diagnostic criteria (e.g., whether or not the individual is distressed or coping well with life).

In recent decades, two lines of evidence have converged to support a continuum model. First, in the late 1970s, psychologists such as Gordon Claridge (1990) at Oxford University and Loren and Jean Chapman at the University of Wisconsin (Chapman et al. 1994; Eckblad and Chapman 1983) (all now retired), discovered that it is possible to detect "schizotypal" experiences or traits in healthy populations of students using simple questionnaires. For example, if asked, a surprising number of students will report hallucinatory or quasi-hallucinatory experiences or bizarre beliefs. This discovery chimed to some extent with the results of early genetic studies (about which I will say more later), which appeared to indicate that the inheritance of schizophrenia was highly non-Mendelian, and that the first-degree relatives of patients with schizophrenia often inherited subsyndromal schizotypal characteristics rather than a full-blown illness. Tying these ideas together, the American psychologist Paul Meehl (1962, 1989) proposed that the children of schizophrenia patients inherit from their parents a cluster of characteristics which he termed "schizotaxia," including anhedonia (a difficulty in experiencing pleasure) and cognitive slippage (a tendency to think in a loosely associated and nonlogical way) but that only a portion of these people, as a consequence of further stressors, become psychotically ill. Since these ideas were first proposed, a cottage industry of research on schizotypy has mushroomed in university psychology departments throughout the world and, in general, students who score highly on these measures have been found to perform analogously to psychotic patients on a wide range of psychological and neuropsychological measures (see Raine 2006 and Lenzenweger 2010 for reviews).

Second, and independently of this discovery, research in the emerging discipline of psychiatric epidemiology has shown that a much larger number of people experience schizophrenic symptoms than might be expected on the basis of admission figures for psychiatric services. For example, in the US Epidemiological Catchment Area Study the number of people experiencing hallucinations at some point in their lives was estimated at about 11% (Tien 1991), and, in the later National Comorbidity Study, 8.5% of those asked reported auditory hallucinations, 7% reported visual hallucinations, and 7% reported tactile hallucinations, with 1.6% reporting all three types (Shevlin, Dorahy, and Adamson 2007).

An implication of these kinds of findings is that there may be large numbers of "happily psychotic" people living unnoticed in the community. This certainly seems to be the case for people who hear hallucinatory voices. Beginning in the 1990s, the Dutch psychiatrist Marius Romme and his partner Sondra Escher (1996) began to use a variety of methods including the mass media to make contact with individuals living in the community who hear voices, and formed *RESONANCE*, a self-help and activist organization for voice hearers, which has subsequently transformed into *INTERVOICE*: The International Hearing Voices Network (http://www.intervoiceonline.org). Anyone who is skeptical about the claims of nonpatient voice hearers might wish to look at the recent TED talk by Eleanor Longden, a young woman who suffered a severe psychotic breakdown before learning to live with her voices, and who now works as a psychological researcher (http://www.ted.com/speakers/eleanor_longden).

Although the idea that it is difficult to draw a line between schizophrenia and normal functioning is now widely accepted, the nature and utility of the schizophrenia spectrum continues to be a topic of debate. Some traditional psychiatrists insist that a dimensional approach to diagnosis is impractical in the psychiatric clinic (Lawrie et al. 2010). Other commentators have argued that, although there can be no doubt that there is a phenomenological continuum (i.e., that many people in the general population report subclinical psychotic experiences), there is nonetheless, as Meehl asserted, a "taxon" or group of individuals who inherit a vulnerability to schizophrenia (Linscott and van Os 2010). This debate has prompted the development of a whole new statistical science of taxometrics, which aims to use sophisticated mathematical techniques to probe beneath apparent continuous distributions of data to see whether different types of people can be identified. Unfortunately, this kind of research has yet to lead to a clear consensus (Beauchaine, Lenzenweger, and Waller 2008; Rawlings et al.

2008) although a recent review found that, on balance, the evidence from the most methodologically rigorous studies supports a continuum model of psychosis (Haslam, Holland, and Kuppens, 2012). As we will see, other kinds of inquiry (particularly in psychiatric genetics) also appear to favor a full structural continuum model.

In defense of the categorical model of psychiatric diagnosis, Lieberman (2015) has recently complained that

> [i]t's common knowledge to every student of medicine and most knowledgeable laypeople that just because you have a symptom doesn't mean that you have an illness. You can have fever without having an infection. You can have shortness of breath without having asthma or heart disease. You can have chest pain without having a heart attack. You can have a headache without having a tumor, so no one has ever conflated a symptom with a diagnosis.

Of course, these comparisons are disingenuous. Diagnoses of infection, asthma, heart disease, and tumor can all be validated against biological measures indicative of types of abnormal physiological functioning that are hazardous to life. There is no lab test or scan that can tell us at what point psychotic experiences turn into schizophrenia.

During periods of scientific revolution, debates about the way forward in science may become heated, and the defenders of a paradigm may feel exasperation at those who question their authority. Lieberman goes on to accuse critics of the categorical model of "challenging the veracity of diagnoses and giving people who have symptoms of a mental disorder, license to doubt that they may have an illness and need treatment."

The important point to note here is that, however the debate about the psychosis continuum is eventually resolved, research shows that large numbers of people who experience psychotic symptoms have indeed taken license to doubt that they have an illness and, as a consequence, lead full lives without any apparent need of psychiatric treatment.

Myth 3: There Is a Clear Dividing Line between Schizophrenia and Other Psychiatric Disorders

At the same time as researchers have begun to question whether there is a clear dividing line between schizophrenia and healthy functioning, others have questioned whether clear distinctions can be drawn between schizophrenia and other psychiatric conditions. The DSM's diagnostic criteria and Lieberman and First's assertion that schizophrenia is a "specific disorder" seem to imply that different kinds of psychiatric disorder can be clearly distinguished or, in the words of Gerald Klerman's (1978) manifesto, that "[t]here are discrete mental illnesses. ... There is not one, but many mental illnesses."

The problem for diagnostic systems presented by patients who experience the symptoms of more than one diagnosis has long been recognized, but the categorical diagnostic system has placed a conceptual stranglehold on attempts to account for this phenomenon. No clearer demonstration of this can be found than in the way that researchers interpreted the data from the US Epidemiological Catchment Area Study.

After eliminating arbitrary exclusion rules in the DSM-III manual (under which, e.g., a diagnosis of bipolar disorder was forbidden if the individual already met the criteria for schizophrenia), the researchers were astonished to find that someone diagnosed as suffering from schizophrenia had a 44 times greater than expected risk of also meeting the diagnostic criteria for mania, and a 13 times greater than chance risk of also being depressed. Rather than concluding that schizophrenia, mania, and depression might not be separate conditions after all, however, the researchers mused that "[t]he most likely explanation for co-occurrence is that having one disorder puts the affected person at risk of developing other disorders" (Robins and Locke 1991). Presumably, they had in mind the idea that the trauma associated with developing schizophrenia was so severe that it would cause bipolar disorder.

In fact, the idea that schizophrenia may blend with other diagnoses goes back a long way. Before the Second World War, the American psychiatrist Joseph Kasanin (1933) proposed the diagnosis of schizoaffective disorder to describe patients who showed a combination of symptoms normally attributed to schizophrenia and those typically attributed to what was then known as manic depression. In the 1970s, the British psychiatrist Robert Kendell argued for a schizoaffective continuum with the majority of patients falling in the middle and relatively few patients presenting with pure schizophrenia or pure bipolar symptoms (Kendell 1991; Kendell and Brockington 1980). Most recently, this idea has been revived by a group of American psychiatrists who have formed the Bipolar and Schizophrenia Network on Intermediate Phenotypes. At the time of writing, this project has collected data from nearly 1,000 patients with DSM-IV diagnoses of schizophrenia, schizoaffective disorder, and bipolar disorder, together with hundreds of their first-degree relatives, and the network has published their initial findings (Tamminga et al. 2014). Overall, the results are more consistent with a continuum between the two diagnoses than with the idea of discrete illnesses. For example, when patients were rated along a ten-point schizophrenia–bipolar continuum, patients with the three diagnoses overlapped, with no evidence that they came from distinct groups (Keshavan et al. 2011). Moreover, when the patients were compared on various measures of brain function and cognitive ability, similarities were much more evident than differences. Reflecting on these findings, Tamminga and her colleagues have concluded, "If preliminary findings hold true, we might need to consider a radical overhaul of our nomenclature for psychosis in the future."

Some researchers have suggested that the extent to which patients meet the criteria for multiple psychiatric diagnoses might provide a clue to a new, empirically based system of diagnosis. This approach was first taken by psychologist Robert Krueger (1999), whose early analyses excluded psychotic symptoms. By examining patterns of *comorbidity* (a term which appears to imply the unfortunate state of suffering from multiple conditions rather than a failure of classification), Krueger found that conditions could be grouped into two main groups or spectra: *internalizing disorders* characterized by problems of mood (typically depression and anxiety) and *externalizing disorders*, in which distress is manifest in behavior (typically conduct problems and substance misuse). This framework has been generally supported in subsequent research, most notably in an analysis of data from over 21,000 people in fourteen countries who were given psychiatric assessments as part of a project known as the World Health Surveys (Kessler et al. 2011). In this study, the researchers not only established whether the participants met the criteria for various psychiatric disorders but also attempted to date at what point in their lives they did so. They found that their data fitted the internalizing–externalizing framework, with comorbidity being observed within each spectrum but not between them. However, within each of the spectra, there was no order discernible in the timing of the diagnoses. For example, some people developed depression before anxiety whereas, for others, the opposite was the case.

Unfortunately, most of the research on the internalizing and externalizing spectra has neglected psychotic disorders. However, in a study using a large sample of psychiatric patients Kotov et al. (2011) found that psychosis formed a third spectrum that was independent of internalizing and externalizing. More recently, a complex analysis of data from a large Australian population sample (Wright et al. 2013) similarly found evidence of a third psychosis spectrum and, moreover, that all three spectra were best described in terms of continua between healthy functioning and disorder.

At first sight, a very different picture of the structure of psychopathology has emerged from a separate and longer line of research, which has examined the covariation between specific symptoms rather than the co-occurrence of diagnoses. This research, which began with studies by Liddle (1987), has used correlational techniques to examine the extent to which behaviors and experiences typically attributed to schizophrenia occur together. The general finding, replicated many times over, has been that psychosis is best described by five separate dimensions: positive symptoms (hallucinations and delusions), negative symptoms (flat affect, social withdrawal, and loss of motivation), cognitive disorganization (including incoherent speech), depression, and mania (Demjaha et al. 2009; Peralta and Cuesta 2001; van Os and Kapur 2009). To add yet another level of complexity, some recent studies have suggested there exists a general unitary psychosis factor (Reininghaus, Priebe, and Bentall 2013) in addition to these five dimensions, or a general psychopathology spectrum in addition to the three internalizing, externalizing, and psychosis spectra (Caspi et al. 2013). On these models, the general factors presumably correspond to a general risk of psychiatric disorder whereas the other factors/spectra determine what kind of symptoms are experienced.

To the uninitiated eye, these findings from quantitative statistical research on psychiatric classification no doubt seem confusing and contradictory. However, it is possible to extract some tentative conclusions from what might seem to be chaos. First, and most strikingly, there is absolutely no support—none whatsoever—for the kind of categorical system of psychiatric classification found in the DSM, and hence for the schizophrenia concept as it is usually understood. Second, on the whole, this research supports both the idea of a continuum (or a number of continua) between psychiatric disorder and healthy functioning and, moreover, between different diagnostic constructs, so that diagnoses such as schizophrenia should be seen as points on a multidimensional landscape that has no fences. Certainly, there is no evidence that schizophrenia is "a specific illness."

Myth 4: Schizophrenia Is Predominantly a Genetic Disease

In their commentary, Lieberman and First state that "the evidence that vulnerability to schizophrenia is at least partly genetic is indisputable." In the sense that all human behavior is influenced by our genetic constitution, this claim is almost a truism, but Lieberman and First probably have something much more particular in mind, namely, the idea that there are specific genes that confer the vulnerability to a schizophrenic illness.

The idea that psychiatric disorders are heritable has driven a large amount of psychiatric research since the unpromising beginnings of psychiatric genetics in the German Third Reich (Proctor 1988). Until recently, this work has largely consisted of family, twin, and adoption studies, which all aim to show that the risk of schizophrenia increases in direct relation to the extent that an individual is genetically related to someone who is already affected. Hence, monozygotic (MZ; identical) twins are expected to have a much higher concordance for schizophrenia than dizygotic (DZ; nonidentical) twins. On the basis of data collected from these kinds of studies, researchers have calculated heritability statistics, which are said to express the proportion of the variation in a trait within a population that can be attributed to differences in genes. There are several different ways of making these calculations, but the simplest is Falconer's (1965) method, which estimates heritability as twice the difference in concordance rates for a disorder between identical and nonidentical twins. Hence, if identical twins are 50% concordant for a disorder (if one twin has the disorder there is a 50% chance of the other's being affected) and nonidentical twins have a 25% concordance rate, the heritability is 50%: [2 × (50 – 25)]. More sophisticated methods use different assumptions but usually generate similar estimates.

For reasons that cannot be discussed in detail here because of limited space, the family and twin studies that are used to generate concordance estimates have been often affected by a variety of methodological limitations which have been overlooked by most researchers. One difficulty is that they assume that the extent to which individuals share environments is unrelated to their genetic closeness, but there is evidence that this assumption is violated, at least in the case of twin studies—if one twin has experienced physical or sexual abuse, for example, the likelihood that the other twin will have experienced similar abuse is higher in MZ twin pairs than in DZ twin pairs (Fosse, Joseph, and Richardson 2015), presumably because children who are more alike are more likely to be treated alike. Another difficulty is that there are several different ways of calculating concordance rates, with genetic researchers typically preferring the methods that give the highest estimates (Marshall 1990). Finally, of course, the unreliability of psychiatric diagnoses provides a further challenge for genetic researchers.

Not surprisingly, earlier, less rigorous studies tend to give higher estimates of genetic effects than more recent studies; when Joseph pooled the data from all available studies, he found an identical twin concordance rate of 40.4% and a nonidentical twin concordance rate of 7.4%, but the pooled data from the nine most recent studies yielded corresponding figures of 22.4% and 4.5% (Joseph 2003; Joseph and Leo, 2006). Although these differences clearly suggest genetic effects, it is notable that three-quarters of the identical twins of people diagnosed with schizophrenia can be expected to avoid being so diagnosed. Using the Falconer method, the estimate of heritability calculated from these numbers is 35.8%, which is much lower than the figures of 70–80% typically reported in psychiatry textbooks. Compounding these problems, heritability estimates, whether low or high, are widely misunderstood, and I will return to this issue in the next section.

In the past few decades, the findings from family studies have been supplemented by developments in molecular genetics. In this kind of research, the aim is to discover particular genes (sequences of DNA) that play a role in conferring risk of psychiatric disorder. The specific methods employed can be complex, but the most widely used approach today is the genome-wide association study (GWAS) in which the entire genome is analyzed and compared between psychiatric patients and controls. However, because there are an enormous number of genes in the human genome, conventional methods of statistical analysis carry a very high risk that apparent differences between the groups will actually be chance observations rather than genuine (what statisticians call type 1 errors). The only way around this problem is to recruit enormous samples—ideally in the tens of thousands—which is why, until recently, in this field of research failed replications were the norm (Crow 2008). Extremely large samples have been required in order to overcome this problem, and these have only been amassed recently.

It is only in the last few years that genetic investigators have become fully aware of the implications of their research for psychiatric classification. For example, the finding that first-degree relatives of schizophrenia patients are at a high risk of also being diagnosed as suffering from the disorder has commonly been interpreted as evidence that the disorder is at least partially inherited (Gottesman 1991), but the further implication of the genetic disease model—that individuals who have a first-degree relative with schizophrenia should *not* have a high risk of other disorders—has been forgotten. A groundbreaking study by Lichtenstein et al. (2009) involved obtaining medical histories from the entire Swedish population, comprising 9 million people in 2 million families, of whom 36,000 had received a diagnosis of schizophrenia and 40,000 had received a diagnosis of bipolar disorder. When examining the first-degree relatives of schizophrenia patients, Lichtenstein and his colleagues found that they were at high risk of being diagnosed with schizophrenia but also of being diagnosed with bipolar disorder; the converse was true of the first-degree relatives of people who had been diagnosed with bipolar disorder.

A similar picture has emerged from recent GWAS studies that have been large enough to produce replicable findings. The results from these studies, far from revealing specific genes for schizophrenia and bipolar disorder, have instead revealed a large number of common genetic variants which each confer a tiny risk of both diagnoses, and indeed other diagnoses such as major depression and autism (Owen 2012; Psychiatric Genomics Consortium 2014). The discovery of such a large number of small and additive genetic influences—many hundred according to some estimates—has prompted one leading genetics researcher to comment that "[t]he genetic risk for schizophrenia is widely distributed in human populations so that we all carry some degree of risk" (Kendler 2015) and is further evidence of a continuum between psychosis and healthy functioning.

Overall, therefore, far from supporting the standard psychiatric conception of schizophrenia, recent genetic research seems to undermine it. What appears to be inherited is nothing like schizophrenia as commonly conceived, but a much more diffuse risk of developing psychiatric disorders in general. Moreover, these effects seem to be much weaker than early research in psychiatric genetics seemed to suggest.

Myth 5: Schizophrenia Is Not Caused by Environmental Factors Such as Childhood Trauma or Parenting

In their *British Medical Journal* editorial, Lieberman and First assert that "[s]chizophrenia is not caused by disturbed psychological development or bad parenting." This claim is consistent with the assumption, widely held among biological psychiatrists, that schizophrenia is primarily a genetic condition, which we have already seen is difficult to justify.

One reason why the role of environmental factors has been hard to spot has been because a strong genetic account of schizophrenia appears to be supported by the heritability statistics. As I described in the last section, these are calculated from data collected in family and twin studies. Technically, they are estimates of the extent to which variations in genes are associated with variations in psychiatric disorder within specific populations; in other words, they are partial correlations calculated between genes and psychiatric disorders while attempting to control for the effect of the environment. As everyone who has ever taken an elementary course in statistics knows, it can be extremely risky to take correlations of this kind as strong evidence of causation.

To understand why this is so, it is helpful to imagine what would happen if variation in disease-causing environmental factors was reduced to zero. In the case of lung cancer, this might happen, for example, if everyone smoked exactly twenty cigarettes a day. Under such circumstances, the main difference between those who succumb to lung cancer and those who remain healthy would presumably be some kind of genetic vulnerability. The heritability of lung cancer in such a world would therefore approach 100%, even though the main cause of illness—smoking—was still environmental.

Some real life phenomena map very well onto this thought experiment. For example, studies of IQ show that intelligence is highly heritable in middle-class families but has very low heritability in working-class families (Turkheimer et al. 2003), presumably because middle-class families are relatively uniform in terms of aspects of the environment that are critical for promoting learning (they all encourage their children to do their homework, read books, etc.). Similarly, a recent study found that the variance in internalizing disorders associated with genes is higher in wealthy families compared to poor families (South and Krueger 2011), presumably because variation in the critical environmental factors is greater in deprived environments. For this and other reasons (Dickins and Flynn 2001) it is wrong to assume that high heritability estimates preclude major environmental contributions to psychiatric disorder.

The only way to estimate the role of the environment in conferring risk of severe psychiatric disorder is to examine environmental factors directly, and this has now been done many times. For example, in a recent meta-analysis of studies of childhood trauma (sexual abuse, physical abuse, bullying by peers, and death of a parent at an early age) and psychosis, my colleagues and I combined data from eight epidemiological studies, eighteen patient versus control comparison studies, and ten prospective studies (Varese et al. 2012). We found very consistent evidence that experiencing childhood trauma approximately triples the risks of psychosis in adulthood, and that children who experience multiple kinds of trauma are at even greater risk. In subsequent studies, we found that specific childhood traumas were associated with specific symptoms of psychosis, so that childhood sexual abuse resulted in a high risk of hallucinations whereas disruptions to early attachment relationships—for example, by being raised in a children's home—led to a high risk of paranoid symptoms (Bentall et al. 2012; Shevlin et al. 2015; Sitko et al. 2014). Recent studies by my research group have also begun to identify some psychological mechanisms that might explain these associations (Varese, Barkus, and Bentall 2011; Wickham, Sitko, and Bentall 2015).

Of course, it is important to remember that these findings do not imply that families are somehow uniquely culpable when their children suffer from psychosis (perpetrators of victimization may not be family members) or that everyone who has experienced psychosis has suffered from a terrible childhood (other factors are important). Moreover, there are subtler and less obviously toxic family influences, which may be just as critical. For example, beginning with the work of Margaret Singer and Lyman Wynne in the early 1960s, a large volume of research has examined the relationship between a particular parental speaking style known as communication deviance and psychosis in offspring (Singer and Wynne 1965a, 1965b). In a meta-analysis of these findings my colleagues and I again found a consistent association between maternal (but, interestingly, not paternal) communication deviance and psychosis in offspring (de Sousa et al. 2014). When this association was examined in a Finnish adoption study, it was found that it could not be explained by genetic effects (Wahlberg et al. 1997).

Other environmental risk factors are extrafamilial. For example, there is consistent evidence that children raised in poverty (Wicks, Hjern, and Daman 2010) or urban environments (Vassos et al. 2012) are at increased risk of psychosis. Migrants and the children of migrants are also at increased risk (Cantor-Graee and Selten 2005), especially if they move into predominantly nonmigrant neighborhoods (Boydell et al. 2001; Veling et al. 2008). Adverse experiences in adulthood have also been consistently associated with risk of a psychotic breakdown (Beards et al. 2013). Hence, although we cannot say that every person who has ever suffered from a severe mental illness has experienced a traumatic event which directly caused their symptoms, the evidence that these kind of events often play a determining role in many cases is, if anything, more compelling than the evidence for genetic risk factors.

Myth 6: Schizophrenia Is a Brain Disease

Finally, of course, the biomedical paradigm assumes that schizophrenia is a brain disease. Hence, Lieberman and First draw attention to the fact that "[c]ompared with normal controls, people with schizophrenia have abnormalities in brain structure and function seen on neuroimaging and electrophysiological tests."

That these differences are observable is beyond doubt, but whether there are specific abnormalities associated with schizophrenia as opposed to other psychiatric disorders seems doubtful. Those studies that have reported apparent differences—for example, by showing enlarged ventricles and reduced gray matter volume in schizophrenia but not bipolar patients (McDonald et al. 2005; McDonald et al. 2006)—have often been compromised by the failure to consider patients with schizoaffective symptoms, a form of sampling bias which is both driven by the dominant paradigm and serves to maintain it. As we have seen, when these patients have been included, similarities in brain function across the schizoaffective continuum have been more striking than differences (Tamminga et al. 2014), and the same has been observed for the kinds of neurocognitive tests that have been designed to pick up more subtle neurological impairments that cannot be detected using scanners, although these deficits are usually more severe at the schizophrenia end of the spectrum (Krabbendam et al. 2005).

In evaluating these findings, however, it is important to put aside the implicit dualism that has guided the majority of research in biological psychiatry, by which risk factors and mechanisms leading to psychiatric distress are assigned to the domains either of psychology or of neuroscience. As Read et al. (2001) pointed out some time ago, abnormal brain structure and function have also been measured in the people who have been victims of trauma, especially childhood abuse, and so it is entirely plausible that the structural and functional abnormalities seen when psychotic patients are placed in a brain scanner are caused by the kinds of environmental factors we considered in the last section.

That this possibility has hardly ever been addressed is, in itself, testament to the grip that the dominant paradigm has over the minds of psychiatric researchers. However, a recent study by Sheffield et al. (2013) compared healthy controls to psychotic patients who reported a history of childhood sexual abuse and those who did not, finding reduced gray matter volume only in the group of patients who had experienced abuse.

Conclusions

As I set out to write this chapter, I did not select the *British Medical Journal* editorial by Lieberman and First for harsh criticism because I thought it particularly foolish or ill intentioned. Rather, I chose it because it seems to represent the mainstream of psychiatric thinking and therefore vividly demonstrates how much that mainstream deviates from what can be concluded from the scientific evidence.

Of course, none of this evidence challenges the view that there are some people who have distressing experiences that appear out of the ordinary and are difficult to understand, nor the moral judgment that these experiences sometimes merit psychological or even medical intervention. However, the evidence does show that the standard biomedical way of thinking about psychiatric conditions is deeply flawed and not fit either for guiding intervention or for the purposes of research.

It is important to note that the research I have reviewed in this chapter is not hidden away. On the contrary, most of it has appeared in highly respected medical journals that are read by psychiatric researchers throughout the world. In some cases (e.g., when interpreting the reliability of diagnoses), the implications have not been recognized because researchers have relaxed previously established rules in an attempt to accommodate uncomfortable data and therefore protect the existing paradigm from challenge. In other cases, the paradigm has stifled research that might further challenge it (particularly research on the role of social and psychological factors in psychosis). But in many cases, it seems, the limitations of the existing paradigm have not been recognized because researchers have simply been blind to data that do not fit their expectations; as I said at the outset, for the researcher lost in a paradigm, its walls are the walls of the world itself. Indeed, particularly striking is the fact that most mental health professionals, whether clinicians or researchers, seem oblivious to an important datum about the utility of conventional psychiatric theory that I have so far omitted to mention: long-term follow-up studies show absolutely no evidence of improvement in schizophrenia patients' outcomes since the 1940s, before the invention of most modern psychiatric therapies (Jääskeläinen et al. 2013). This lack of therapeutic progress—surely the most egregious consequence of clinging to a paradigm that is past its use-by date—contrasts with the dramatic advances in reducing morbidity and mortality achieved by other branches of medicine such as oncology and cardiology (Bentall 2009).

When Thomas Kuhn (1970) proposed his theory of scientific paradigms, he highlighted the importance of sociological factors in understanding why science sometimes progresses and sometimes fails to progress. On this view, progress is impeded not only by the cognitive limitations imposed on researchers by the dominant paradigm, which prevents them from identifying when that paradigm is failing, but also by powerful social forces that keep the paradigm in place.

I will leave it for others to comment in detail on what those forces might be in the case of modern psychiatry, but they undoubtedly include professional hierarchies that are concerned to preserve the claims to expertise made by mental health professionals (for a naked example of this kind of claim, see Craddock et al. 2008), a pharmaceutical industry that aggressively seeks markets in which to peddle its psychiatric drugs (Moncrieff 2003), governments that seek to justify coercive practices for the control of troublesome citizens (Molodynski, Rugkasa, and Burns 2010), and media industries that pander to all of these concerns in order to sell copy (Coverdale, Nairn, and Claasen 2002; Philo et al. 1994).

But dysfunctional paradigms cannot last forever. Eventually, their inadequacies must become apparent to even the most closed-minded of observers. We may be approaching such a point in the history of psychiatry.

References

American Psychiatric Association. 1980. *Diagnostic and Statistical Manual of Mental Disorders*. 3rd ed. Washington, DC: American Psychiatric Association.

American Psychiatric Association. 2013. *Diagnostic and Statistical Manual of Mental Disorders*. 5th ed. Arlington, VA: American Psychiatric Association.

Beards, S., C. Gayer-Anderson, S. Borges, M. E. Dewey, H. L. Fisher, and C. Morgan. 2013. Life events and psychosis: A review and meta-analysis. *Schizophrenia Bulletin* 39 (4): 740–747. doi:10.1093/schbul/sbt065.

Beauchaine, T. P., M. F. Lenzenweger, and N. G. Waller. 2008. Schizotypy, taxometrics, and disconfirming theories in soft science: Comment on Rawlings, Williams, Haslam, and Claridge. *Personality and Individual Differences* 44:1652–1662.

Bentall, R. P. 2003. *Madness Explained: Psychosis and Human Nature*. London: Penguin.

Bentall, R. P. 2009. *Doctoring the Mind: Why Psychiatric Treatments Fail*. London: Penguin.

Bentall, R. P., S. Wickham, M. Shevlin, and F. Varese. 2012. Do specific early life adversities lead to specific symptoms of psychosis? A study from the 2007 The Adult Psychiatric Morbidity Survey. *Schizophrenia Bulletin* 38:734–740.

Bleuler, E. 1911/1950. *Dementia Praecox or the Group of Schizophrenias*. Trans. E. Zinkin. New York: International Universities Press.

Boydell, J., J. van Os, J. McKenzie, J. Allardyce, R. Goel, R. G. McCreadie, and R. M. Murray. 2001. Incidence of schizophrenia in ethnic minorities in London: Ecological study into interactions with environment. *British Medical Journal* 323:1–4.

Boyle, M. 1990. *Schizophrenia: A Scientific Delusion*. London: Routledge.

Cantor-Graee, E., and J. P. Selten. 2005. Schizophrenia and migration: A meta-analysis and review. *American Journal of Psychiatry* 163:478–487.

Caspi, A., R. M. Houts, D. W. Belsky, S. J. Goldman-Mellor, H. Harrington, S. Israel, M. Meier, et al. 2013. The p factor: One general psychopathology factor in the structure of psychiatric diorders? *Clinical Psychological Science* 2 (2): 119–137.

Chapman, L. J., J. P. Chapman, T. R. Kwapil, M. Eckblad, and M. C. Zinser. 1994. Putatively psychosis-prone subjects 10 years later. *Journal of Abnormal Psychology* 103:171–183.

Claridge, G. S. 1990. Can a disease model of schizophrenia survive? In *Reconstructing Schizophrenia*, ed. R. P. Bentall, 157–183. London: Routledge.

Coverdale, J., R. Nairn, and D. Claasen. 2002. Depiction of mental illness in print media: A prospective national sample. *Australian and New Zealand Journal of Psychiatry* 36 (5): 697–700.

Craddock, N., D. Antebi, M.-J. Attenburrow, A. Bailey, A. Carson, P. Cowen, B. Craddock, et al. 2008. Wake-up call for British psychiatry. *British Journal of Psychiatry* 193:6–9.

Crow, T. J. 2008. The emperors of the schizophrenia polygene have no clothes. *Psychological Medicine* 38:1679–1680.

David, A. S. 2010. Why we need more debate on whether psychotic symptoms lie on a continuum with normality. *Psychological Medicine* 40:1935–1942.

Demjaha, A., K. Morgan, C. Morgan, S. Landau, K. Dean, A. Reichenberg, P. Sham, et al. 2009. Combining dimensional and categorical representation of psychosis: The way forward for DSM-V and ICD-11? *Psychological Medicine* 39 (12): 1943–1955. doi:10.1017/S0033291709990651.

de Sousa, P., F. Varese, W. Sellwood, and R. P. Bentall. 2014. Parental communication deviance and psychosis: A meta-analysis. *Schizophrenia Bulletin* 40:756–768. doi:10.1093/schbul/sbt088.

Dickins, W. T., and J. R. Flynn. 2001. Heritability estimates versus large environmental effects: The IQ paradox resolved. *Psychological Review* 108:346–369.

Eckblad, M., and L. J. Chapman. 1983. Magical ideation as an indicator of schizotypy. *Journal of Consulting and Clinical Psychology* 51:215–225.

Falconer, D. S. 1965. The inheritance of liability to certain diseases, estimated from the incidence among relatives. *Annals of Human Genetics* 29:51–76.

Fosse, R., J. Joseph, and K. Richardson. 2015. A critical assessment of the equal-environment assumption of the twin method for schizophrenia. *Frontiers in Psychiatry* 6:62. doi:10.3389/fpsyt.2015.00062.

Freedman, R., D. A. Lewis, R. Michels, D. S. Pine, S. K. Schultz, C. A. Tammiga, G. O. Gabbard, et al. 2013. The initial field trials of DSM-5: New blooms and old thorns. *American Journal of Psychiatry* 170:1–5.

Gottesman, I. I. 1991. *Schizophrenia Genesis: The Origins of Madness*. New York: Freeman.

Guze, S. 1989. Biological psychiatry: Is there any other kind? *Psychological Medicine* 19:315–323.

Haslam, N., E. Holland, and P. Kuppens. 2012. Categories versus dimensions in personality and psychopathology: A quantitative review of taxometric research. *Psychological Medicine* 42:903–920.

Healy, D. 2011. *Mania: A Short History of Bipolar Disorder*. Baltimore: Johns Hopkins University Press.

Hyler, S., J. Williams, and R. Spitzer. 1982. Reliability in the DSM-III field trials. *Archives of General Psychiatry* 39:1275–1278.

Insel, T., B. Cuthbert, M. Garvey, R. Heissen, D. S. Pine, K. Quinn, C. Sanislow, and P. Wang. 2010. Research Domain Criteria (RDoC): Toward a new classification framework for research on mental disorders. *American Journal of Psychiatry* 167:748–751.

Jääskeläinen, E., P. Juola, N. Hirvonen, J. J. McGrath, S. Saha, M. Isohanni, and J. Miettunen. 2013. A systematic review and meta-analysis of recovery in schizophrenia. *Schizophrenia Bulletin* 39:1296–1306.

Joseph, J. 2003. *The Gene Illusion: Genetic Research in Psychology and Psychiatry under the Microscope*. Ross-on-Wye, UK: PCCS Books.

Joseph, J., and J. Leo. 2006. Genetic relatedness and the lifetime risk for being diagnosed with schizophrenia: Gottesman's 1991 figure 10 reconsidered. *Journal of Mind and Behavior* 27:73–90.

Kasanin, J. 1933. The acute schizoaffective psychoses. *American Journal of Psychiatry* 90:97–126.

Kendell, R. E. 1991. The major functional psychoses: Are they independent entities or part of a continuum? Philosophical and conceptual issues underlying the debate. In *Concepts of Mental Disorder: A Continuing Debate*, ed. A. Kerr and H. McClelland, 1–16. London: Gaskell.

Kendell, R. E., and I. F. Brockington. 1980. The identification of disease entities and the relationship between schizophrenic and affective psychoses. *British Journal of Psychiatry* 137:324–331.

Kendler, K. S. 2015. A joint history of the nature of genetic variation and the nature of schizophrenia. *Molecular Psychiatry* 20:77–83. doi:10.1038/mp.2014.94.

Keshavan, M. S., D. W. Morris, J. A. Sweeney, G. Pearlson, G. Thanker, L. J. Seidman, S. M. Eack, and C. Tamminga. 2011. A dimensional approach to the psychosis spectrum between bipolar disorder and schizophrenia: The Schizo-Bipolar Scale. *Schizophrenia Bulletin* 133:250–254.

Kessler, R. C., J. Ormel, M. Petukhova, K. A. McLaughlin, J. G. Green, L. J. Russo, D. J. Stein, et al. 2011. Development of lifetime comorbidity in the World Health Organization world mental health surveys. *Archives of General Psychiatry* 68 (1): 90–100. doi:10.1001/archgenpsychiatry.2010.180.

Klerman, G. 1986. Historical perspectives on contemporary schools of psychopathology. In *Contemporary Directions in Psychopathology: Towards DSM-IV*, ed. T. Millon and G. Klerman, 3–28. New York: Guilford Press.

Klerman, G. L. 1978. The evolution of a scientific nosology. In *Schizophrenia: Science and Practice*, ed. J. C. Shershow, 99–121. Cambridge, MA: Harvard University Press.

Kotov, R., S. W. Chang, L. J. Fochtmann, R. Mojtabai, G. A. Carlson, M. J. Sedler, and E. J. Bromet. 2011. Schizophrenia in the internalizing-externalizing framework: A third dimension? *Schizophrenia Bulletin* 37 (6): 1168–1178. doi:10.1093/schbul/sbq024.

Krabbendam, L., B. Arts, J. van Os, and A. Aleman. 2005. Cognitive functioning in patients with schizophrenia and bipolar disorder: A quantitative review. *Schizophrenia Research* 80:137–149.

Kraepelin, E. 1907. *Textbook of Psychiatry*. 7th ed. Trans. A. R. Diefendorf. London: Macmillan.

Kraepelin, E. 1990. *Psychiatry: A Textbook for Students and Physicians. Vol. 1, General Psychiatry*. Canton, MA: Watson Publishing International. (1899).

Krueger, R. 1999. The structure of common mental disorders. *Archives of General Psychiatry* 56:921–926.

Kuhn, T. 1970. *The Structure of Scientific Revolutions*. 2nd ed. Chicago: University of Chicago Press.

Kutchins, K., and S. A. Kirk. 1997. *Making Us Crazy: DSM—The Psychiatric Bible and the Creation of Mental Disorders*. New York: Free Press.

Lawrie, S. M., J. Hall, D. G. C. Owens, and E. C. Johnstone. 2010. The 'continuum of psychosis': Scientifically unproven and clinically impractical. *British Journal of Psychiatry* 197:423–425.

Lenzenweger, M. F. 2010. *Schizotypy and Schizophrenia*. New York: Guilford Press.

Lichtenstein, P., B. H. Yip, C. Bjork, Y. Pawitan, T. D. Cannon, P. F. Sullivan, and C. M. Hultman. 2009. Common genetic determinants of schizophrenia and bipolar disorder in Swedish families: A population-based study. *Lancet* 373: 234–239.

Liddle, P. F. 1987. The symptoms of chronic schizophrenia: A reexamination of the positive-negative dichotomy. *British Journal of Psychiatry* 151:145–151.

Lieberman, J. 2013. Caught between mental illness stigma and anti-psychiatry prejudice. *Scientific American Mind.* http://blogs.scientificamerican.com/mind-guest-blog/2013/05/20/dsm-5-caught-between-mental-illness-stigma-and-anti-psychiatry-prejudice.

Lieberman, J. 2015. What does the New York Times have against psychiatry? *New York Times*, January 17, 2015. http://www.medscape.com/viewarticle/838764/.

Lieberman, J. A., and M. B. First. 2007. Renaming schizophrenia: Diagnosis and treatment are more important than semantics. *British Medical Journal* 334:108.

Linscott, R. J., and J. van Os. 2010. Systematic reviews of categorical versus continuum models in psychosis: Evidence for discontinuous subpopulations underlying a psychometric continuum. Implications for DSM-V, DSM-VI, and DSM-VII. *Annual Review of Clinical Psychology* 6:391–419.

Marshall, R. 1990. The genetics of schizophrenia: Axiom or hypothesis? In *Reconstructing Schizophrenia*, ed. R. P. Bentall, 89–117. London: Routledge.

McDonald, C., E. Bullmore, P. Sham, X. Chitnis, J. Suckling, J. MacCabe, M. Walshe, and R. M. Murray. 2005. Regional volume deviations of brain structure in schizophrenia and psychotic bipolar disorder: Computational morphometry study. *British Journal of Psychiatry* 186:369–377.

McDonald, C., N. Marshall, P. Sham, E. T. Bullimore, K. Schultze, B. Chapple, E. Bramon, et al. 2006. Regional brain morphometry in patients with schizophrenia or bipolar disorder and their unaffected relatives. *American Journal of Psychiatry* 163:478–487.

Meehl, P. 1962. Schizotaxia, schizotypia, schizophrenia. *American Psychologist* 17:827–838.

Meehl, P. 1989. Schizotaxia revisited. *Archives of General Psychiatry* 46:935–944.

Meyer, A. 1951. *The Collected Papers of Adolf Meyer.* Baltimore: Johns Hopkins Press.

Molodynski, A., J. Rugkasa, and T. Burns. 2010. Coercion and compulsion in community mental health care. *British Medical Bulletin* 95:105–119.

Moncrieff, J. 2003. *Is Psychiatry for Sale?* London: Institute of Psychiatry.

Owen, M. J. 2012. Implications of genetic findings for understanding schizophrenia. *Schizophrenia Bulletin* 38 (5): 904–907. doi:10.1093/schbul/sbs103.

Peralta, V., and M. J. Cuesta. 2001. How many and which are the psychopathological dimensions in schizophrenia? Issues influencing their ascertainment. *Schizophrenia Research* 49:269–285.

Philo, G., J. Secker, S. Platt, L. Henderson, G. McLaughlin, and J. Burnside. 1994. The impact of the mass media on public images of mental illness: Media content and audience belief. *Health Education Journal* 53:271–282.

Popper, K. 1963. *Conjectures and Refutations: The Growth of Scientific Knowledge*. London: Routledge.

Proctor, R. N. 1988. *Racial Hygiene: Medicine under the Nazis*. Cambridge, MA: Harvard University Press.

Psychiatric Genomics Consortium. 2014. Biological insights from 108 schizophrenia-associated genetic loci. *Nature* 511:421–427.

Raine, A. 2006. Schizotypal personality: Neurodevelopmental and psychological trajectories. *Annual Review of Clinical Psychology* 2:291–326.

Rawlings, D., B. Williams, N. Haslam, and G. Claridge. 2008. Taxometric analysis supports a dimensional latent structure for schizotypy. *Personality and Individual Differences* 44:1640–1651.

Read, J., B. D. Perry, A. Moskowitz, and J. Connolly. 2001. A traumagenic neurodevelopmental model of schizophrenia. *Psychiatry* 64:319–345.

Regier, D. A., W. E. Narrow, D. E. Clarke, H. C. Kraemer, S. J. Kuramoto, E. A. Kuhl, and D. J. Kupfer. 2013. DSM-5 field trials in the United States and Canada. II. Test-retest reliability of selected categorical diagnoses. *American Journal of Psychiatry* 170:59–70.

Reininghaus, U., S. Priebe, and R. P. Bentall. 2013. Testing the psychopathology of psychosis: Evidence for a general psychosis dimension. *Schizophrenia Bulletin* 39:884–895.

Robins, L. N., and B. Z. Locke, eds. 1991. *Psychiatric Disorders in America*. New York: Free Press.

Romme, M., and A. Escher. 1996. Empowering people who hear voices. In *Cognitive Behavioural Interventions with Psychotic Disorders*, ed. G. Haddock and P. D. Slade, 137–150. London: Routledge.

Schneider, K. 1959. *Clinical Psychopathology*. New York: Grune & Stratton.

Sheffield, J. M., L. F. Williams, N. D. Woodward, and S. Heckers. 2013. Reduced gray matter volume in psychotic disorder patients with a history of childhood sexual abuse. *Schizophrenia Research* 143:185–191.

Shevlin, M., M. Dorahy, and G. Adamson. 2007. Childhood traumas and hallucinations: An analysis of the National Comorbidity Survey. *Journal of Psychiatric Research* 41:222–228.

Shevlin, M., G. McAnee, R. P. Bentall, and J. Murphy. 2015. Specificity of association between adversities and the occurrence and co-occurrence paranoia and hallucinations: Evaluating the stability of childhood risk in an adverse adult environment. *Psychosis: Psychological, Social and Integrative Approaches* 7 (3): 206–216. doi:10.1080/17522439.2014.980308.

Singer, M. T., and L. C. Wynne. 1965a. Thought disorder and family relations of schizophrenics. III. Methodology using projective techniques. *Archives of General Psychiatry* 12:187–200.

Singer, M. T., and L. C. Wynne. 1965b. Thought disorder and family relations of schizophrenics. IV. Results and implications. *Archives of General Psychiatry* 12:201–212.

Sitko, K., R. P. Bentall, M. Shevlin, N. O'Sullivan, and W. Sellwood. 2014. Associations between specific psychotic symptoms and specific childhood adversities are mediated by attachment styles: An analysis of the National Comorbidity Survey. *Psychiatry Research* 217:202–209. doi:10.1016/j.psychres.2014.03.019.

South, S. C., and R. Krueger. 2011. Genetic and environmental influences on internalizing psychopathology vary as a function of economic status. *Psychological Medicine* 41:107–117.

Spitzer, R. L., and J. L. Fliess. 1974. A reanalysis of the reliability of psychiatric diagnosis. *British Journal of Psychiatry* 125:341–347.

Tamminga, C. A., G. Pearlson, M. Keshavan, J. Sweeney, B. Clementz, and G. Thaker. 2014. Bipolar and Schizophrenia Network for Intermediate Phenotypes: Outcomes across the psychosis continuum. *Schizophrenia Bulletin* 40 (Suppl. 2): S131–S137. doi:10.1093/schbul/sbt179.

Tien, A. Y. 1991. Distribution of hallucinations in the population. *Social Psychiatry and Psychiatric Epidemiology* 26:287–292.

Turkheimer, E., A. Haley, M. Waldron, B. D'Onofio, and I. I. Gottesman. 2003. Socioeconomic status modifies heritability of IQ in young children. *Psychological Science* 14:623–628.

van Os, J., and S. Kapur. 2009. Schizophrenia. *Lancet* 374:635–645.

Varese, F., E. Barkus, and R. P. Bentall. 2011. Dissociation mediates the relationship between childhood trauma and hallucination-proneness. *Psychological Medicine* 42:1025–1036.

Varese, F., F. Smeets, M. Drukker, R. Lieverse, T. Lataster, W. Viechtbauer, J. Read, et al. 2012. Childhood adversities increase the risk of psychosis: A meta-analysis of patient-control, prospective and cross-sectional cohort studies. *Schizophrenia Bulletin* 38:661–671. doi:10.1093/schbul/sbs050.

Vassos, E., C. B. Pedersen, R. M. Murray, D. A. Collier, and C. M. Lewis. 2012. Meta-analysis of the association of urbanicity with schizophrenia. *Schizophrenia Bulletin* 38:1118–1123.

Veling, W., E. Susser, J. van Os, J. P. Mackenbach, J. P. Selten, and H. W. Hoek. 2008. Ethnic density of neighborhoods and incidence of psychotic disorders among immigrants. *American Journal of Psychiatry* 165:66–73.

Wahlberg, K.-E., L. C. Wynne, H. Oja, P. Keskitalo, L. Pykalainen, I. Lahti, J. Moring, et al. 1997. Gene-environment interaction in vulnerability to schizophrenia: Findings from the Finnish Adoptive Family Study of Schizophrenia. *American Journal of Psychiatry* 154:355–362.

Wickham, S., K. Sitko, and R. P. Bentall. 2015. Insecure attachment is associated with paranoia but not hallucinations in psychotic patients: The mediating role of negative self-esteem. *Psychological Medicine* 45:1495–1507. doi:10.1017/S0033291714002633.

Wicks, S., A. Hjern, and C. Daman. 2010. Social risk or genetic liability for psychosis? A study of children born in Sweden and reared by adoptive parents. *American Journal of Psychiatry* 167:1240–1246.

Wright, A. G. C., R. Krueger, M. J. Hobbs, K. E. Markon, N. R. Eaton, and T. Slade. 2013. The structure of psychopathology: Toward an expanded quantitative empirical model. *Journal of Abnormal Psychology* 122:281–294.

11 Looking for the Self in Psychiatry: Perils and Promises of Phenomenology–Neuroscience Partnership in Schizophrenia Research

Şerife Tekin

Schizophrenia and Extraordinary Science

Schizophrenia is a mental disorder with high rates of prevalence in the United States and elsewhere (Jablensky 1999). It is listed as the ninth leading cause of disability worldwide (Thaker and Carpenter 2001). Yet, precisely what schizophrenia is, how its etiology unfolds, and which treatments are most effective in treating it remain largely controversial. It is diagnosed primarily according to the criteria provided by the *Diagnostic and Statistical Manual of Mental Disorders* (DSM). However, these particular criteria have been the target of a number of criticisms, resulting in a Kuhnian crisis in the DSM-led schizophrenia research. There are a number of anomalous research findings inconsistent with the dominant DSM paradigm. Consider a few. First, DSM's phenomenology-oriented critics suggest that the symptoms and signs listed in the DSM's schizophrenia category do not match the clinical realities of the patients (e.g., Parnas 2000; Parnas and Handest 2003). There are also environmental, cultural, and gender-related variations in the expression of the symptoms (American Psychiatric Association 2013, 103). Second, there are concerns about the DSM's reliability; there is no uniformity between the DSM and the *International Classification of Diseases* (ICD) with respect to schizophrenia diagnostic criteria (Jansson et al. 2002). In fact, based on such findings, some philosophers and psychologists including Richard P. Bentall (1993; see also this volume), Mary Boyle (1990), and Jeffrey Poland (2007) have argued against considering schizophrenia as a discrete illness. For instance, Bentall challenges the view that what are considered the symptoms of this condition fall neatly under the label "schizophrenia," and that hallucinations and delusions associated with the condition are meaningless. In this regard, the concept of "schizophrenia" is similar to a number of other concepts; for example, "phlogiston" and "the luminiferous ether" were widely employed by scientists for a time but turned out to be scientifically misleading (Bentall 1993, 227). These concerns are mirrored also in the psychiatric community, especially in the United Kingdom and continental Europe, where there is an international debate on what to replace the concept of schizophrenia with. Third, there are cultural variations in recovery rates; for example, third-world countries have higher recovery rates than first-world countries (Warner 2009). Finally, there is skepticism raised by the National Institute of Mental Health (NIMH) about the DSM-led research program's efficacy in encouraging research into the genetic and neural etiology of mental disorders; these concerns are applicable to schizophrenia (Insel 2013). It remains to be seen how schizophrenia will be targeted by the NIMH's Research Domain Criteria project—the proposed research alternative to the DSM-5.

Psychiatric research on schizophrenia is currently undergoing a period of extraordinary science, to apply Kuhn's terminology to the current situation in psychiatry, with many alternative research programs investigating the illness using different assumptions and methodologies. As the struggles the DSM-led research faces are now "more generally recognized as such by the profession," trust in the dominant DSM-led research paradigm is shaken, and "numerous partial solutions to the problem" are made available (Kuhn 1962, 82–83). I use philosophical tools in this chapter to evaluate one of these alternative research approaches that I call "phenomenology–neuroscience partnership" (PNP). First, in the "Phenomenological Approach to Schizophrenia" section, I lay out the phenomenological approach to schizophrenia that is critical of the DSM-led research. Next, in the "Phenomenology–Neuroscience Partnership in Schizophrenia Research" section, I focus on the PNP that takes this phenomenological approach as a starting point to investigate schizophrenia, and I address its shortcomings. Then, in the "Adjudication of Phenomenology–Neuroscience Partnership Paradigm" section, I conclude by pointing out the strengths of the PNP and offer prescriptions for its improvement.

Phenomenological Approach to Schizophrenia

The phenomenological approach to schizophrenia takes issue with the DSM description of schizophrenia. According to the DSM, the illness is individuated by the following signs and symptoms (American Psychiatric Association 2013): delusions or hallucinations; disorganized speech (e.g., frequent derailment or incoherence); grossly disorganized or catatonic behavior; affective flattening; alogia (poverty of speech); and avolition (inability to initiate or persist in goal-directed activities) For a diagnosis, two (or more) of the above need to be present for a significant portion of time during a one-month period. Social/occupational dysfunction must be present as well, and the symptoms need to be evident for a *six-month* period. This description plays a central role in diagnosis, research, treatment, and administrative contexts in North America, given the DSM's monopoly over these contexts.

The DSM framework, specifically DSM-III, DSM-IV, and DSM-5 (American Psychiatric Association 1980, 1994, 2013), has received criticism for its symptom-based criteria from phenomenologically oriented psychiatrists (e.g., Sass and Parnas 2003; Parnas et al. 1998). One specific concern is that self-experience-related anomalies, such as a subject's diminished sense of ownership of his or her own cognitive and emotional experiences and a loss of presence in his or her first-person experience of the world, are among the most frequently encountered features of schizophrenia, yet they are not part of the DSM taxonomy. Some of these psychiatrists even argue that all schizophrenia symptoms can be traced to self-experience-related anomalies, construing, thereby, schizophrenia as a pathology in self-experience (Parnas et al. 1998; Nelson et al. 2009; McGorry, Campbell, and Copolov 1987). If the DSM taxonomy that is instrumental for research and clinical intervention inaccurately represents schizophrenia, so the criticism goes, the goals of research and intervention are necessarily compromised.

Considering schizophrenia as a self-experience-related disorder is not novel. In fact, since the early days of theorizing about schizophrenia, researchers have recognized that the condition involves profound transformations of the self. For instance, an earlier theoretician, Emil Kraepelin considered loss of inner unity of consciousness, an "orchestra without a conductor" to be a core feature of schizophrenia (Sass and Parnas 2003, 427). Early in the twentieth century, Eugen Bleuler (1911/1950, 143) noted the patient's ego tends to undergo "the most manifold alterations," including "splitting of the self" and "loss of the feeling of activity or the ability to direct thoughts." More recently, phenomenologically oriented psychiatrists define schizophrenia as a disorder involving "subtle but pervasive and persistent aspects of subjective experience," where subjective experience is defined as the sense of ownership of the experience, and the feeling of being fully present as the subject of experience (Parnas, Bovet, and Zahavi 2002, 428). Such a definition is mostly based on the first-person reports of those with schizophrenia and clinical observations. These clinicians and theoreticians take self-experience pathologies as early signs of schizophrenia and operationalize the concept as a tool for early diagnosis. They primarily rely on their clinical experience with patients, as well as their historical work on early conceptualizations of schizophrenia, which also feature first-person reports. To my knowledge, they have not conducted a general study among individuals with schizophrenia to see if they all share such disturbances in their first-person experiences. Nor is there any work that evaluates whether such anomalies may also be prevalent in the nonschizophrenic population.

Phenomenologists consider what I call self-experience^{subjecthood} to be pathological in schizophrenia. Self-experience^{subjecthood} refers to the subject's experience of himself or herself as the *subject* of cognition and emotion, *through* which the individual attains *first-person perspective* on the world. Put otherwise, self-experience^{subjecthood} is experiencing oneself as the vital *subject* of awareness, emotion, and cognition. It is pathological in individuals with schizophrenia according to phenomenologists because these subjects fail to consider themselves as the vital subjects of awareness, emotion, and cognition, as I discuss below.

Self-experience^{subjecthood} is taken to be manifest in all forms of consciousness, for example, perceiving objects, classifying pictures, remembering the past, and so forth. In our self-experience^{subjecthood}, we are *directly*, that is, noninferentially or nonreflectively, conscious of our own thoughts, perceptions, feelings, or pains as uniquely ours. These experiences appear in a first-person mode of presentation and immediately reveal themselves as our own. Phenomenologists call this the "mineness" of first-person experience (Parnas and Sass 2011). When I see the book on my desk, I am instantly aware that the perception of the book is mine; I am the subject of the perception. In this sense, self-experience^{subjecthood} is world directed; it can be thought of as the unarticulated constituent of subjective experience (Perry 1998).

In contrast, self-experience^{objecthood} refers to the individual's experience of himself or herself as the *object* of cognition, and emotion, through which he or she adopts a *third-person perspective* toward himself or herself. In other words, self-experience^{objecthood} is experiencing oneself as the very vital *object* of one's own awareness, emotion, and cognition. Unlike self-experience^{subjecthood}, which is world directed, self-experience^{objecthood} is self-directed. When I see my face in the mirror, I recognize the face I see as my face. The *object* of my perception is my self. The individual may consider himself or herself as an object where the individual represents some mental or physical feature as a feature of himself or herself; this may happen during perceptual self-recognition, for example, when the individual identifies a hand he or she perceives as his or her own hand; during introspection, for example, when the individual reports his or her emotional responses to visual stimuli; during personal self-reference, for example, when deciding whether a personality trait adjective applies to oneself.

Phenomenologists characterize schizophrenia as disturbance or pathology in self-experience^{subjecthood}, as explained in the following:

> Schizophrenia, we propose, is a self-disorder or, more specifically, an ipseity disturbance in which one finds certain characteristic distortions of the act of awareness. *Ipseity* refers to the experiential sense of being a vital and self-coinciding *subject* of experience or *first person perspective on the world*. (authors' note: *ipse* is Latin for "self or "itself" (Sass and Parnas 2003; emphasis in original)

In this understanding, individuals with schizophrenia have diminished intensity or vitality of their own subjective self-presence, in that they do *not* feel themselves as the subjects of their own emotions and cognition. In fact, they report feeling the loss of the sense of inhabiting their own actions, thoughts, feelings, impulses, bodily sensations, or perceptions, sometimes to the point of feeling these are actually in the possession of some alien being (Parnas and Sass 2011). Along with this diminishment, the distinction between self and other disappears. A patient may report, for instance, that he is no longer able to distinguish how much of himself is in him and how much is in others (Freeman, Cameron, and McGhie 1958, 54). Disturbance in self- experience^{subjecthood} ranges from seemingly ordinary utterances such as "I don't feel myself" or "I am not myself," "I am losing contact with myself," or "Something inside me turned inhuman," to "occupied by my own inner world," "feeling like a spectator to my own life," "in painful distance to self" (Parnas and Handest 2003). Psychiatrists report the patient's sense of an "inner void" or "lack of inner nucleus" (Parnas and Handest 2003). They say such things as the following: "I have no consciousness"; "My consciousness is not as whole as it should be"; "I am half-awake"; "My I-feeling is diminished"; "My I is disappearing for me"; "It is a continuous universal blocking" (Parnas and Sass 2011). These psychiatrists have even developed a scale to measure disruptions in the sense of self to help in clinical assessment and treatment of the patients (Parnas et al. 2005).

Parnas reviews the case of Robert, a 21-year-old high school graduate, from a phenomenological stance (Parnas 2000). Robert, Parnas reports, has complained for over a year that he has been feeling cut off from the world. He has lost his initiative-taking energy, with disruptions also in his sleep patterns. He felt as if he was not really present or fully alive and that he did not feel as if he was participating in interaction with his surroundings. He reported an enhanced tendency to observe his inner life. His first-personal life, he tells, has been lost and is replaced by a third-person perspective. To illustrate, Robert describes how, in listening to music on his stereo, he sometimes has the impression that the musical tune lacks its natural fullness. He reports that he is somehow watching his own receptivity to the music, his own mind's receiving or registering of musical tunes. Periodically, Robert experiences his own movements as reflected upon and de-automatized. His thinking processes acquire a distressingly acoustic quality. From a phenomenological perspective, Parnas sees distortions in the I-experience:

> Robert has lost the normally tacit and prereflective "myness" of experience that is a condition and medium of spontaneous, absorbed intentionality; instead there is a sense of "phenomenological distance" within both perception and action. The perceived object appears somehow filtered, deprived of its fullness of presence—largely, we would argue, because the sensory process lacks the tonality of auto-affection. Perception now seems a mechanical, purely receptive sensory process, unaccompanied by its normal feeling-tone and deformed by now-intrusive processes of knowing ... Robert, in fact, seems to experience a general transformation of the implicit/explicit organization of the act of awareness, with normally foundational and constituting processes becoming objectified. Thus he reports inner speech being increasingly transformed from a *medium* of thinking into an object-like entity having quasi-perceptual, acoustic-like characteristics (Parnas 2000, 124–125).

Some clinical reports cohere with more recently published first-person memoirs of those with schizophrenia. Elyn Saks, for instance, writes,

> Then something odd happens. My awareness of myself, of my father, of the room, of the physical reality around and beyond us instantly grows fuzzy. Or wobbly. I think I am dissolving, I feel—my mind feels—like a sand castle with all the sand sliding away in the receding surf. ... Consciousness gradually loses its coherence. One's center gives way ... [it] cannot hold. The "me" becomes a haze, and the solid center from which one experiences reality breaks up. ... There is no longer a sturdy vantage point from which to look out, take things in, assess. ... No core holds things together, providing the lens through which we see the world. (Saks 2007, 12)

Saks experiences some distance from her subjecthood, in a way similar to Robert. In both cases, we learn of a decreased vitality in the first-person perspective, replaced by a sense of being a mere object of one's own experiences.

Some of the typical symptoms of schizophrenia, as identified in the DSM, such as hearing voices, are considered a form of self-experience^{subjecthood} disturbance. Voice hearing involves hearing one's own thoughts as if they were spoken aloud and simultaneously available to other persons (Sass 2010). The subject seems to have disappeared, in that the individuals are not aware that *they* are the author of those voices.

The phenomenological research program is one of the alternative paradigms developed in response to the crisis in the DSM-led research paradigm; however, it is yet unclear whether it is able to solve the puzzles and address the controversies faced therein. Among others, for instance, it is unclear whether self-experience^{subjecthood} anomalies can be generalized across the entire schizophrenia population, or whether self-experience^{subjecthood} disturbance *may* affect self-experience^{objecthood}. Yet, its main commitments had inspired the development of the PNP paradigm, which takes the phenomenological research as a starting point and integrates it into neuroscientific research on schizophrenia. I turn to that, now, to evaluate its promises and challenges. Note that I do not endorse the phenomenologically oriented characterization of schizophrenia. My goal is merely to show how this characterization is appropriated and used in the PNP paradigm and to enumerate its strengths and shortcomings.

Phenomenology–Neuroscience Partnership in Schizophrenia Research

PNP is the integration of two traditionally opposing paradigms that investigate mental disorders, namely, phenomenological approaches to mental disorders and scientific approaches. Phenomenological approaches are often characterized as subjective, both in scope and methodology. As discussed above, their scope includes the first-person experience of mental disorder and particular life experiences that make the patient's illness experience unique. Their methodology often involves a clinician's engagement with a single individual's self-reports, and the inferences the clinician draws based on these reports, using his or her clinical expertise. In contrast, scientific approaches are considered objective, insofar as they aim to make generalizable observations about mental disorders, with a focus on the population of the mentally ill, as opposed to a single individual. Methodologically, they target the easily measurable symptoms and signs of mental disorders, with the purpose of designing studies amenable to replication. Examples include clinical trials, neuroimaging studies, genetics research, and so forth. Proponents of the scientific approaches to mental disorders typically want psychiatry to resemble basic sciences, while those advocating phenomenological approaches suggest that psychopathology is complex and that it involves experiences that are unique to individuals, and thus it cannot be captured by basic sciences. In the last decade or so, the tension has become more relaxed, with philosophers, clinicians, and scientists acknowledging that phenomenology *versus* science is not a true, or, at least, not a productive dichotomy, and we need both to amalgamate the approaches to investigate mental disorders. The suggestion is that they provide different levels of analysis of psychopathology; phenomenology targeting the subjective level, and science targeting the objective level. Nonetheless, integrating them is challenging, as certain concepts are not commensurate, which is one of the challenges that the PNP is faced with.

The PNP paradigm is being developed by some neuroscientists (e.g., Nelson et al. 2008; Yung, Phillips, and McGorry, 2004) who take phenomenologists' characterization of schizophrenia as a self-experience anomaly as a starting point and attempt to trace its etiology to atypical activity in the brain's default network system (DNS)—the anatomically defined brain system that is active when individuals are not focused on the external environment. Findings on the correlations between atypical activity in the DNS and the symptoms of schizophrenia have increased optimism that DNS research will shed light on the neurological underpinnings of schizophrenia (e.g., Whitfield-Gabrieli et al., 2009; Buckner, Andrews, and Schachter 2008; Nelson et al. 2009). Under the PNP paradigm, schizophrenia is construed as a DNS activity anomaly, with some researchers proposing to use DNS activity as a diagnostic tool to identify the at-risk population and facilitate early intervention (Nelson et al. 2009). More specifically, the goal is to detect DNS anomalies in individuals who are in the prodromal phase of schizophrenia, that is, who do not experience all typical symptoms of schizophrenia but merely show some early signs of psychosis, and "treat" them before the disorder is entrenched (Nelson et al. 2009). It is envisioned that this will improve the likelihood of long-term recovery or even prevent the illness onset (Yung et al. 1996; Yung 2003; Yung, Phillips, and McGorry 2004). For instance, one early intervention strategy is to start psychopharmacological treatment on the prodromal population before they fully develop schizophrenia. This, of course, raises ethical problems about whether to treat an individual before he or she fully develops the illness, not to mention other problems including the following: nonpharmaceutical interventions are not contemplated and their efficacy remains unexplored, the side effects of the pharmaceutical interventions, toxic effects of neuroleptics, the likelihood of false positives, and so forth. While these are obviously important issues, I have neither the time nor the space to consider them here. Nor do I take issue with the assumption in the PNP paradigm that schizophrenia is a self-experience disorder. As noted above I do not endorse this phenomenological view of schizophrenia, but for present purposes, I leave the assumption unquestioned. After all, during extraordinary science where the DSM-led research paradigm is in crisis, a range of stances regarding psychopathology research may coexist. Rather, I tackle the assumption that self-experience can be individuated by DNS activity in the brain, the starting point for the proposals about early intervention.

Anomalies in DNS activity are believed to reveal the neurological underpinnings of the disturbance of self-experience in schizophrenia; evidence of the traction of self-experience through DNS activity comes from a number of functional magnetic resonance imaging studies (Northoff 2015; Qin and Northoff 2011; Northoff et al. 2006). However, in these studies, as we shall see, self-experience is not construed as phenomenologists construe it. To be clear: phenomenologists track anomalies in self-experience^{subjecthood} in schizophrenia whereas DNS researchers track self-experience^{objecthood}. These noncommensurate conceptualizations of self-experience stifle progress in schizophrenia research. What I shall call the problem of "wandering terminology" makes it challenging, if not impossible, to draw reliable conclusions about the correlation between DNS anomalies and schizophrenia.[1]

To substantiate my argument, I should start with an overview of DNS research. Imaging studies have traditionally focused on measuring brain activity when subjects are absorbed in an attention-demanding task, such as solving a math problem, classifying pictures, and so on. In the last 35 years or so, a growing number of studies have examined brain activity (spontaneous fluctuations in the blood-oxygen-level-dependent signal) during resting-state conditions, that is, when subjects are *not* engaged in an attention-demanding task and are left to think undisturbed by the external environment (Fox and Raichle 2007; Buckner, Andrews, and Schachter 2008). One significant finding is that the resting-state activity is organized into a dynamic network connected both anatomically and functionally, the DNS (Fox and Raichle 2007). Anatomically, the DNS involves posterior cingulate/precuneus, medial frontal cortex, and bilateral temporoparietal regions.

In most individuals, DNS activity alternates dynamically between task-dependent, external-world-oriented, and world-directed states, such as solving a puzzle or classifying pictures, and task-independent, internal-world-oriented, and self-directed states, such as remembering the past, envisioning future events, or considering the thoughts and perspectives of other people. In the former, DNS activity decreases, while in the latter, it increases. The latter is often referred to as a "self-directed state" in the sense of being engaged within the individual's internal states as opposed to being engaged with a nonself. For this reason, some neuroscientists claim

DNS activity individuates, or at least, is highly correlated with "self," "self-related thoughts," "self-experience," or "self-related processing," often using these concepts interchangeably (Qin and Northoff 2011; Nelson et al. 2008; Northoff et al. 2006). In individuals with schizophrenia, during the task-dependent, external-world-oriented, and world-directed states, DNS activity remains high, unlike the reducing activity found in typical non-schizophrenics. During the task-independent, internal-world-oriented, and self-directed states, DNS becomes even more active among schizophrenics than among typical individuals without schizophrenia. Susan Whitfield-Gabrieli, a researcher of DNS activity and schizophrenia, says the "dial" on DNS does not turn down as it should in schizophrenia patients; the DNS is overconnected and overactive (Whitfield-Gabrieli et al. 2009).

Such findings have led some researchers (Nelson et al. 2009; Yung et al. 1996; Yung 2003) to combine the phenomenological framework of schizophrenia with the DNS framework in neuroscience, developing the PNP paradigm. Because schizophrenia is a self-experience disorder and because self-experience is individuated by DNS activity, they assume schizophrenia etiology can be traced in anomalous DNS activity. However, as I show below, this inference has been made too quickly and contains conceptual fallacies.

When phenomenologists suggest schizophrenia is a self-experience disorder, they take self-experience to be self-experience^{subjecthood}. Meanwhile, the PNP paradigm operationalizes self-experience^{objecthood} when its proponents claim that DNS individuates or approximates self-experience. A wide variety of studies measure how DNS activity changes as a function of tasks that can be expected either to suppress or not suppress introspective processes. These studies are confined to cognition during self-directed states (as opposed to world-directed states). DNS activity is measured when subjects are engaged in perceptual and cognitive tasks that involve representing some mental or physical feature as a feature of themselves. In a frequently cited study, tasks that purportedly track self-experience include "trait adjective judgment," where subjects are asked if a particular adjective defines their personality trait, and "face and body recognition," where subjects are asked to pick themselves out in photographs (Qin and Northoff 2011). These tasks require perceptual self-recognition, for example, when an individual identifies a hand that the individual perceives as his or her own hand; introspection, for example, when an individual reports his or her emotional responses to visual stimuli; personal self-reference, for example, when an individual decides whether a personality trait adjective applies to himself or herself. All tasks ask subjects to engage in self-directed cognitive states; thus, self-experience here refers to self-experience^{objecthood}. It is wrong, therefore, based on this particular research, to infer that because schizophrenia is a self-experience disorder and because self-experience is individuated by DNS activity, schizophrenia etiology can be traced in anomalous DNS activity. Self-experience does not denote the same phenomenon in phenomenological and neuroscientific concepts.

The major conceptual limitation of the studies claiming to locate self-experience in the brain is the exclusive focus on the individual's experience of himself or herself as the *object* of emotion and cognition (Legrand 2007; Legrand and Ruby 2009). The self as the *subject* of emotion and cognition is neglected. At their best, these studies show correlations between DNS activity and self-experience^{objecthood}. Simply stated, DNS activity does not track self-experience^{subjecthood}. Self-experience^{subjecthood} is present, even in attention-demanding tasks; it is not "absent" as is often claimed.

Limiting self-experience to self-experience^{objecthood} has negative implications for the PNP paradigm. What I call the problem of wandering terminology renders fallacious the inference that schizophrenia is a DNS anomaly. Thus, the proposal to treat individuals at risk of developing schizophrenia based on DNS anomalies is misguided because the concept of self-experience operationalized by the PNP paradigm and the concept of self-experience experienced in schizophrenia are incongruent.

Note that the PNP paradigm is among the many research programs that explore the relationship between schizophrenia and DNS activity. For instance, the DNS is also involved in other attention-demanding tasks, such as remembering past events, and there are a number of studies that compare schizophrenia patients' performance in working memory tasks to the control group's (e.g., Whitfield-Gabrieli et al. 2009). My criticism of wandering terminology does not apply to these research programs; I primarily take issue with those studies that operationalize self-experience to individuate schizophrenia in the brain. Thus, there may be other resourceful research venues that investigate DNS involvement in schizophrenia which avoid the conceptual problems I discuss here.

Adjudication of Phenomenology–Neuroscience Partnership Paradigm

Is anything salvageable in the PNP paradigm? More importantly, if it is among the paradigms put forward during psychiatry's extraordinary science period, does it make more progress in schizophrenia research in comparison to the DSM-led research program? I argue that while PNP has some advantages over the DSM-led research, insofar as it makes central to research the elements of psychopathology that were previously ignored, that is, self-experience, it is hard to infer that it makes more progress, simply because it suffers from a number of conceptual problems that stifle progress in empirical research. Moving forward, it has to pay more attention to these.

The biggest promise of PNP is the acknowledgment of and engagement with the concept of the self, the subject of mental disorder, in schizophrenia research. This is significant because the concept of self has been missing from scientific frameworks that investigate mental disorders since the publication of DSM-III (American Psychiatric Association 1980). A core feature of the last three editions of the DSM (i.e., DSM-III, DSM-IV, and DSM-5; hereinafter DSM-III+) is the operational approach, according to which mental disorders are individuated through an operational criterion consisting of a sufficient number of symptoms (experienced by the patient) and signs (observed by the observer). What is also called the descriptive or atheoretical approach developed as a reaction to earlier etiological approaches grounded in psychoanalytic theory; these relied on empirically undefended theoretical assumptions and involved a narrative prototype description and a process of matching the individual patient to such prototypes. Operationalism was considered a necessary step to make psychiatry more scientific, allowing researchers to identify and investigate its readily measurable targets, that is, the clusters of symptoms and signs serving as outwardly observable correlates of disease and as bases for genetic and neural research into illness etiology. Operational criteria were also deemed useful in clinical contexts where the DSMs are used by psychiatrists, medical doctors of different specializations, nurses, counselors, and so forth, easing the process of diagnosis and treatment. DSM-III+'s operationalism has been a target of significant criticism concerning its efficacy in meeting psychiatry's scientific and clinical goals (Poland, Von Eckardt, and Spaulding 1994; Sadler 2005; Murphy 2006; Fulford, Thornton, and Graham 2006; Tekin 2014; Pearce 2014; Parnas and Bovet 2014; Schaffner and Tabb 2014).

One particular criticism is the neglect of the complexity of the self in the operational descriptions of mental disorders such as depression and schizophrenia (Sadler 2005; Dean 2012; Parnas and Bovet 2015; Schaffner and Tabb 2015; Parnas and Sass 2003; Tekin 2015). Under operationalism, the self was not found to be a suitable scientific target, because it was considered too abstract or not readily measurable to allow the scientific investigation of mental disorders.[2] In an attempt to move away from the psychoanalytic framework, operationalism left out important self-related features of mental disorders from the scientific discussions. More specifically, under the operational criteria guiding scientific research, four suppositions about mental disorders stand out. Mental disorders are characterized as (1) behavioral anomalies, thus leaving out their phenomenological features; (2) atemporal events, thus leaving out their gradual development over time; (3) emergent phenomena, thus divorced from underlying causal factors; and (4) things that happen to solitary individuals disengaged from the social and cultural world, thus omitting intersubjective contexts that may contribute to their development. These four have led to what I dub the problem of the missing self in psychiatric taxonomy.

First, as an outcome of (1), the first-person-specific dimension of the encounter with mental illness is not part of the DSM descriptions, even though it is crucial to understanding the nature of a mental disorder. Such first-person-specific phenomena include the content of what the individual hears when hearing voices or the distortions in the sense of self prior to the full development of psychotic episodes. Second, as an outcome of (2), (3), and (4), historical-narrative aspects of mental disorders are omitted from scientific scrutiny. These include the individual's particular life history, interpersonal relationships, biological and environmental risk factors, gender, race, class, and status, and the developmental trajectory of mental disorder in the individual from childhood to adulthood. This feature of the DSM is called "hyponarrativity," or the abstraction of the illness category from the particular experiences and contingencies of the individual patient (Sadler 2005). Elsewhere I address the negative implications of the limited representation of mental disorders for the clinical context (see, e.g., Tekin 2011, 2013, 2014, 2015; Tekin and Mosko 2015). It also has implications for research, as we have an incomplete picture of a complex phenomenon, and we need the full picture to understand etiology.

In this respect, PNP's interest in the phenomenology of schizophrenia, and its attempt to include self-experience in the research program, is a positive step forward. In particular, it is more progressive than the DSM-led research in two ways. First, it acknowledges that the concepts of self or self-experience are at least potentially empirically tractable, challenging the DSM's assumption that the self is not a suitable scientific target. There is an attempt to enumerate self-experience empirically, based on first-person reports and measurements of DNS activity. Second, it challenges the first presupposition of the DSM's operational criteria in characterizing schizophrenia, namely, that schizophrenia is not merely a behavioral anomaly, when its phenomenological features are taken into account. Whether the individual encounters any oddities in their self-experience is considered to be an important domain of research.

That said, however, inconsistent and wandering definitions of self-experience lead to serious problems in the first of these two steps forward, where PNP has promise. The attempts to track self-experience are stifled by the problem of wandering terminology; PNP scientists must carefully reconsider their definitions of schizophrenia, as well as self-experience, and examine whether their scientific methodologies and tools accurately probe these.

Acknowledgments

I thank Jeffrey Poland, Owen Flanagan, George Graham, Jennifer Radden, Kristin Andrews, and Brian Keeley for their feedback on this chapter.

Notes

1. Note that the disorders of consciousness that are the targets of either sort of research are not specific to schizophrenia; the assumption that such disorders are core features of schizophrenia is at least questionable. However, neither of these points undermines my analysis here; they just point out that talk of schizophrenia as a discrete illness is arguably gratuitous. The methodological morals I draw may well survive a reframing of the research that does not employ the diagnostic category of schizophrenia, and my hope is that the research will benefit from such a reframing. Thanks to Jeffrey Poland for drawing my attention to this point.

2. Desire for leaving the self out of the psychiatric taxonomy seems to have stemmed from several—not mutually exclusive—points of view, including the influence of logical positivist views of science on psychiatry and increased resistance to psychodynamic psychiatry, the American Psychiatric Association's desire to move away from Freudianism and psychoanalysis in general and replace them with Kraepelin's operational criteria, Carl Hempel's influence on the image of science in psychiatry, pragmatic goals to find reliable universal criteria for diagnosis for epidemiological measurements, and so forth. For reasons of space I do not include this discussion in the current chapter.

References

American Psychiatric Association. 1980. *Diagnostic and Statistical Manual of Mental Disorders*. 3rd ed. Washington, DC: American Psychiatric Association.

American Psychiatric Association. 1994. *Diagnostic and Statistical Manual of Mental Disorders*. 4th ed. Washington, DC: American Psychiatric Association.

American Psychiatric Association. 2013. *Diagnostic and Statistical Manual of Mental Disorders*. 5th ed. Arlington, VA: American Psychiatric Association.

Bentall, R. P. 1993. Deconstructing the concept of schizophrenia. *Journal of Mental Health* 2:223–238.

Bleuler, E. 1911/1950. *Dementia Praecox or the Group of Schizophrenias. Trans. J. Zinkin.* New York: International Universities Press.

Boyle, M. 1990. *Schizophrenia: A Scientific Delusion?* London: Routledge.

Buckner, R. L., J. A. Andrews, and D. Schachter. 2008. The brain's default network: Anatomy, function, and relevance to disease. *Annals of the New York Academy of Sciences* 1124:1–39.

Dean, C. 2012. The death of specificity in psychiatry: Cheers or tears. *Perspectives in Biology and Medicine* 55:443–460.

Fox, M. D., and M. E. Raichle. 2007. Spontaneous fluctuations in brain activity observed with functional magnetic resonance imaging. *Nature Reviews. Neuroscience* 8:700–711.

Freeman, T., J. L. Cameron, and A. McGhie. 1958. *Chronic Schizophrenia*. New York: International Universities Press.

Fulford, K. W. M., T. Thornton, and G. Graham. 2006. *Oxford Textbook of Philosophy and Psychiatry*. Oxford: Oxford University Press.

Insel, T. (2013). Director's Blog: Transforming Diagnosis. http://www.nimh.nih.gov/about/director/2013/transforming-diagnosis.shtml.

Jablensky, A. 1999. The concept of schizophrenia: Pro et contra. *Epidemiologia e Psichiatria Sociale* 8 (4): 242–247.

Jansson, L., P. Handest, J. Nielsen, D. Saebye, and J. Parnas. 2002. Exploring boundaries of schizophrenia: A comparison of ICD–10 with other diagnostic systems. *World Psychiatry: Official Journal of the World Psychiatric Association (WPA)* 1 (2): 109–114.

Kuhn, T. 1962. *The Structure of Scientific Revolutions*. Chicago: University of Chicago Press.

Legrand, D. 2007. Pre-reflective self-as-subject from experiential and empirical perspectives. *Consciousness and Cognition* 16:583–599.

Legrand, D., and P. Ruby. 2009. What is self-specific? A theoretical investigation and critical review of neuroimaging results. *Psychological Review* 116:252–282.

McGorry, P. D., R. Campbell, and D. L. Copolov. 1987. The Zelig phenomenon: A specific form of identity disturbance. *Australian and New Zealand Journal of Psychiatry* 21 (4): 532–538.

Murphy, D. 2006. *Psychiatry in the Scientific Image*. Cambridge, MA: MIT Press.

Nelson, A., B. Fornito, B. Harrison, M. Yucel, L. A. Sass, A. R. Yung, A. Thompson, S. J. Wood, C. Pantelis, and P. D. McGorry. 2009. A disturbed sense of self in the psychosis prodrome: Linking phenomenology and neurobiology. *Neuroscience and Biobehavioral Reviews* 33:807–817.

Nelson, B., A. R. Yung, A. Bechdolf, and P. D. McGorry. 2008. The phenomenological critique and self-disturbance: Implications for ultra-high risk ("prodrome") research. *Schizophrenia Bulletin* 34 (2): 381–392.

Northoff, G. 2015. Resting state activity and the "stream of consciousness" in schizophrenia—neurophenomenal hypotheses. *Schizophrenia Bulletin* 41 (1): 280–290.

Northoff, G., A. Heinzel, M. de Greck, F. Bermpohl, H. Dobrowolny, and J. Panksepp. 2006. Self-referential processing in our brain—a meta-analysis of imaging studies on the self. *NeuroImage* 31:440–457.

Parnas, J. 2000. The self and intentionality in the pre-psychotic stages of schizophrenia: A phenomenological study. In *Exploring the Self: Philosophical and Psychopathological Perspectives on Self-experience*, ed. D. Zahavi, 115–147. Philadelphia: John Benjamins.

Parnas, J., and P. Bovet. 2014. Psychiatry made easy: Operationalism and some of its consequences. In *Philosophical Issues in Psychiatry III: The Nature and Sources of Historical Change*, ed. K. S. Kendler and J. Parnas, 190–212. Oxford: Oxford University Press.

Parnas, J., P. Bovet, and D. Zahavi. 2002. Schizophrenic autism: Clinical phenomenology and pathogenetic implications. *World Psychiatry: Official Journal of the World Psychiatric Association (WPA)* 1 (3): 131–135.

Parnas, J., and P. Handest. 2003. Phenomenology of anomalous self-experience in early schizophrenia. *Comprehensive Psychiatry* 44 (2): 121–134.

Parnas, J., L. Jansson, L. A. Sass, and P. Handest. 1998. Self-experience in the prodromal phases of schizophrenia: A pilot study of first-admissions. *Neurology, Psychiatry & Brain Research* 6 (2): 97–106.

Parnas, J., P. Møller, T. Kircher, J. Thalbitzer, L. Jansson, P. Handest, and D. Zahavi. 2005. EASE: Examination of anomalous self-experience. *Psychopathology* 5:236–258.

Parnas, J., and L. Sass. 2003. Schizophrenia, consciousness, and the self. *Schizophrenia Bulletin* 29 (3): 427–444.

Parnas, J., and L. Sass. 2011. The structure of self-consciousness in schizophrenia. In *The Oxford Handbook of the Self*, ed. S. Gallagher, 521–546. Oxford: Oxford University Press.

Pearce, S. 2014. DSM-5 and the rise of the diagnostic checklist. *Journal of Medical Ethics* 40:515–516.

Perry, J. 1998. Indexicals, contexts and unarticulated constituents. In *Proceedings of the 1995 CSLI-Amsterdam Logic, Language and Computation Conference*, 1–16. Stanford: CSLI Publications.

Poland, J. 2007. How to move beyond the concept of schizophrenia. In *Reconceiving Schizophrenia*, ed. M. Chung, K. W. M. Fulford, and G. Graham, 167–191. Oxford: Oxford University Press.

Poland, J., B. Von Eckardt, and W. Spaulding. 1994. Problems with the DSM approach to classification of psychopathology. In *Philosophical Psychopathology*, ed. G. Graham and L. Stevens, 235–260. Cambridge, MA: MIT Press.

Qin, P., and G. Northoff. 2011. How is our self related to midline regions and the default-mode network? *NeuroImage* 57:1221–1233.

Sadler, J. 2005. *Values and Psychiatric Diagnosis*. Oxford: Oxford University Press.

Saks, E. 2007. *The Center Cannot Hold: My Journey through Madness*. New York: Hyperion.

Sass, L. 2010. Phenomenology as description and as explanation: The case of schizophrenia. In *Handbook of Phenomenology and the Cognitive Sciences*, ed. S. Gallagher and D. Schmicking, 635–654. Berlin: Springer-Verlag.

Sass, L., and J. Parnas. 2003. Schizophrenia, consciousness, and the self. *Schizophrenia Bulletin* 29 (3): 427–444.

Schaffner, K. F., and K. Tabb. 2014. Hempel as a critic of Bridgman's operationalism: Lessons for psychiatry from the history of science (a response to Bovet and Parnas). In *Philosophical Issues in Psychiatry III: The Nature and Sources of Historical Change*, ed. K. S. Kendler and J. Parnas, 213–230. Oxford: Oxford University Press.

Tekin, Ş. 2011. Self-concept through the diagnostic looking glass: Narratives and mental disorder. *Philosophical Psychology* 24 (3): 357–380.

Tekin, Ş. 2013. Will I be pretty, will I be rich? The missing self in antidepressant commercials. *American Journal of Bioethics* 13 (5): 19–21.

Tekin, Ş. 2014. Psychiatric taxonomy: At the crossroads of science and ethics. *Journal of Medical Ethics* 40:513–514.

Tekin, Ş. 2015. Against hyponarrating grief: Incompatible research and treatment interests in the DSM-5. In *The DSM-5 in Perspective: Philosophical Reflections on the Psychiatric Babel*, ed. P. Singy and S. Demazeux, 179–197, History, Philosophy and the Theory of the Life Sciences Series. Dordrecht, the Netherlands: Springer.

Tekin, Ş., and M. Mosko. 2015. Hyponarrativity and context-specific limitations of the DSM-5. *Public Affairs Quarterly* 29 (1): 111–136.

Thaker, G. K., and W. T. Carpenter. 2001. Advances in schizophrenia. *Nature Medicine* 7:667–671.

Warner, R. 2009. Recovery from schizophrenia and the recovery model. *Current Opinion in Psychiatry* 22 (4): 374–380.

Whitfield-Gabrieli, S., H. W. Thermenos, S. Milanovic, M. T. Tsuang, S. V. Faraone, R. W. McCarley, M. E. Shenton, A. I. Green, A. Nieto-Castanon, P. LaViolette, J. Wojcik, J. D. E. Gabrieli, and L. J. Seidman. 2009. Hyperactivity and hyperconnectivity of the default network in schizophrenia and in first-degree relatives of persons with schizophrenia. *Proceedings of the National Academy of Sciences of the United States of America* 106:1279–1284.

Yung, A. R. 2003. The schizophrenia prodrome: A high risk concept. *Schizophrenia Bulletin* 29:857–863.

Yung, A. R., P. D. McGorry, C. A. McFarlane, H. J. Jackson, G. C. Patton, and A. Rakkar. 1996. Monitoring and care of young people at incipient risk of psychosis. *Schizophrenia Bulletin* 22 (2): 283–303.

Yung, A. R., L. J. Phillips, and P. D. McGorry. 2004. *Treating Schizophrenia in the Prodromal Phase*. London: Taylor & Francis.

12 DSM Applications to Young Children: Are There Really Bipolar and Depressed Two-Year-Olds?

Harold Kincaid

Is it reasonable to think that young children have psychiatric disorders such as depression or bipolar disorder as these are characterized by the *Diagnostic and Statistical Manual of Mental Disorders* (DSM) classification system? The commonsensical answer is negative. Small children do not have the level of development to express the complex characteristics of these disorders—adult disorders often involve failure of executive function and diminished activity of the prefrontal cortex, but that is the natural state of small children. However, turning this commonsensical intuition into an argument requires looking in detail at evidence and research behind specific classifications in children. Doing so will hopefully provide some interesting detail about how the DSM works in practice and how it can go wrong.

The chapter is divided into two parts. The first gives a general perspective on DSM that will be applied in looking at childhood psychiatric diagnoses and should be of some interest in its own right. I don't believe that everything in DSM is fundamentally flawed. In particular, I think there are some DSM-based categorizations—those of major depressive disorder and bipolar disorder—that can and have grounded substantial research findings. I argue briefly for that conclusion while showing how it is consistent with thinking that large parts of the DSM practice is not scientifically fruitful. The second part of this chapter then discusses in detail how classifications have been applied in pediatric psychiatric research in the case of depression and bipolar disorder. By focusing on two classifications in children with some real validity in adult populations, the intention is to focus on the best case for pediatric psychiatric disorders. Of course, if the best case fails, and I argue that it largely does at our current state of knowledge, then these results are significant for pediatric psychiatric disorders in general. The interest in all this has implications beyond the quality of DSM-based research since small children are increasingly being given powerful psychoactive drugs on the grounds that they have major depressive or bipolar disorder.[1]

A General Perspective on DSM Classifications

What do we want from a classification system of psychological problems? For research we want to know that we can systematically pick out behaviors and individuals that objectively group phenomena and individuals in such a way that we can study causes, courses, and interventions. For patient care, we want to pick out significant problems in people's lives that are amenable to the kinds of interventions we have at our disposal. Ideally, those diagnoses and interventions will be based on classifications and information that research has given us. This seems obvious enough, even if it is vague in various ways (what are significant psychological problems?). The question is the extent to which DSM delivers.

Delivers in what respect? In keeping with the theme of this volume, my interest is in its value for research, though obviously this question also has implications for clinical practice. The key thing we want from a classification system for research is the ability to pick out objective groupings in nature, where objective means at least that distinctions exist in nature and are not mere impositions by the researcher. The main routes to finding objective groupings are through multiple independent measures and through embedding categories in what Cronbach and Meehl (1955) call a nomological net. So temperature, for example, can be measured by various independently working devices, and the concept of temperature is involved in various cause-and-effect relations such as those described by the gas laws.

The actual practices of measuring and using concepts of temperature (Chang 2004) reveal some important morals for how we should go about evaluating the DSM in research. Those morals are that successful scientific concepts get tied down to reality through a series of piecemeal and case-specific auxiliary devices and assumptions as Wilson (2007) has shown in wonderful detail for parts of applied physics. There is an interplay between how concepts are defined and how they are used in empirical work. It is not a case of first getting clear on the concept and then to go about applying it. Chang makes just such a case for temperature. The actual history of the concept of temperature illustrates this complex interplay. Scales were conducted without any clear definition or theory of what heat was. The fixed points of boiling and freezing were not so fixed and admitted multiple definitions. Linearity across the range was largely assumed, not justified. Dealing with temperatures of the very hot and very cold required different scales not easily related to each other. The diverse ways that physics dealt with such problems are essential to understanding how the concept of temperature works.

I would suggest that these morals apply to understanding DSM and evaluating its success. Tying DSM categories to reality is partially done with the help of various screens, especially in research contexts involving large population sizes. The screens involve sets of questions which are supposed to allow researchers and clinicians to determine whether a specific disorder is present. In practice the screens face a number of problems. Most directly, they often have a tenuous connection to the DSM criteria for specific classifications. What follows are two examples that show that there is some distance between the DSM criteria and the screens used to look for these disorders.

Table 12.1 lists side by side the DSM-IV[2] criteria for major depressive disorder and the items from the Hamilton Rating Scale for Depression, a commonly used measure of symptom severity that is also sometimes used as a screen. Obviously there are differences between the two.

Similarly, the most common screen for addictive gambling, an area where I have done empirical research (Kincaid et al. 2013), is the Problem Gambling Screening Index (PGSI). Its items and the DSM-IV criteria are listed in table 12.2. It is obvious that some criteria are not captured by the items and some items are only weakly correlated with the criteria.

In both cases a comparison shows that it is pretty clear that there is some distance between the DSM criteria and the screens used to look for these disorders. This is true in terms of the items asked and in their scoring: the items in the screens differ from the criteria in various ways, and the criteria are all or nothing while the screen items have 4- or 5-point Likert scale responses.

In the ideal case the screens are verified by comparison with diagnoses from full clinical interviews. In practice screens are often tested against each other—different screens are assessed in terms of their statistical intercorrelations with each other. In either case, there is a clear instantiation of what is known as the "experimenter's regress"—the circular nature of validating a set of criteria by showing they pick out the right things when determining what are "the right things" relies on yet another set of criteria, as illustrated by the case of temperature mentioned earlier where different methods of measurement were often calibrated against each other without any clear independent verification of either. In the abstract this is the antifoundationalist situation that faces all testing in science. Yet there is testing and there is testing. Some experimenter's regresses are very short circles indeed, and that is surely the case for some DSM screens that are pretty much entirely tested against other, similar screens. Even when they are tested against clinical interviews, the looseness of the DSM criteria and

Table 12.1
DSM-IV Criteria for Depression and Hamilton Screen Compared

DSM-IV Criteria	Hamilton Items
Depressed mood or irritable most of the day, nearly every day, as indicated by either subjective report or observation made by others	Feeling sad
Decreased interest or pleasure in most activities	Decreased appetite
Significant weight change (5%) or change in appetite	Weight loss
Change in sleep: Insomnia or hypersomnia	Early insomnia (e.g., trouble falling asleep) Insomnia in the form of wakefulness after falling asleep Insomnia in the form of restlessness
Change in activity: Psychomotor agitation or retardation	Agitation
Fatigue or loss of energy	Decreased functioning in work and other activities
Guilt/worthlessness: Feelings of worthlessness or excessive or inappropriate guilt	Feelings of guilt
Concentration: Diminished ability to think or concentrate, or more indecisiveness	Retarded thought and speech
Suicidality	Suicidal thoughts
	Anxiety—psychic
	Anxiety—somatic
	Loss of libido
	Fatigue, headaches, body aches
	Hypochondria
	Poor insight into condition

Note. DSM-IV, *Diagnostic and Statistical Manual of Mental Disorders*, fourth edition.

Table 12.2
Comparison of DSM-IV Criteria for Problem Gambling and PGSI Screen

DSM-IV Criteria	PGSI Items
Restless or irritable when trying to cut back gambling	Bet more than could afford to lose
Need to bet larger amounts to feel excited	Need to bet larger amounts to feel excited
Go back another day to recoup losses	Go back another day to recoup losses
Borrowed to fund gambling	Borrowed or sold things to fund gambling
Preoccupied with gambling	Felt to have problem with gambling
Made repeated failed attempts to control gambling	Gambling causes health, stress, anxiety problems
People have criticized your gambling	People have criticized your gambling
Lies to conceal the extent of gambling	Gambling has caused financial problems
Gambling has endangered relations, jobs, career	Feel guilty about gambling
Has committed illegal acts to fund gambling	

Note. DSM-IV, *Diagnostic and Statistical Manual of Mental Disorders*, fourth edition; PGSI, Problem Gambling Screening Index.

the subjectivity in clinical interviews mean that experimenter's regress creates serious worries. A main worry is that the slack or looseness in the tie between reported diagnoses and the kind of subject responses—in both clinical interviews, screens, and the correlation between them—allows for various kinds of nonepistemic factors such as disciplinary trends and fashion, financial interests, and so forth to play a significant role.

However, in understanding actual scientific research on psychiatric disorders, I would also draw on some other general morals about scientific classification. A useful framework for thinking about how DSM and other classification approaches label psychopathology can be found in several "pragmatist" philosophical frameworks. I have in mind work by Quine (1969), Hacking (1993), the "promiscuous realism" of Dupré (1993), and the "rainforest realism" of Dennett (1991) and Ross (2004). A basic insight here is that data, evidence, and phenomena are always approached "under a description." The idea that data are theory laden is one version of this claim, but not the best. The thought is that we approach data and phenomena with descriptions and categories, and those may or may not be descriptions or categories that come from some organized body of interlocking laws. The pragmatism and promiscuous and rainforest realism slogans assert that there may be multiple descriptions that are equally good in various senses (such as the purposes we want categorizations for), where predictive success is balanced against other epistemic values such as simplicity, consistency with background knowledge, fruitfulness in intervening, and so forth.

How does this bear on the DSM and the problem of categorizing psychopathology? Put simply, the task of classification in psychopathology has two key steps: first, collect data on individuals from surveys, interviews, and observations, where observations may run the range from clinical to behavioral experimental to neurobiological, and second, organize those data into categories in a way that is alleged to promote scientific and practical goals. In the second step, the slogan "under a description" is fairly obvious, for we have to find ways of grouping the data, and there may well be multiple ways to do so. What we count as the data in the first place—what our questionnaires ask, how they categorize, and so forth—no doubt also are under a description and multiply approachable. Thus, this vision suggests that the data relevant to psychopathology—answers on screens and results of structured questionnaires, for example—have to be categorized and that there may be multiple fruitful ways of doing so.

This sort of pluralism does not mean that anything goes. That there are multiple ways of categorizing does not entail that all ways of categorizing are equally good. As suggested above, good categorizations need independent, convergent methods of measurement as well as evidence that categories fit into a confirmed nomological net describing causes, effects, and outcomes.

In a way, the polythetic nature of DSM criteria can be seen as frank acknowledgment of this kind of pluralism of dividing up disorders, with the crucial concession being made with DSM-III. On its own that is not an inherent problem I would argue. However, there has been very little systematic attempt to determine whether the different ways of dividing up symptoms actually ground successful prediction. There are few studies that ask whether particular subsets of criteria for a given disorder, rather than the aggregate of all cases meeting the minimum number needed for diagnosis, provide convergent and discriminant validity.

The looseness of screens in connection with DSM and the polythetic nature of DSM definitions certainly open the door to worries that many DSM classifications are socially constructed labels for various problems in living or, even more skeptically, for behaviors society deems unacceptable.

The label of gender identity disorder in DSM-IV seems an obvious case of the latter. It is clear that DSM was developed to shore up the scientific standing of psychiatry and to facilitate insurance billing for psychiatric care. Even relatively well-established categories such as major depressive disorder can be overdiagnosed,[3] an argument that Horwitz and Wakefield (2007) have made for depression specifically. I would argue that there is a core syndrome of major depressive disorder that is an objectively identifiable psychopathology, but that practitioners and the DSM extend the diagnosis to cases that are understandable problems in living.

So far, I have argued the following:

1. Some DSM categories have a very loose relation to the screens that measure them.
2. But that does not necessarily tell against them because it is generally true in science that fundamental concepts have a complex relation to the phenomena and data that are supposed to support them.
3. The polythetic nature of the DSM categories is not inevitably a flaw because it is not uncommon in science for there to be multiple ways of categorizing or dividing up the data.

Thus, my point here is that it is a mistake to dismiss the DSM approach and practice altogether. As I will suggest below, some DSM categorizations have something going for them. However, it is also clear that there are serious problems with large parts of DSM, and I turn next to those.

Another problem with the DSM is that it frames the project of classifying psychopathology in terms of medical models of psychopathology. DSM explicitly claims that it is picking out diseases or disorders.[4] The various criteria sets for the entries are there to make diagnoses. Despite efforts in the last round of DSM revisions to introduce dimensional elements, DSM remains categorical—either you have or do not have the various conditions described. With the disease framing also comes the idea that there is some kind of biological lesion or malfunction within the individual that explains disease status and course and that medical, especially pharmacological, intervention is called for. Maybe environmental or social factors are distal causes of mental disease, but proximal causes are internal biological problems, though we still have to discover those causes in most cases. The faith behind the medical model is that functional magnetic resonance imaging (fMRI) studies and other methods will eventually identify the lesions in question.[5]

However, the DSM does not have a coherent, defensible notion of disease. It invokes two distinct concepts of disease: disease as a dysfunction and disease as symptoms or behavior outside what is normal. So DSM-5 says, as have other previous versions, that "a mental disorder is a syndrome characterized by clinically significant disturbance in an individual's cognition, emotion regulation, or behavior that reflects a dysfunction in the psychological, biological, or developmental processes underlying mental functioning" (American Psychiatric Association 2013, 20). Elsewhere it says mental illness is a "psychopathological condition in which physical signs and symptoms exceed normal ranges" (American Psychiatric Association 2013, 19). The deviation from normal ranges is invoked often in the criteria for specific psychopathologies.

The first conception of disease relies on the idea that diseases involve breakdown in the proper functioning of specific systems in the individual. The second conception equates disease with deviation from average functioning. It is well-known that these two conceptions can easily come apart—that they will give conflicting answers on specific cases. Rupturing of an appendix is not normal and thus a disease state, yet the appendix has no function and thus its rupturing cannot be a disease on the dysfunction view. Running a fever is not normal but is probably an adaptive biological response to infection. Not only can the two definitions come apart, but there is also a well-known set of apparent counterexamples to either definition of disease. Osteoarthritis in old age and prostate cancer in elderly men are normal or average; sepsis is the proper functioning of the immune system but a disease nonetheless (Murphy 2015).

However, the framework of medical models of psychopathology is in large part a legitimizing rhetoric for the complex of practices in which the DSM is embedded. The idea that mental problems involve dysfunctions of systems carries very little weight in the real application of the DSM and the way DSM classifies behaviors. There is very little research into the evolutionary adaptive role of psychological processes, and nearly none of that work is used to justify the DSM categories. The idea of grounding DSM classifications in the abnormal functioning of biological, psychological, or developmental processes certainly makes more sense—who, except extreme followers of the antipsychiatry movement, can doubt that severe schizophrenia involves abnormal functioning of these systems. Yet such considerations are distant from the actual classifications made by the DSM. Thus, the idea of mental disorders largely does little work in the DSM classificatory system. This is no surprise given the aggressively atheoretical nature of the DSM approach. Removing this unnecessary baggage is a first step to defending the prospect that some DSM categories may pick out objectively identifiable and predictive groupings of behavior.

Another way in which DSM in practice does not reflect the medical model results from the essential place given to deficits in interpersonal or social functioning in making diagnoses. Interestingly, exactly what kind of deficits these are vary from classification to classification. For depression it is "impairment in social, occupational, or other important areas of functioning" (American Psychiatric Association 2013, 125) while for the manic part of bipolar disorder it is "impairment in social or occupational functioning" (American Psychiatric Association 2013, 124). This is a clear break from the strict medical model which generally does not make degree of impairment a criterion for disease status.

The medical model behind DSM does have real effects in that the DSM classifications are all categorical in nature. This continues to be the case in DSM-5 despite the strong push in its development to make a place for a dimensional component. Indeed the impairment requirement just described is motivated in DSM-5 as a way to include subthreshold, that is, continuous, manifestations. Is the categorical nature of DSM classifications a major problem? I would argue largely in the affirmative, but not always.

There are various reasons not to treat continuous phenomena as categorical. For research purposes, doing so loses information when variation is eliminated. For clinical purposes, doing so encourages (1) the medicalization of cases that may be best thought of as problems in living and/or (2) not regarding nonmedical conditions as worthy of help. Probably the largest part of the DSM classifications are really describing problems that vary in degree rather than in kind and thus are promoting all such errors.

However, I would argue that there are a number of bad reasons for criticizing DSM on the grounds of its categorical approach, as was done in the run up to DSM-5 (Helzer et al. 2008):

1. That a categorical approach fits much pyschopathology poorly does not entail that it is uniformly a mistake.
2. Classifying in terms of categorical distinctions does not mean that degrees of symptoms and problems cannot be allowed. Either you have Huntington's disease or you do not, but the disease definitely varies in severity.
3. Classifying in terms of categorical distinctions does not commit one to an exhaustive, mutually exclusive classification system. In particular, there is nothing incoherent in there being individuals with multiple categorical diagnoses and those diagnoses sharing some of the same characteristics. Individuals can have AIDS and leukemia at the same time, and

they have some overlapping symptoms. In some cases of psychopathology we know enough about the relevant brain systems involved that it would be surprising if there were not individuals with multiple conditions and if the conditions shared some common features. I have argued elsewhere (Kincaid 2014) that this is the case for depression and anxiety.

4. The main critics of DSM on the grounds of its categorical nature come from the psychometric, abnormal psychology tradition in clinical psychology. However the standard kind of evidence used in psychometric studies—factor analysis, latent trait analysis, and so forth—presupposes that phenomena are dimensional rather than testing that hypothesis. Treating everything as dimensional is just as dogmatic as treating everything as categorical. It is worth noting that dimensional assumptions threaten to greatly expand what behaviors get labeled as needing treatment.
5. Treating categorical phenomena as continuous or dimensional also results in lost statistical power for research studies and can result in a one-approach-fits-all strategy in clinical settings where it is not justified. If categorical phenomena are treated as continuous, then we have in effect omitted variable bias, for a variable—disorder or not—is left out. This is equivalent, for example, to leaving out race or sex when they make a difference in social science studies. In the clinic, treating a disorder that is categorical as dimensional means that interventions are not tailored to the differences in problems.

Therefore, I would argue that whether any particular DSM categorical classification actually picks out an objective distinction in nature that allows for understanding causes, course, and possible treatment is an empirical issue that has to be argued case by case. The general steps that I think are needed to defend a conclusion that we have a distinct defensible classification are two: that there are evidentially independent criteria or measures that point to the same objective grouping and that there are a series of relatively well-confirmed claims about the causes and effects of those groupings, what Meehl aptly called a nomological net. Such distinctions can potentially be made while shedding the medical model rhetoric, recognizing the looseness of screens, and admitting possible different but not conflicting ways to identify specific disorders. Thus, in short, while there are many problems in the DSM system, some DSM classifications can pick out objective and predictive groupings of psychopathology.

I believe there are some types of adult psychopathology that are approximately picked out by the DSM classifications that ground objective categorical style classifications, making it possible to identify causal, course, and treatment judgments. I want to argue that there is a prima facie case that major depressive disorder and bipolar disorder are two such cases. The taxonomic, neurobiological, physiological and cognitive functioning evidence provide a wide enough experimenter's regress that we can have some confidence that the DSM classifications are picking out a real, objective grouping of individuals. These results will then motivate my investigations of the possibilities of the same disorders in young children.

Let me begin with major depressive disorder. I have argued elsewhere that the major depressive disorder (Kincaid 2014) classification can pick out an objective and predictive grouping of individuals and behavior. For major depressive disorder, evidence of this sort comes from the following:

1. Recent taxometric studies (Ahmed, Stahl, and McFarland 2011) showing that questionnaire data on depressive symptoms from the general population are best explained by postulating a distinct categorical group of depressed individuals. Taxometic methods (Ruscio, Haslam, and Ruscio 2006) are statistical methods that have distinct advantages over factor analysis and latent class analysis, which do not directly test the hypothesis of a distinct grouping but instead assume the phenomena are dimensional and probe how many dimensions there are. Taxometric methods work by taking repeated samples of different compositions of individual scores on indicators and looking for correlations that only begin to appear as the samples approach 50–50 composition of the two putative groups. Baldness and height have no correlation in pure samples of men and women, but as the samples approach 50–50, correlations increase. These methods have been widely applied to psychopathology, finding that most, but not all, putative DSM disorders are dimensional, not categorical (Haslam, Holland, and Kuppens 2012). There are various methods for assessing a dimensional versus categorical assumption, among them finding distinct, inverted U-shaped curves in plots of indicators against each other and the comparison of simulated taxonic and dimensional data with research data by means of the comparison curve fit index (CCFI).
2. A host of studies using different measures shows that those with major depressive disorder respond differently than controls. This includes fMRI studies (Price and Drevets 2012), cortisol stress responses (Drevets 2002), increased behavior sensitivity to negative feedback and decreased sensitivity to rewards (Henriques, Glowacki, and Davidson 1994; Pizzagalli, Jahn, and O'Shea 2005; Pizzagalli et al. 2008), greater discounting of

future rewards (Takahashi et al. 2008), and histopathological differences (Drevets 2008).

3. Carefully done structural equation models of the causal antecedents and consequences for those falling into the major depressive disorder category (Bronte-Tinkew et al. 2007). These provide empirically defensible causal models of the causes and consequences associated with the depression construct.

Bipolar disorders[6] inherit these successes, and thus the question is the extent to which classifications of mania can have comparable strengths. I would argue that they do on similar grounds to those backing the objectivity of depression classifications:

1. Recent taxometric studies (Ahmed et al. 2011) show that questionnaire data on mania symptoms from the general population are best explained by postulating a distinct categorical group of individuals with bipolar disorders.[7]
2. Individuals classified as bipolar respond to lithium, whereas individuals classified as schizophrenic, the other disorder with symptoms that may be analogous to mania, do not (Leucht, Kissling, and McGrath 2004).
3. There is little evidence that individuals classified as bipolar respond to conventional antipsychotics while as a group individuals classified as schizophrenic certainly do (Strakowski et al. 2003).
4. Concordance in twins has been reported as high as 90% in recent studies (Maletic and Raison 2014), and genome-wide association studies find polymorphisms unique to biopolar disorder but not found in schizophrenia, perhaps its nearest cousin among psychopathologies.
5. Various brain differences are found in bipolar patients. Ventricle volumes differ. fMRI studies of areas activated by the presentation of happy or sad faces differentiate bipolar from unipolar depression, with unipolar showing greater amygdala activation for sad faces and vice versa for bipolar (Maletic and Raison 2014).
6. Bipolar patients exhibit specific deficits in executive function and verbal memory (Robinson et al. 2006).

Of course, more than I have done here and elsewhere would be needed to make a strong case that major depressive disorder and bipolar disorder pick out objective groupings that allow for successful prediction. However, what I have given provides at least a prima facie case for this claim, which is still compatible with diagnoses sometimes being wrongly made in research studies. Moreover, I think the case that I have made justifies focusing on depression and bipolar classifications in children because they are paradigm cases of adult disorders.

So the overall picture of DSM that I paint here is of a diagnostic system of very heterogeneous validity. The medical model framework is largely a mishmash that does little to no work in the actual classifications aside from rationalizing the categorical nature of the diagnoses and justifying pharmacological interventions (nontrivial consequences for sure). The categorical character of many DSM classifications is doubtful. Some classifications are overdiagnosed, some are probably best thought of as problems in living, and others are simply behaviors that are socially constructed and often disapproved behaviors (gender identity disorder in DSM-IV and probably gender dysphoria in DSM-5 are cases). However, those deficiencies do not prevent some DSM classifications from approximately picking out objective groupings of individuals that allow for some understanding of the causes, consequences, and treatment prospects. There is evidence that depression and bipolar classifications are two such cases.

With this conclusion and the framework developed above, I turn to ask whether we have reason to believe that the classifications of depression and bipolar disorder in young children have similar evidence going for them. My argument is that while adult major depressive disorder and bipolar disorder can identify objective and predictive groupings of adult individuals (shorn of overdiagnoses), even these best case examples are not warranted in thinking about the problems of small children.

DSM, Psychopathology, and Children

My goal in this section is to critically analyze the use of DSM categories of depression and bipolar disorders in research on young children. By "young" I mean preschool children. There are numerous confident assertions in the literature that these disorders are well established in this age group (e.g., Stalets and Luby 2006). Yet a careful assessment of the evidence shows no such thing, as I will detail below. Diagnostic criteria are revised in ways that would make Popper turn over in his grave, exhibiting very short and manipulated experimenter's regresses. Results are over- or misinterpreted in various ways. Obvious alternative explanations are ignored. Key claims are made based on unpublished data. While making a full case would require more careful historical and sociological analysis than I can do here, there is a prima facie case that most current applications of DSM depression and bipolar disorders in young children do not pick out an objective grouping but are rather a human imposition on the phenomena—social constructions if you like that phraseology. It may be that there are some children who really meet the full adult criteria for bipolar and depression, but so far the literature does not establish that, and it is surely true that there is significant overdiagnosis.

Let me begin with depression. The taxometric evidence on childhood depression does not support the claim that there is a categorical group with a diagnosable disorder. Hankin and colleagues (2005) used a sample of 845 nine- to seventeen-year-olds. The Child and Adolescent Psychopathology Scale (CAPS) was used. The scale asks multiple questions about the same DSM depression criteria; the scores on those questions for each of the criteria were combined to form the indicators for taxometric analysis. The CAPS questionnaire was administered both to the children and to their parents. Taxometric analyses were done for both sets and were also done separately for nine- to thirteen-year-olds and the fourteen to seventeen age group.

None of the taxometric analyses supported a categorical interpretation of the data—they found no evidence that there is a distinct group of young children identified by the criteria for major depressive disorder. However, those conclusions are tentative for two reasons. Assessment was made through the visual comparison of research and simulated data curves. Ideally, the evidence would have included CCFI measures. Moreover, since the youngest subjects were nine years old, this is still only indirect evidence about preschoolers.

In another taxometric study Richey and coauthors (2009) report on evidence for a taxon of "child depression." However, their work exemplifies the low standards that are a common problem on my view for pediatric psychiatric research. They do not really study preschoolers—the mean age of their sample is 13.37 and the standard deviation is 3.48, so their sample is largely an adolescent one. Their taxometric results entail that the base rate for bipolar disorder in children is 13%, an entirely unbelievable number that calls into question the entire study. Their indicators come from the Children's Depression Inventory, a revision of the Beck Depression Inventory which is widely thought only to measure negative affect, not depression. Their taxometric methods in this sample are limited to MAXCOV and MAXEIG, which are two different algorithms looking for randomly drawn subsamples of the population where correlation of indicators increases as samples approach 50–50 distributions of putative category members and noncategory members. However, these are mathematically equivalent approaches, and pretending that they provide independent lines of evidence is just false and violates well-known standards of taxometric research (Ruscio et al. 2006). They use only a visual inspection criterion to determine whether a taxon exists when the clear standard in the literature is the much more objective comparison curve fit analysis. Finally, the data they report do not really support the taxonic conclusion even if all the above problems did not exist: a full third of their curves do not show the typical peaked curves that provide evidence for a categorical interpretation of their data.

Preschool depression might still be a real phenomenon if it is only dimensional, not taxonic. However, in general, research and clinical practice are based on the categorical assumption. Admitting that an alleged psychopathology is really a more or less normally distributed trait in the population raises doubts about thinking in terms of psychopathology and the medical model. That, of course, does not preclude other approaches which might find certain behaviors worthy of intervention.

Given our earlier discussion of the loose connection between DSM and research screens, it is also not surprising that there is dubious evidence that screens are actually picking out depression in young children. The doubts are several. Sometimes authors simply misstate what evidence reported by others shows. Stalets and Luby (2006, 900) is a telling example. They cite literature which shows "the basic validity and prevalence of depressive disorders in a large, community based sample of preschoolers (Egger et al. 2006)." However, a close look at Egger et al. shows they do nothing of the sort. Their study concerns the reliability of the Preschool Age Psychiatric Assessment (PAPA). Reliability measures the extent to which independent raters using the screen agree on diagnoses. That researchers agree on applying a screen on its own does not provide much evidence that the screen is picking out an objective disorder, for such agreement can also be explained as a social consensus producing a pure social construct. Egger et al. make no claims about the validity of this instrument, contra what Stalets and Luby very misleadingly claim. While Egger et al. do find some evidence for the reliability of the PAPA, it comes from agreement on eight cases out of thirteen, not exactly a large sample. They also report the comparative reliability of other commonly used screens for preschool depression and find that they have very poor reliability, with agreement rates as low as 50%. The Egger et al. article provides virtually no evidence for the validity of preschool depression and, in fact, seems to be evidence against it. Stalets and Luby also do what is common in the literature on preschool psychiatric disorders: in arguing for the reality of preschool depression, they consistently cite evidence that turns out to be about older children and adolescents, not preschoolers.

A further doubt about screens is that the DSM criteria for depression in children have been revised in light of the fact that children seldom show depressed mood. Instead, irritability can replace depressed mood in the diagnosis of children, and studies show that it is the core feature in most extant diagnoses of childhood depression. Key studies (Luby, Heffelfinger, and Mrakotsky 2003a) also drop the two-week-duration requirement of adult depression, with 80% of children diagnosed not meeting that standard (Stalets and Luby 2006). Essential adult criteria are dropped in an effort to find depression in preschoolers. This is an instance of the experimenter's regress, but revision is sufficiently major and undermotivated that one wonders about the falsifiability[8] of the claims these researchers are making about prepubertal depression. Advocates of these modifications cite studies showing that childhood depression as so diagnosed predicts childhood depression twenty-four months later (Luby et al. 2009), claiming this shows the reality of childhood depression. Of course, depression at both periods is measured by screens that deviate significantly from core factors of adult depression, and thus it is debatable that this consistency provides much evidence at all.

Nor is there unambiguous genetic, neurobiological, and cognitive evidence that there is a unique group of depressed prepubertal children:

- Rice (2010) reviews studies of genetics and familial trends in prepubertal children and does not find the high genetic load reported in adult depression and finds there is little continuity or predictive value of prepubertal diagnoses vis-à-vis adult depression.
- Stalets and Luby (2006) report evidence that there are deficits in spatial skills in depressed children. Yet they also report that their skills are in the normal range for children of their age. Also, and quite strikingly, their claims here are supported by what they call "unpublished data" which are not revealed in the paper in question and which thus have no statistics. It is quite exceptional for a journal to allow major claims in an article to be supported by data that are not presented.
- fMRI studies are inconsistent and report some findings that are opposite in direction to those for adults. Depressed youth have been shown to have lower amygdala activity in fear protocols while the opposite is true in adult depression (Klein et al. 2013).

Furthermore, there is compelling evidence that children diagnosed with depression show high "comorbidity" with other conditions. Attention deficit/hyperactivity disorder (ADHD) (42%), oppositional defiant disorder (ODD) (62%), and both ADHD and ODD (41%) are found in children diagnosed with depression, yet anxiety is diagnosed much less often in children (Luby et al. 2003b). The opposite pattern is found in adult depression.

Given that most children diagnosed with depression exhibit not depressed mood but irritability, the natural hypothesis suggests itself that if there is an objective grouping here that we want to treat as a medical condition, it is a condition with much more similarity to these two alleged disorders than depression.

A final piece of evidence worth noting is that for the role of social context in these diagnoses. It is worth distinguishing social context from what we might call predisposing social conditions. I mean by the latter the kinds of factors that there is evidence for vulnerability of adult depression, for example, major life events in childhood. These are distal social causes. By social context I mean ongoing proximal social and familial factors. There is evidence that these are associated with children who get diagnosed with childhood psychiatric disorders (Mash and Barkley 2014 survey the literature). The medical model rhetoric of DSM of course transfers over to its childhood applications, and writing about childhood depression is framed in terms of dysfunctional causes internal to the child. However, it is entirely possible that some part of the phenomena that get labeled as childhood depression are really ongoing problems with family and friends, not internal defects.

So the moral of the discussion just presented is that there is very little evidence for major depressive disorder in young children. Much of the cited evidence turns out to be evidence about adolescents, not young children (young children are the target of my analysis, and I am taking no explicit stand on the evidence for depression and bipolar diagnoses in adolescents). Childhood diagnoses depart significantly from the criteria used for the adult disorder. There is not the kind of genetic, neurobiological, and cognitive evidence like that found in adult major depressive disorder to support the claim that there is a unique group of depressed prepubertal children. The taxometric evidence does not support the existence of such a grouping. The level of comorbidity with ADHD raises worries that if there is a disorder present, it is the latter rather than major depressive disorder. Finally, there is some evidence childhood diagnoses of major depressive disorder are really picking out social and familial problems these children are facing, not an underlying psychopathological disorder.

I turn next to make a similar case for childhood bipolar disorder. A first thing to note is that, so far as I can find, there have been no taxometric studies of bipolar disorder in children. Of course, positive results in such studies are among the strongest available evidence that a classification is picking out an objective grouping. There is no such evidence in the case of bipolar disorder in children, unlike the case in adult bipolar.

Soutullo et al. (2005) summarizes some of the evidence concerning differences in the estimates of the prevalence of bipolar disorder in preschool children. The results raise serious doubts about the objectivity of the alleged disorder. US studies find that the prevalence of bipolar disorder in preadolescent youth is 1.4%. However, a large UK epidemiological study (Taylor, Dopfner, and Sergeant 2004) found no cases; a study in psychiatric hospitals in Finland found that 0.0006% of patients had bipolar disorder (Sourander 2004). A large epidemiological study in the UK found no cases, 2,500 clinical referrals at Manchester Children's Hospital also found no cases, and the same result was found in Maudsley Hospital in London over a twenty-two-year period (Richey et al. 2009). These results are supported by the findings of Dubicka et al. (2008). They gave identical vignettes to US and UK physicians representing pediatric behavior and got very different levels of bipolar diagnosis. All of these studies are based on DSM criteria. They suggest that the reliability of the various screens is very low, raising the worry that there is no objective distinction in the phenomena to support bipolar classification in children. The vast difference in US vs. UK diagnosis rates suggests that US diagnoses of bipolar are being imposed (socially constructed) from a very general set of behaviors in young children that do not map neatly on to any well-confirmed adult disorder, a conclusion also supported by the evidence I report next that there is severe overlap of symptoms between bipolar disorder in children and other childhood psychiatric classifications.

There is little evidence for familial patterns in bipolar disorder for young children, unlike the situation with adult bipolar where there are very strong family associations. Birmaher et al. (2010) studied the children of a large sample of bipolar adults and did not find statistically significant rates of bipolar disorder in their children.

Not surprisingly, bipolar diagnoses in children overlap very significantly with other diagnoses. A meta-analysis of seven studies found an average of 62% overlap between bipolar and ADHD diagnosis, with some studies showing as high as 98% overlap (Youngstrom and Algorta 2014). Another study (Geller et al. 2002) found there was no difference in rate of irritability (98% bipolar vs. 72% ADHD), accelerated speech (97% vs. 82%), distractibility (94% vs. 96%), and unusual energy (100% vs. 95%). Irritability is a key diagnostic feature of pediatric bipolar disorder, but it is also a diagnostic feature of depression, generalized anxiety disorder, ODD, post-traumatic stress disorder, ADHD, and intermittent explosive disorder. Likewise, risk factors and neurocognitive symptoms in bipolar disorder in children also overlap significantly with those for other diagnoses. Candidate genes for bipolar disorder also show correlations with ADHD and schizophrenia (Youngstrom and Algorta 2014).

As in childhood depression, there has been a consistent move to transform the criteria for bipolar disorder from those of the original definition of bipolar disorder in adults when confronted with evidence that children do not manifest adult bipolar symptoms. The DSM-5 (American Psychiatric Association 2013) criteria for mania in adult bipolar disorder require a "distinct period of abnormal and persistently elevated, expansive, or irritable mood" (124). The distinct period requires seven days, with symptoms most of the time. For pediatric bipolar diagnoses, it is just irritable mood that is characteristic of bipolar disorder,[9] and researchers diagnose the condition in children who do not meet the criterion of seven days most of the time. This practice was the result of a National Institute of Mental Health expert committee consensus recommendation (Nottelman 2001), not of strong evidence that these phenomena were somehow still really bipolar disorder. Stalets and Luby justify this on the grounds that young children typically show irritability off and on. However, that is reason for requiring a longer duration for a diagnosis of mania in children, because that would be needed to avoid the false positives arising from chance runs of mania-like symptoms. Furthermore, irritability in these children is a chronic condition, not a deviation from their normal functioning as is required in the adult bipolar criteria. All of these points raise serious doubts about the existence of bipolar disorder in young children.

There is good evidence in the case of adult bipolar disorders that lithium is effective in treating mania. To my knowledge there is one positive result for lithium in a small randomized trial involving adolescents (Moreno et al. 2007). That lithium works for mania in bipolar adults but has no efficacy in treating depression or schizophrenia is convincing evidence that the disorder is a distinct phenomenon. That kind of evidence is nonexistent in children labeled as bipolar.

The neurobiological evidence for bipolar disorder in children is in large negative. However, some influential researchers work hard to reinterpret that data to support the bipolar diagnosis. Chang (2007), publishing in a journal with a high impact factor, exemplifies the circularity of these moves. He notes that decreased frontal brain volumes are found in adult bipolar disorder but not in children, that studies of prefrontal neuronal density show decreased levels in adult diagnoses but not in children, and that prefrontal activation in fMRI scans in adults shows a decrease but an increase in children. Rather than drawing the obvious conclusion that these neurobiological findings are evidence against bipolar disorder in children, he concludes that they support the reality of bipolar disorder. How so? They support a "neurodevelopmental progressive model of BD." One is hard pressed to see what would refute that model if normal brain function in children is evidence for bipolar disorder.

Finally, there is a sociological story to be told about the massive increase in diagnoses of bipolar disorder in children. Kaplan (2011) documents the media coverage that resulted in enormous increases in parents' asking their doctors whether their child had bipolar disorder. Papalos (2007) published *The Bipolar Child*, which sold 200,000 copies and was featured on Oprah and other US television programs. Scientifically, the book is weak, claiming that an enormous number of typical childhood characteristics are evidence of bipolar disorder in children. The authors have started two foundations around childhood bipolar disorder and have a newsletter with 20,000 subscribers and a web page on bipolar disorder in children. It is hard to avoid the suspicion that while the empirical evidence for bipolar and major depressive disorder in young children is very thin, social factors unconnected to the evidence are leading clinicians and researchers to take these diagnoses seriously. Exactly how these factors work is no doubt a complex story in need of much further elaboration.[10]

Conclusion

I have tried to examine the best case for DSM psychopathology classifications in young children. I have not assumed that all of DSM is fatally flawed. Rather, I have looked at two kinds of classifications that in adults probably have the best prospects for picking objective groupings that allow for predictions on causes, effects, and course of a condition. I have found little evidence that these classifications do that in young children but have not argued that the prospect is impossible—in the end it is still an empirical question, but empirical prospects so far are bleak. In the process, I have tried to show that assessments of claims about the categorization of psychopathology have to be treated case by case rather than looking for global defenses or criticisms of psychiatric practice, and that it is essential to look in detail at the actual standards of evidence and strategies used to warrant diagnostic categories. Good work in psychopathological categorization, like categorization more generally in the sciences, provides multiple lines of relatively independent evidence and shows that proposed categorizations allow for identifying causal antecedents and consequents.

Acknowledgments

Jeffrey Poland, Şerife Tekin, and Dan Stein made very helpful comments on this paper.

Notes

1. One US study found that antidepressants are the second most common psychotropic medication given to children ages 2–4 and their use doubled between 1991 and 1994 (Zito, Safer, and dos Reis 2000), with 3,000 prescriptions given to children younger than one year of age in 1994.

2. I use DSM-IV in the two following examples because these screens were developed or revised at the time of DSM-IV. DSM-5 has not yet had an effect on these screens that I know of.

3. "Overdiagnosed" means false positives. That is entirely consistent with large parts of a population going undiagnosed because of lack of screening.

4. DSM talks of disorders, but their definition of "disorder" is clearly equivalent to standard notions of disease.

5. The recent Research Domain Criteria project of moving away from the DSM categories nonetheless remains a medical model of dysfunction, and it is still very peripheral to current research and practice.

6. There are multiple subspecies of bipolar disorder in the DSM, with the Bipolar I requiring mania for at least a week but not requiring depression (though most adults with Bipolar I have depression) and Bipolar II requiring mania symptoms for only four days and requiring depression. There is also a "not otherwise specified" version, which in the DSM means that patients do not meet the full criteria of either type but have similar symptoms. The differences in these subspecies play no direct role in my argument.

7. There is a second study arguing for dimensionality (Prisciandaro and Roberts 2011). However, the study is very weak. Taxons are much harder to find when the expected base in the population is less than 10%; this study is done in a general population where estimates of bipolar prevalence would not be more than 2%. The indicators used are binary, and binary indicators generally work poorly in finding taxons. Thus, this data is strongly biased against finding a taxon if one existed. The paper claims to have found evidence for dimensionality, but on one of the two taxometric procedures run, the CCFI—the single best measure of taxonic versus dimensional solutions—was 0.45, which is neutral evidence, supporting neither taxonic nor dimensional interpretations.

8. I argue that there are issues of falsifiability for both childhood depression research and bipolar research. In doing so I am not buying into Popper's full philosophical framework. However, one can still acknowledge that as the science is practiced there is real difficulty in seeing what would count as disconfirming evidence.

9. Strictly speaking, only Bipolar II in the DSM has any direct criterion for children in that major depressive disorder is required and can be indicated in children by extreme irritability.

10. One wonders, for example, what percentage of the parents of children with these diagnoses are themselves on psychotropic medication, making their use in young children seem less drastic a step to them.

References

Ahmed, A. O., K. C. Stahl, and M. E. McFarland. 2011. Latent structure of unipolar and bipolar mood symptoms. *Bipolar Disorders* 13 (5–6): 522–536.

American Psychiatric Association. 2013. *Diagnostic and Statistical Manual of Mental Disorders*. 5th ed. Arlington, VA: American Psychiatric Association.

Birmaher, B., D. Axelson, M. Goldstein, K. Monk, C. Kalas, M. Obreja, M. Hickey, et al. 2010. Psychiatric disorders in preschool offspring of parents with bipolar disorder: The Pittsburgh Bipolar Offspring Study (BIOS). *American Journal of Psychiatry* 167:321–330.

Bronte-Tinkew, J., M. Zaslow, M. Capps, A. Horowitz, and M. McNamara. 2007. Food insecurity works through depression, parenting, and infant feeding to influence overweight and health in toddlers. *Journal of Nutrition Community and International Nutrition* 137:2160–2165.

Chang, H. 2004. *Inventing Temperature Measurement and Scientific Progress*. Cambridge: Cambridge University Press.

Chang, K. 2007. Adult bipolar disorder is continuous with pediatric bipolar disorder. *Canadian Journal of Psychiatry* 52 (7): 418–424.

Cronbach, L. J., and P. E. Meehl. 1955. Construct validity in psychological tests. *Psychological Bulletin* 52 (4): 281–302.

Dennett, D. 1991. Real patterns. *Journal of Philosophy* 88 (1): 27–51.

Drevets, W. C. 2002. Glucose metabolism in the amygdala in depression: Relationship to diagnostic subtype and plasma cortisol levels. *Pharmacology, Biochemistry, and Behavior* 71:431–447.

Drevets, W. C. 2008. Brain structural and functional abnormalities in mood disorders: Implications for neurocircuitry models of depression. *Brain Structure & Function* 213:93–118.

Dubicka, B., G. Carlson, A. Vail, and R. Harrington. 2008. Prepubertal mania: Diagnostic differences between US and UK clinicians. *European Child & Adolescent Psychiatry* 17:153–161.

Dupré, J. 1993. *The Disorder of Things*. Cambridge, MA: Harvard University Press.

Egger, H., A. Erkanli, G. Keeler, E. Potts, B. Walter, and A. Angold. 2006. Test-retest reliability of the Preschool Age Psychiatric Assessment (PAPA). *Journal of the American Academy of Child and Adolescent Psychiatry* 45 (5): 906–917.

Geller, B., B. Zimerman, M. Williams, M. P. Delbello, K. Bolhofner, J. L. Craney, J. Frazier, L. Beringer, and M. J. Nickelsburg. 2002. DSM-IV mania symptoms in a prepubertal and early adolescent bipolar disorder phenotype compared to attention-deficit hyperactive and normal controls. *Journal of Child and Adolescent Psychopharmacology* 12 (1): 11–25.

Hacking, I. 1993. Working in a new world: The taxonomic solution. In *World Changes: Thomas Kuhn and the Nature of Science,* ed. Paul Horwich, 275–310. Cambridge, MA: MIT Press.

Hankin, B., C. Fraley, and I. Waldman. 2005. Is depression best viewed as a continuum or discrete category? A taxometric analysis of childhood and adolescent depression in a population-based sample. *Journal of Abnormal Psychology* 114:96–110.

Haslam, N., E. Holland, and P. Kuppens. 2012. Categories versus dimensions in personality and psychopathology: A quantitative review of taxometric research. *Psychological Medicine* 42:903–920.

Helzer, J., H. Kraemer, R. Krueger, H. Wittchen, H. Sirovatka, and D. Regier. 2008. *Dimensional Approaches in Diagnostic Classification: Redefining the Research Agenda for DSM-V*. Arlington, VA: American Psychiatric Publishing.

Henriques, J. B., J. M. Glowacki, and R. J. Davidson. 1994. Reward fails to alter response bias in depression. *Journal of Abnormal Psychology* 103:460–466.

Horwitz, A., and J. Wakefield. 2007. *The Loss of Sadness: How Psychiatry Transformed Normal Sorrow into Depressive Disorder*. Oxford: Oxford University Press.

Kaplan, S. 2011. *Your Child Does Not Have Bipolar Disorder*. New York: Praeger.

Kincaid, H. 2014. Defensible natural kinds in the study of psychopathology. In *Classifying Psychopathology: Mental Illness and Natural Kinds,* ed. H. Kincaid and J. Sullivan, 145–173. Cambridge, MA: MIT Press.

Kincaid, H., R. Daniels, A. Dellis, A. Hofmeyr, J. Rousseau, C. Sharp, and D. Ross. 2013. A taxometric analysis of the performance of the problem gambling severity index in a South African national urban sample. *Journal of Gambling Studies* 29:377–392.

Klein, D., A. Kujawa, S. Black, and A. Pennoch. 2013. Depressive disorders. In *Child and Adolescent Psychopathology*, ed. T. Beauchaine and S. Hinshaw, 543–547. Hoboken, NJ: Wiley.

Leucht, S., W. Kissling, and J. McGrath. 2004. Lithium for schizophrenia revisited: A systematic review and meta-analysis of randomized controlled trials. *Journal of Clinical Psychiatry* 65 (2): 177–186.

Luby, J., A. Heffelfinger, and C. Mrakotsky. 2003a. The clinical picture of depression in preschool children. *Journal of the American Academy of Child and Adolescent Psychiatry* 42 (3): 340–348.

Luby, J., C. Mrakotsky, A. Heffelfinger, A. Brown, M. Hessler, and E. Spitznagel. 2003b. Modification of DSM-IV criteria for depressed preschool children. *American Journal of Psychiatry* 160:1169–1172.

Luby, J., X. Si, A. Belden, M. Tandon, and E. Spitznagel. 2009. Preschool depression: Homotypic continuity and course over 24 months. *Archives of General Psychiatry* 66 (8): 897–905.

Maletic, V., and C. Raison. 2014. Integrated neurobiology of bipolar disorder. *Frontiers in Psychiatry* 25 (5): 1–24.

Mash, E. J., and R. A. Barkley. 2014. *Child Psychopathology*. 3rd ed. New York: Guilford Press.

Moreno, C., G. Laje, C. Blanco, H. Jiang, A. Schmidt, and M. Olfson. 2007. National trends in the outpatient diagnosis and treatment of bipolar disorder in youth. *Archives of General Psychiatry* 64 (9): 1032–1039.

Murphy, D. 2015. *Concepts of disease and health*. Stanford Online Encyclopedia of Philosophy. http://plato.stanford.edu/entries/health-disease/.

Nottelman, E. 2001. National Institute of Mental Health research roundtable on prepubertal bipolar disorder. *Journal of the American Academy of Child and Adolescent Psychiatry* 40 (8): 871–878.

Papalos, D. 2007. *The Bipolar Child*. New York: Broadway Books.

Pizzagalli, D. A., D. Iosifescu, L. A. Hallett, K. G. Ratner, and M. Fava. 2008. Reduced hedonic capacity in major depressive disorder: Evidence from a probabilistic reward task. *Journal of Psychiatric Research* 43:76–87.

Pizzagalli, D. A., A. L. Jahn, and J. P. O'Shea. 2005. Toward an objective characterization of an anhedonic phenotype: A signal-detection approach. *Biological Psychiatry* 57:319–327.

Price, J., and W. Drevets. 2012. Neural circuits underlying the pathophysiology of mood disorders. *Trends in Cognitive Sciences* 16 (1): 61–71.

Prisciandaro, J., and J. Roberts. 2011. Evidence for the continuous latent structure of mania in the Epidemiologic Catchment Area from multiple latent structure and construct validation methodologies. *Psychological Medicine* 41:575–588.

Quine, W. 1969. *Ontological Relativity and Other Essays*. New York: Columbia University Press.

Rice, F. 2010. Genetics of childhood and adolescent depression: Insights into etiological heterogeneity and challenges for future genomic research. *Genome Medicine* 2 (68): 1–6.

Richey, J., N. Schmidt, C. Lonigan, B. Phillips, S. Catanzaro, J. Laurent, R. Gerhardstein, and R. Kotov. 2009. The latent structure of child depression: A taxometric analysis. *Journal of Child Psychology and Psychiatry, and Allied Disciplines* 50 (9): 1147–1155.

Robinson, L., J. M. Thompson, P. Gallagher, U. Goswami, A. H. Young, I. N. Ferrier, and P. B. Moore. 2006. A meta-analysis of cognitive deficits in euthymic patients with bipolar disorder. *Journal of Affective Disorders* 93:105–115.

Ross, D. 2004. Rainforest realism. In *Dennett's Philosophy: A Comprehensive Assessment*, ed. A. Brook, D. Ross, and D. Thompson, 147–168. Cambridge, MA: MIT Press.

Ruscio, J., N. Haslam, and A. Ruscio. 2006. *Introduction to the Taxometric Method: A Practical Guide*. Mahwah, NJ: Erlbaum.

Sourander, A. 2004. Combined psychopharmacological treatment among child and adolescent inpatients in Finland. *European Child & Adolescent Psychiatry* 13:179–184.

Soutullo, C., K. Chang, A. Dez-Suarez, A. Figueroa-Quintana, I. Escamilla-Canales, M. Rapado-Castro, and F. Ortuno. 2005. Bipolar disorder in children and adolescents: International perspective on epidemiology and phenomenology. *Bipolar Disorders* 7:497–506.

Stalets, M., and J. Luby. 2006. Preschool depression. *Child and Adolescent Psychiatric Clinics of North America* 15:899–917.

Strakowski, S. M., M. P. Del Bello, C. M. Adler, and P. E. Keck. 2003. Atypical antipsychotics in the treatment of bipolar disorder. *Expert Opinion on Pharmacotherapy* 4 (5): 751–756.

Takahashi, T., H. Oono, T. Inoue, S. Boku, Y. Kako, Y. Kitaichi, I. Kasumi, et al. 2008. Depressive patients are more impulsive and inconsistent in intertemporal choice behavior for monetary gain and loss than healthy subjects—an analysis based on Tsallis' statistics. *Neuroendocrinology Letters* 29 (3): 291–390.

Taylor E., M. Dopfner, and J. Sergeant . 2004. European clinical guidelines for hyperkinetic disorder—first upgrade. *European Child and Adolescent Psychiatry* 13 (Suppl. 1): i7–i30.

Wilson, M. 2007. *Wandering Significance*. Oxford: Oxford University Press.

Youngstrom, E., and G. Algorta. 2014. Pediatric bipolar disorder. In *Child Psychopathology*, ed. E. Mash and R. Barkeley, Kindle 10520–12509. New York: Guilford Press.

Zito, J., D. Safer, and S. dos Reis. 2000. Trends in the prescribing of psychotropic medications to preschoolers. *Journal of the American Medical Association* 283 (8): 1025–1030.

13 Truth and Sanity: Positive Illusions, Spiritual Delusions, and Metaphysical Hallucinations

Owen Flanagan and George Graham

> "The truth, the whole truth, and nothing but the truth" [is] a perverse and paralyzing policy for any world maker (Goodman 1978, 19).

Saving Normal

Contemporary psychiatry diagnostically overreaches. It pathologizes—or acts as if it has permission to pathologize—too much of what are perfectly acceptable forms of living and being. In *Saving Normal*, Allen Frances (2013, xix–xx), a psychiatrist and chair of the DSM-IV Task Force, laments his own past contribution to the "wholesale medicalization of normality" that culminated in DSM-5 (American Psychiatric Association 2013).[1] According to Frances, a perfect storm of the interests of medical health professionals, the ascendency of therapeutic culture to treat ordinary human suffering, a class of "worried well" with money, and the rapacious hunger of "Big Pharma" have led to hyperinflation of mental illness diagnoses, overtreatment, and misallocation of medical resources. Those who are really sick, who will not regain existential footing by the healing powers of human companionship and ordinary resilience and time, are not treated, while those who have perfectly ordinary, perennial problems of living are led to believe they have mental illnesses and take psychotropic drugs to alter their moods, but often not their lives.

In this chapter, we criticize a worrisome trend in contemporary psychiatry that pathologizes normalcy on dubious epistemic grounds, on the naive premise that mental health has some sort of clear, precise, and firm link to true belief and, conversely, that mental disease or disorder has some clear, precise, and firm link to false or misbegotten belief. We deny this premise and show how it should make us worry that we understand what makes illusions, delusions, and hallucinations unhealthy or abnormal. In fact, we deny that illusions, delusions, and hallucinations are categorically or even typically unhealthy or abnormal.[2]

We give three examples of ways of worldmaking that are sensible and acceptable, even normal and healthy, but that are pathologized or pathologizable by cooperation among the expansive regimen of psychiatry, segments of postmodern culture that accept and encourage its normative regimen, and norms of both philosophy and science that would ask us to domesticate human imagination and meaning making in all zones of life.

The project of living a good and meaningful life is an extraordinarily high-stakes project and may well require states or conditions of mind and ways of being a person that are transgressive, even, a bit, as they used to say, mad or crazy. We describe certain states of mind or, better, ways of normal worldmaking, which are sometimes pathologized but which are, from other perspectives, experientially enjoyable, beautiful, and truth seeking. They are at the epistemic edge, sometimes beyond that edge, but existentially inspiring and morally uplifting.

Examples of states of mind that tempt but do not merit being pathologized include (1) positive illusions, empirically false beliefs or unrealistic attitudes that make individuals happier and nicer than individuals who are narrow-minded, truth-centered realists; (2) some potentially classifiable spiritual delusions, such as unshakeable religious attitudes that serve to bind peoples ("religio" means to bind); and (3) some metaphysical hallucinations, attitudes toward ultimate reality that can easily be induced by hallucinogens and that involve experiences of ego diminishment or dissolution as well as feelings such as that love is all that matters, or that all is one, and that can have good personal and moral effects. All three kinds of examples require reflection on how circumscribed norms of mentally healthy belief ought to be. Certain trends in psychiatry, secular scientific culture, and philosophy pull for norms of "being in touch with reality as it is" that would, if abided, impoverish human life. At the same time many secular philosophies press for epistemic belief-forming discipline that would theoretically prohibit certain widespread ways of conceiving of meaningful and demanding forms of being human.

Positive Illusions

According to the standard analysis, so-called positive illusions are false beliefs that have good making features (Taylor and Brown 1988). Ordinary people who are taught that the average person has a certain objective chance of getting a certain disease, being in a bad accident, or being involved in a painful betrayal, and who think that the odds do not apply to them, are generally happier and more pleasant to be around than people who think that the poor odds apply to them. The people who believe that not-so-good objective probabilities apply to them (they get that they are average) tend to be moderately depressed and self-centered. Thus, they are dubbed depressive realists (Alloy and Abramson 1979; Golin, Terrell, and Johnson 1977; Bradley 1978). People who believe that they are above average in looks, talents, and virtue are happier and nicer (arguably, no one has tested real virtue) to be around than accurate self-assessors. The standard view is that positive illusions are epistemically or evidentially negative, but existentially positive.

Positive illusions have an interesting feature from a mental health point of view. Positive illusions are said to involve false beliefs, primarily about the self, which contribute nonetheless to personal happiness and interpersonal niceness. If we think that the best world is one in which mental health comes from living at the intersection of the true, the good, and the beautiful, where virtue, mental health, subjective happiness, and a sense of meaning and purpose go together, then the existence of positive illusions is worrisome. Positive illusions are a real-life example where the true and the good (and the "pretty," if not the full-on beautiful) come apart, and not just once in a while. They are cases where realistic assessment about one's self, on the one side, and happiness, well-being, niceness, and feeling pleasantly about oneself regularly and reliably go their separate ways. If there are positive illusions, they are systemic among the relatively happy and the relatively nice.

According to a comprehensive survey of dominant views of mental health in the mid-twentieth century, Marie Jahoda (1958) claimed that the expectation of accurate appraisal of reality is a central component in all extant models of the mentally healthy person. She writes, "The perception of reality is called mentally healthy when what the individual sees *corresponds with what is actually there*" (Jahoda 1958, 6). In an earlier paper she wrote, "Mentally healthy perception means a process of viewing the world so that one is able to take in matters one wishes were different without distilling them to fit those wishes" (Jahoda 1953, 349).

The dialectic changes with Taylor and Brown's (1988) important meta-analysis, which is entitled "Illusion and Well-Being: A Social Psychological Perspective on Mental Health." Taylor and Brown write that one consequence of the existence of positive illusions is that "in establishing criteria of mental health, then, we must subtract this particular one [accurate self-assessment]" (Taylor and Brown 1988, 197). Of course, one could choose to go the other way and maintain the norm of accurate self-assessment but judge most people as a bit off mentally. In any case, by the last decade of the last century, we have three threads in the dialectic and in tension with each other: a classical norm of mental health that requires thinking that corresponds "*with what is actually there*," evidence that depression is related to realism, and the claim that positive illusions are related to optimism and kindness.

One could take a nonindividualistic view of well-being, think this supposed rupture between the true and the good is bad, and look for structural or systemic causes of the disconnect, refusing to let the epistemic condition in the classical view of mental health slide. One might gain some confidence in this approach by noting that there is evidence from cultural psychology that one class of alleged positive illusions, the self-serving ones (one is in the top 5–10% in terms of looks, talent, virtue, etc.) is not common outside of the West (Flanagan 1991, 2007; Henrich et al. 2010). One might then, based on such evidence, claim that excessive emphasis on self-esteem, self-marketing, and boasting in North America produces the disconnect, and that such practices ought to be modified, which might then diminish current problems in our North American culture of narcissism.

We do not pursue this worthwhile culturally holistic and comparative idea here, but instead we question assimilating the entire class of positive illusions to a type of false belief. This avoids, right out of the gate, two common mistakes: first, categorizing mental states that are not plausibly classified as beliefs as beliefs, as attempts at representing or mirroring what is there; second, tying mental well-being too closely to a truth-centered epistemology, where health is assessed in terms of success at mirroring the way things really are. To the degree that so-called positive illusions involve hopes, expectations, and an optimistic attitude, then false belief is not an essential component or key ingredient and no epistemic norm is violated. If that is right, then positive illusions do not necessarily violate the classical mental health norm of failing to see things as they really are (although, as we will indicate shortly, we doubt this is the most helpful norm).

Here is a proposal: accept that positive illusions are states of mind that benefit the consumer, but reject the claim that they (all, most, many) are best interpreted as essentially requiring or being holistically constituted by false beliefs, as opposed to having positive attitudes, expectations, and hopes, as their vehicles. Hopes and a can-do attitude are not best conceived as beliefs or as belief-like states or structures, and they need not involve any false belief as even minor components (Flanagan 2007, 2009; Graham 2013, 221–225).

One needs to be careful distinguishing beliefs from hopes (Flanagan 1992, 2007, 2009, 2011; Graham 1998, 2013, 2015). Hope is "a more evidentially slack attitude than [empirical] belief." "Belief consists in attending to how things seem: to where the truth appears to reside. Hope, on the other hand, can subsist on a more evidentially Spartan diet" (Graham 1998, 33). So, whereas I ought not to believe that base rates don't apply to me, it is perfectly sensible to hope that they don't. It is nice (self-esteem wise) to think that I am very good looking, talented, and good. But thinking this is not the same as actually believing, especially on reflection, that this is so. It is not very well worked out in the positive illusions literature whether certain kinds of "the cup is half full/half empty" temperament explain the positive illusion/negative illusion results, in which case a general attitude or orientation toward life, optimism or pessimism, is mistakenly described in terms of beliefs. The general attitude would be better described as a kind of hopefulness or confidence, which, of course, would still need to abide by certain norms, lest it become hope against all possibility or crazy overconfidence. Such norms may involve having certain sensible beliefs, but the states of mind themselves are not best described holistically as states of belief or sets of beliefs. "In hope, we are invited to trust in possibilities that we cannot defend or perhaps even describe adequately just because they answer to our aspirations, desires, and needs" (Graham 1998, 33).

When Muhammad Ali famously remarked before his final fight with Smokin' Joe Frazier—the "Thrilla in Manila"—that "[i]t will be akilla and achilla ... and athrilla when I get the gorilla in Manila," did he believe that he would kick Smokin' Joe's ass? Or is he best understood as doing something, performing an action that was, in effect, part of the fight before the first bell sounded? Both boxers presumably believed that they could win and hoped that they would win. So far, there is no epistemic mistake regardless of outcome. "Can" does not entail "will." The epistemic standards governing hopes, desires, and the like are different from those that govern beliefs. It would be very odd to say that the losers in zero-sum games always have false beliefs going in—that I will certainly win. In fact, Ali might have believed that he could not win unless he made Smokin' Joe worry that he might know how to beat him. Furthermore, Smokin' Joe need not have believed he would lose after Ali's provocation. The effect might work this way: Ali knows how to do things with words. He speaks with the intention of undermining Smokin' Joe's confidence, and does so. In this case, the mechanisms at work do not operate via beliefs at all, although they might commonly be assimilated to that class of states when specified folk psychologically. The point is that many things we do with words and thoughts can be viewed as strategic—engendering self-confidence, undermining the competitor's abilities—and not as straightforwardly epistemic.

Consider this from Aristotle: "We ought not to follow the proverb-writers, and 'think human, since you are human', or 'think mortal, since you are mortal.' Rather, as far as we can, we ought to be pro-immortal, and go to all lengths to live a life that expresses our supreme element; for however this element may lack in bulk, by much more it surpasses everything in power and value" (*Nicomachean Ethics*, X: 13.37). Interpreted in one way, Aristotle can be read as encouraging two false beliefs—I am not human (but rather god-like), and I am not mortal. Interpreted in another way, however, he can be read as encouraging a complex attitude that one can achieve something excellent if one sets one's eyes on surpassing ordinary limits caused (in our case) by our animal nature and time's insurmountable regimen. Coaches often speak this way to their charges. A professional tennis match always produces one winner and one loser. Both players, if they are any good, go into the match believing that they can win, indeed that they will win. Believing one can win is a true belief. Hoping that one will win is a sensible expectation. In neither case is there a mistake.

A sensible test for whether a person in fact holds a belief or is in some associated epistemic state in a strong and objectionable way would be this: Does the state-in-question yield, and if so how quickly, easily, and so on, when there is strong countervailing evidence? If I go bald, get prostate cancer, divorce, or get in a car accident despite saying that I think I won't, I will quickly yield my initial thought or claim that these calamities will not befall me. This signals that the initial state was less a conviction than a hope.

Taylor and Brown (1988, 197) write, "[T]he extreme optimism individuals display [about such probabilities] appears to be illusory." But this is not obvious. Optimism can be unrealistic, perhaps—illusory is a different matter. There is no evidence that individuals who are prone to positive illusions fail to give up the relevant thoughts when they are provided with strong countervailing evidence. If people did dig in their heels and sincerely say that they are not really divorced, bald, and so forth when they are, and when it is obvious that they are, we might say that they are deluded, which is a different and, some would say, genuinely serious mental problem.

The upshot is that if there are positive illusions and if they are (1) common, correlated with (2) moral decency and (3) happiness, positive affect, optimism, as well as with (4) the capacity to engage in profitable, creative, productive work, then (5) there is a problem with the view that mental health and human flourishing require, or demand, overcoming the tendency to harbor false beliefs.

The way around these conflicts or troubles is to deny that most or all so-called positive illusions are beliefs.[3] Positive illusions are typically something much more interesting and important than that, running a gamut from hopes, wishes, optimistic attitudes, to holistic temperamental orientations. Once we reconceive the kinds as multifarious and not as suitable objects to be assessed by a truth-oriented epistemology, it is easier to consider the question of whether particular kinds of "positive illusions" are defective and, if so, across which dimensions, and whether they enhance or detract from psychological well-being (Young 2014).

We now turn to a standard mental state kind that is almost always judged as a kind of insanity, delusions. Delusions are almost always conceived in psychiatry and philosophy as beliefs or belief complexes (Bortolotti 2010). Unlike positive illusions, delusions truly do typically involve beliefs. But this does not mean that the problems the deluded person suffers are primarily doxastic or that the problem with the deluded person's doxastic attitudes are that they are more distant from reality or less likely true than other widely shared sets of beliefs.

Delusions and Moral Grandeur

Consider these cases:

Claire lives in the suburbs of a large American city. She works in the city. She commutes on a public transit bus. Once seated in the bus, she prays to God silently and fervently. She petitions that whenever each and every person on the bus dies, including Claire herself, they will go to Heaven. "God save us all," she says to herself.

The other people on the bus are ignorant of her prayers. The driver and passengers regard Claire as a quiet person who is polite to anyone who sits next to her. Not given to idle talk, Claire is emotionally heavily invested in the activity of praying. No matter how unlikely the possibility that her prayers will be instrumental in anyone's salvation, they occupy her silence on the bus.

Religious rituals in general, not just prayer, are dear to Claire's heart. She is a devout Roman Catholic. One reason that she is wedded to Catholicism is the great variety of behaviors that this version of Christianity identifies as helpful rituals. Is Claire deluded in any way, shape, or form?

Wenqing is Chinese. She lives in a district of a major city with many temples, some Confucian, some Daoist, and some Buddhist. These all survived Maoist China's official atheism. Wenqing doesn't really know the intricacies of these different traditions. But she knows that she can go to any temple, pray, light incense, and ask her ancestors to bless her and her family and to care for their own lineage going forward. She believes that her ancestors can intervene in the world now and make day-to-day life go better for her and her family. Wenqing doesn't believe in a creator God or, better, the idea hasn't really ever crossed her mind. But she believes that her ancestors abide in the community of beloved souls who have passed away. She sometimes experiences the presence of her grandmother and her great-grandfather, whom she remembers from when she was a little girl, and she judges these to be actual visitations from them. Wenqing is a good mother and expects to be able to help her family going forward, long after she has passed away. Is Wenqing deluded in any way, shape, or form?

Now consider Roberto and Tiwana. Roberto thinks that his wife Camilla is not really Camilla, but is Camilla's body with a malevolent alien zombie imposter inside. Roberto suffers from Capgras's delusion.

Tiwana wonders when she will be buried since she is dead and does not exist.[4] Tiwana suffers from Cotard's delusion. How do Claire and Wenqing differ from Roberto and Tiwana? How do great saints, sages, prophets, and philosophers—Moses, Abraham, Confucius, Buddha, Plato, Mary, Jesus, Augustine, Mohammed, Francis of Assisi, Teresa of Avila, and Thomas Aquinas—differ from Claire, Wenqing, Roberto, and Tiwana?

According to DSM-IV and DSM-5, they all—not just Claire and Wenqing, Tiwana and Roberto, but all the saints and sages above—arguably suffer from delusions, mainly because they violate some set of epistemic conditions endorsed in those manuals. According to DSM-IV, a delusion is in part "a false belief based on incorrect inference about external reality that is firmly sustained despite what almost everyone believes and despite what constitutes incontrovertible and obvious proof or evidence to the contrary" (American Psychiatric Association 2000, 765), whereas in DSM-5, delusions are said to be, in part, "fixed beliefs that are not amenable to change in the light of conflicting evidence" (American Psychiatric Association 2013, 87).

Now it is standard in mental health practice to give any widespread spiritual belief a free pass as not a delusion. The DSM-IV description of delusion is conjunctive: most people do not believe it AND there is obvious and decisive or incontrovertible evidence to the contrary. Any widespread religious belief will get a pass on the most/many people (a community) believe it clause. So Christians will now get a pass because Christianity is widespread, but Jesus Christ will not get a pass since it was not when he preached his gospel. And any unfalsifiable belief—God exists; There are spirits everywhere; I am immortal—will get a pass because there is no (conceivable) incontrovertible evidence against it.

Cotard's delusion might better fit the DSM bill since arguably Tiwana cannot assert, or have the belief, that she is both dead and does not exist while she is alive and thinking these very thoughts. There is a performative inconsistency first noted by Augustine and made famous by Descartes, in trying to doubt that I exist, or to think that I do not exist, while thinking that very thought (Kennedy and Graham 2007).

Roberto's thought that his wife is a zombie isn't quite so simple since most philosophers think that it is a logical possibility that there are no other minds, and thus that there is no logical or performative fallacy in thinking this. That said, Capgras's delusion is a delusion because (in part) it fails the "what most think" test, and even skeptical philosophers cannot sustain the thought that others are zombies in the real world. However, these are mostly points about social psychology and pragmatics, not about established epistemic certainties.

DSM-5's reference to fixed beliefs that are not amenable to change despite conflicting evidence helps a bit with Roberto's and Tiwana's cases. But that criterion covers way too much since almost all worldviews, political and spiritual, will show such features. And then some. Political and spiritual worldviews are also often cluttered with vast, variable, and trivial attendant beliefs and attitudes—when to salute the flag, when not to pray aloud in church, or how best to avoid the distracting influence of contrarian views or ideologies.

The main feature that explains our practices of dubbing some ways of worldmaking or self-conceiving as delusional have, we suggest, at least as much to do with the negative personal and social meaning-making features and their moral consequences as with any distinctive epistemic features they have (Graham 2013, 2015). The beliefs are harmful, subjectively and interpersonally. They are not necessarily dangerous although danger is another nonepistemic feature that counts on when we judge a delusion as a problem, a public health problem. To be sure, Roberto and Tiwana differ from Claire and Wenqing along the dimensions of possessing nonshared beliefs (and thus they are both insensitive to certain standards of peer epistemics, or what might be called, less kindly, groupthink), as well as being extremely resistant to certain local epistemic facts that bear on their beliefs, for example, Roberto was with Camilla when the zombie takeover took place; Tiwana is thinking right now that she does not exist and simultaneously believes that she is having that very thought. But they also have beliefs that undermine radically their personal and interpersonal well-being. Roberto cannot love his wife; instead he is terrified by the alien inside her and is thus denied by his beliefs one of the greatest sources of meaning that life can offer. Tiwana cannot love or be loved because she no longer exists; she can neither act nor do anything because she is not. Her death and nonexistence end her chances to love and work and thus to find meaning in standard ways.

Most of the professional psychiatric and philosophical literature on delusion is committed to thinking of delusions as being or involving primarily epistemic failure—false or evidentially misbegotten beliefs. There are such cases, but as our examples show, being false or evidentially misbegotten is not normally what is wrong with the deluded person. A good theory of delusion must be expanded to include nonepistemic failures, as well as epistemic ones (Graham 2015).

Building a general theory of delusions, if such a thing is possible, requires at the start denying the dogma, a sort of epistemologist's fetish, that beliefs are the definitive and dominant mental attitude by way of which humans make their worlds, and by which sanity and insanity are assessed (Graham 2013, 2015; Stephens and Graham 2004, 2007). The line between delusional and nondelusional states is not epistemically tractable and precise. And insofar as there are rough-and-ready heuristics for sorting the true, the false, and the misbegotten, delusions of the debilitating sort do not reliably fall on the failed or misbegotten belief side of the ledger. Failure to find a neat formula for sorting beliefs and other attitudes into the delusional and the nondelusional suggests the need for a more ecumenical approach (Graham 2013, 2015). Hallucinations, for example, are precipitants of some delusions—but not all delusions are sourced by hallucinations. Some hallucinations (as we shall see) are not associated with pathology. It has long been known, for example, that there are similarities between spiritual or mystical experiences and psychotic or delusional conditions. Some commentators have wanted to collapse such experiences into the category of hallucinations by claiming that they are symptomatic of some pathology (see Brett 2003 for an analysis and critique of such a claim).

But this tactic won't work. We now consider good hallucinations, what we call metaphysical hallucinations—of which spiritual hallucinations are a subset or a close sibling.

Metaphysical Hallucinations

Our third class of mental state kinds that might be considered necessarily pathological but that are not are metaphysical hallucinations (Flanagan

2015). Metaphysical hallucinations are experiences. Metaphysical hallucinations are, involve, or seed unusual, typically epistemically radically underdetermined thoughts about *being*, about *what there is*, which (the kind we are discussing) have good existential effects, personal and/or moral. They are similar to some positive illusions and spiritual delusions in this respect. They differ from standard illusions and delusions insofar as they are sometimes intentionally induced by individuals in real time to produce (possibly) the very effects they have. Two standard ways to produce metaphysical hallucinations are the following:

1. Hallucinogens (e.g., peyote, ayahuasca, LSD, psilocybin)
2. Meditative or Yogic absorption (*jhānas*).

In a *New Yorker* article (February 9, 2015) Michael Pollan reports on renewed research on hallucinogens at top medical centers like Johns Hopkins and NYU. The first paper on the new research is by R. R. Griffiths et al. (2006) in *Psychopharmacology* entitled "Psilocybin Can Occasion Mystical-Type Experiences Having Substantial and Sustained Personal Meaning and Spiritual Significance." Psilocybin, the key ingredient in magic mushrooms, is now being given to patients with terminal illnesses, and the results so far reveal that the well-controlled daylong trips are normally pleasant, interesting, and enjoyable—not at all like the bad trips of the days of yore with unpleasant flashbacks. Unlike dreams during REM (rapid eye movement) sleep, the trips are well remembered, and thus they are subsequently available for revisitation and fine-grained analysis. Most importantly, as far as the patients go, the trips reduce fear and anxiety about dying and produce a kind of acceptance, even contentment, about their impending death. Remarkably, even for individuals at death's door, the experience is judged as in the very top group of existentially meaningful experiences in their lives.

A common feature of the phenomenology is described in terms of a sense of completeness, where this involves feelings of unity, sacredness, ineffability, peace, joy, as well as the impression of having transcended space and time and the "noetic sense" that the experience has disclosed some deep truth about reality. A "complete" metaphysical experience is one that exhibits all seven characteristics.

The so-called "astronaut effect" of seeing the world from above, where one feels extremely small and experiences awe, ego dissolution, oneness, and expansive love, is another way that the experiences are commonly described. Interestingly, around the same time as the *New Yorker* article, Oliver Sacks (2015) wrote a moving op-ed in the *New York Times* (February 19, 2015) about receiving news that he was terminally ill. He writes, "[O]ver the last few days, I have been able to see my life as from a great altitude, as a sort of landscape, and with a deepening sense of the connection of all its parts."

Buddhists, among others, think that well-being requires getting over a certain view about the self, perhaps several views about the self: that each one of us possesses a permanent, eternal essence that is our self, and that the main project of life is to feed this self. There is a metaphysical and a moral mistake involved in believing in the self of a certain sort. It engenders egoism. One route to getting over the incorrect views about self is to meditate, achieve an altered state of consciousness (*jhāna*) in which one sees that metaphysically one really is *no-self*. This metaphysical insight, it is said, will reduce radically moral egoism and seed compassion and lovingkindness. Ideally, the meditator thus enlightened is existentially compelled to follow the bodhisattva path bringing compassion and lovingkindness to all sentient beings. She has experienced her own maximally compassionate selfless personhood, and she is committed to enacting her Buddha nature for the sake of all sentient beings.

The philosopher Miri Albahari describes the relevant phenomenology of achieving "insight" this way:

> [Her] theoretical understanding of the proposition that "there is no self" (and by implication that she is not such a self) is being coupled with the overcoming of a powerful and pervasive delusion—the delusion that she is a self. Overcoming this delusion imbues her with a genuinely accurate feeling of noetic resonance: of having dispelled a cognitive error—analogous, it is sometimes said, to awakening from a dream. The depth and pervasiveness of the error overcome explains and grounds her feeling that the insight is profound and irreversible, resulting in a more accurate mode of cognition. (Albahari 2014, 14)

The sort of confidence that Alhabari describes in terms of "noetic resonance" is remarkably similar to the way the psilocybin patients possess unshakeable insight into the way things really are or, what is different, the way they ought to be, when they experience ego dissolution and a sense of oneness.[5]

Now here's the rub: Buddhists will say that *no-self* is true, although there is vast controversy inside the Buddhisms about what *no-self* means and how to express it and thus numerous distinctive projects of providing evidence for the truth of *no-self*. Others will say that *no-self* is not true, at least not in any interesting form that is stronger than something like a psychobiological continuity view familiar from thinkers who deny that humans possess eternal Platonic or immortal Hindu (*atman*) or Abrahamic souls, claiming instead that humans are finite sentient gregarious animals (Flanagan 2011). One and done—and all that.

However, believing that *no-self* is false is compatible with thinking it good to believe (or as we should say "make-believe" or imagine) *no-self,* and that it is even better, morally good, to hallucinate *no-self,* and then to live as if the hallucination were true. If hallucinating *no-self,* when *no-self* is false, is good, then it is an example of one kind of metaphysical hallucination, a false metaphysical belief, or better, a complex way of envisioning things that does not mirror or represent the way things are, that can be inculcated, and that has good effects.[6]

One might think that various confirmation biases overdetermine both the drug-induced hallucinatory experience and meditative insight and thus that noetic confidence is best explained in terms of leading the witness or in terms of self-hypnosis. But this is entirely acceptable on the interpretation that what is happening does not require truth for the relevant insights, but rather inspiring uplifting experiences, positive imagination, and good effects, some of which possibly seed or motivate good action and good being in the world.[7]

Pollan (2015) asks,

> How are we to judge the veracity of the insights gleaned during a psychedelic tour? It's one thing to conclude that love is all that matters, but quite another to come away from a therapy convinced that "there is another reality" awaiting us after death, as one volunteer put it, or that there is more to the universe—and consciousness—than a purely materialistic view of the world would have us believe. Is psychedelic therapy simply foisting a comforting delusion on the sick and dying?

Pollan goes on to tentatively endorse William James's view that we can judge mystical experiences not by their objective truth value, but by their fruits, by whether they have positive effects, results (see also Graham 2015). The class of fruitful experiences, good-making ways of conceiving the world, is vast once we start to look for instances.

Here is an example. Bertrand Russell (1950, 52–53) wrote this about overcoming the fear of death:

> The best way to overcome it ... is to make your interests gradually wider and more impersonal, until bit by bit the walls of the ego recede, and your life becomes increasingly merged in the universal life. An individual human existence should be like a river: small at first, narrowly contained within its banks, and rushing passionately past rocks and over waterfalls. Gradually the river grows wider, the banks recede, the waters flow more quietly, and in the end, without any visible break, they become merged in the sea, and painlessly lose their individual being.

This seems like good advice. However, note that Russell is not quite speaking about adopting a particular belief or set of beliefs, but is speaking about adopting a certain attitude, an image, a picture that helps one accept that death, in all likelihood, is the end of me for all eternity, but makes this feel fitting. I am the kind of creature who is made of stardust and will return to stardust. The cosmos is my mother, and I return soon to her bosom. Russell may also be understood, not incompatibly, as speaking about what it feels or seems like to adopt that attitude, and thus in a certain sense as a careful phenomenologist. Is he saying anything about the way consciousness normally is or the way the world is, the way the metaphysical facts line up? We don't think so.

One might worry that the attitudes of "make-believe" required for (or better, by) a genuine metaphysical hallucination are familiar in children but unusual for grown-ups and are frowned upon for good reasons. They involve some sort of creedal attitude (but perhaps not any kind of ordinary belief) toward propositions that are logically possible, but that, like creedal attitudes toward the tooth fairy or Santa Claus, are highly implausible, much more likely literally false than true. For example, a metaphysical hallucinator might say, "All is love" when it is obvious that at least right now all is not love.

This is another reason it is best, probably, not to conceive of the hallucinatory state(s) as involving primarily belief, but something more like full-on imagination and a powerful desire to make something that is not yet real, real. So the hallucinator who says that "all is love" might say, or be most charitably interpreted as thinking, that "all is love deep-down inside" in the sense that reality has love as its *telos*, or that "love is the answer" in the sense that everything would be better if there was love everywhere.

Metaphysical hallucinations involve having certain experiences, embracing how things seem while having those experiences, and then trying to imaginatively project oneself into a world in which the relevant experiences or thoughts seem as real as real can be, as worthwhile as worthwhile can be, and are thus spirit constituting and action guiding. They involve working one's way into a certain kind of strong noetic confidence that reveals itself in how one experiences and lives one's life. One comes to think that a hallucinated attitude toward reality is worth adopting and then one tries to make it—the way things seem while hallucinating—so. The noetic confidence attaches perhaps not to believing that things are in fact such and so (although it might involve some of that), but wanting the world to be a certain way, a way one experiences as good, better, excellent.

Most religions and most philosophies one could live by, philosophies that attempt to provide a genuine way of life, a comprehensive way of being in the world (and thus not most contemporary philosophy), link a metaphysics, a story about what there is, how it is, and what things would be at their best, with endorsement of an ethical vision, a picture of a good person, and an excellent human life. Once in place, the typical relationship between the metaphysic and the morals is one of mutual support.

Imagine someone who hallucinates that "all is one" in some way that motivates her to want to bring love, compassion, and forgiveness whenever and wherever there is hate, resentment, and desire for revenge. Or imagine someone hallucinates that everything is alive or living (vitalism) or that everything is sentient (panpsychism), and this motivates an ethic of maximal love. Is this bad? Is there a mistake? If the hallucination is not understood as a set of beliefs that mirror or are intended to mirror the ways things in fact are (now), it is hard to see what the mistake is.

The Ethics of Belief

For those familiar with the debate between William Clifford and William James about the ethics of belief in the last quarter of the nineteenth century, you might think we are endorsing James's view. Actually we are endorsing—well, at least seriously considering—a stronger view. A much stronger view. We are endorsing make-believe, hallucination, metaphysical fantasy, and self-hypnosis that will result in feeling attuned to a way of conceiving things that is unlikely true, probably false, or at a minimum, radically underdetermined by the evidence. We are endorsing metaphysical hallucinations that involve experiences that are or seed noble projection when it might have really good-making moral, personal, and social effects.

Clifford (1877) argued, "It is wrong always, everywhere, and for anyone, to believe anything upon insufficient evidence." And in addition "[i]t is wrong always, everywhere, and for anyone, to form beliefs without seeking any readily available evidence that is relevant to them." James, meanwhile, argued that there are certain momentous beliefs that will always be underdetermined by the evidence, but that nonetheless a person can will rationally to believe because sometimes the meaning and significance of life for that individual depends on the belief. In the case of beliefs of the sorts that "all is one" or "love is the answer" that might engender maximally expansive moral thinking and acting, the evidence is not just insufficient, it is not really there at all. So you shouldn't believe that "all is one" or that "love is the answer" or in vitalism or panpsychism on Clifford's stringent standards, and you shouldn't believe in them on Jamesean standards either because, although each of vitalism and panpsychism are logically possibly true, they are quite empirically incredible given the evidence. But, it might be a good idea to project yourself into a notional reality that would make them seem as if they are worth making true.[8] One might want to have metaphysical hallucinations for instrumental reasons, but also at the same time because they are intrinsically pleasant, peak experiences. However, the end, the aim of the hallucination, is maximizing personal and moral excellence, which is—on the view we are considering—good for its own sake, noninstrumentally good.

Conclusion

Current psychiatric practices of classification, as evidenced in both DSM-IV and DSM-5, threaten to pathologize many perfectly normal, sometimes perfectly healthy varieties of being-in-the-world. We have made this case by focusing on positive illusions, spiritual delusions, and metaphysical hallucinations that resist being corralled into the realm of the pathological. The impulse of psychiatric overreach is fueled in part by interpreting some varieties of ways of worldmaking as primarily or mostly epistemic when they are not, and then disciplining acceptable ways of worldmaking according to narrow norms of true belief. Progressive forms of mental health practice need to be informed by deep understanding of what people are doing when they absorb a form of life, when they adopt, adapt, and abide one among the multiplicity of ways of being a person, of finding meaning, and of living well. An ecumenical form of mental health practice needs to be governed by sensitive, philosophically deep understanding of the elements of a good life. A major challenge to psychiatry will be to adapt research policies and clinical practice to reflect such pluralistic, normatively nuanced frameworks.

The project of living a good life is primarily about making things better, anew, more caring, compassionate, beautiful, and good. The apposite kind of truth is not correspondence. It involves ways of worldmaking that are prospective, that seek in multifarious ways to make real what hope and imagination reveal as worthy. Psychiatry should resist the impulse to pathologize or to squeeze the normal out of normalcy by aligning itself with a picture of the mind as primarily involved in the business of accurately mirroring the way things are. That is hardly a major, or worthy, or interesting overall aim for most human lives.

A little known fact about Ullin Place, one of the early staunch defenders of the physicalist view of mind (Place 1956/2004), is that his mother was a direct descendant of Margaret Fell, the Mother of Quakerism, who, after the death of her first husband, married George Fox, the founder of the Society of Friends. As a young Quaker man, Place was attracted to mysticism because it appeared to offer him "a personality transformation" and "inner strength" (Place 2004, 22). Although his personal sympathy with mysticism evaporated over time, Place did appreciate the possibility of distinguishing "between ... experiences of the mystic and those of the psychotic by their fruits." "[Those] of the mystic [classified as] morally and socially adaptive, and those of the psychotic [classified as] morally and socially maladaptive" (24).

That, in a nutshell, is our view about certain illusions, delusions, and hallucinations. They are perfectly acceptable, sometimes praiseworthy ways of being hopeful, committed to imagining and enacting a better world for oneself and others, possibly only future generations. We are all engaged in the high-stakes project of making moral and meaningful lives. Epistemic rectitude is only a very minor part of a life well lived. And it is really no business of medical psychiatry to enforce a certain positivistic epistemic regimen or a view of worldmaking as involving primarily truth as correspondence. Some mental health professions and scientists would like to arrive at psychiatric taxonomy akin to the periodic table of elements, wherein the character, content, and cognitive-motivational structure of each disorder could be identified narrowly in the mind–brain. But that is itself a crazy idea. Absent sensitive, empathic understanding of the personal and communal purposes and consequences that a way of thinking and being serves or fails to serve, possibly frustrates, there is no health or illness, no mental well-being or ill-being. Truth, like beauty and goodness, is a key component of a good human life. But the kind of truth that matters to human flourishing is not remotely the kind of narrow truth that mere epistemology theorizes.

Acknowledgments

We are indebted to this volume's coeditors, Jeff Poland and Şerife Tekin, for helpful comments on an earlier draft of this chapter.

Notes

1. Speaking of DSM (the *Diagnostic and Statistical Manual of Mental Disorders*), diagnostic overreach is a popular target in critiques of the manual. First published in 1952, under the influence of psychodynamic psychology and containing approximately 106 diagnostic categories, DSM's most recent edition (DSM-5), with its

1950s Freudian influence long discarded, contains approximately 300 categories of disorder.

2. The true and false beliefs that we are discussing in this chapter are so-called empirical beliefs or beliefs about empirical facts of the matter. The delusions that we believe are not categorically or necessarily unhealthy are delusions of the sort described in DSM-IV and DSM-5, namely, delusory beliefs that (among other things) are empirically false or otherwise fail to fit the empirical facts. Perhaps such delusions or states of mind should not even be called "delusions" once stripped of pathology—a topic for other contexts (Graham 2013, 217–218; see also Graham 2014).

3. There is a cottage industry in philosophy, motivated by recognizing the limits of belief–desire psychology to expand the lexicon of the mind sciences. New hybrid concepts like "alief" and "bimagination" are proposed (see Gendler 2008; Egan 2009).

4. These two beliefs are separable, of course. People may believe that they have died, biologically, but have successfully survived the death and decay of their body.

5. Alhabari describes the effects of the altered state of consciousness, the hallucination, as "overcoming of a powerful and pervasive delusion."

6. There are strong veins inside the Abrahamic traditions, as well as inside Hinduism, Jainism, and neo-Confucianism, which are not as deconstructive about the self as some varieties of Buddhism, but go directly for altering by prayer and meditation normal states of ego-consciousness, thinking that my weal and woe is most important, and so on.

7. Conventional psychiatry puts too little emphasis on what is right for the patient and too much emphasis on empirical belief acquisition and management. Richard Bentall aptly complains, "In Western [psychiatry] ... the need to distinguish what is 'real' from what is 'imaginary' seems self-evident" (Bentall 2003, 356). But it is not self-evident. Some modest suggestions for therapy for religious voice hearing experiences, in particular, may be found in Graham (2015).

8. Our proposal could be read as making a different point than the one debated by Clifford and James on grounds that we are not endorsing belief at all but rather such states as vision, imagination, hope, and possibility.

References

Albahari, M. 2014. Insight knowledge of no self in Buddhism: An epistemic analysis. *Philosophers' Imprint* 14 (21): 1–30.

Alloy, L., and L. Abramson. 1979. Judgment of contingency in depressed and nondepressed students. *Journal of Experimental Psychology. General* 108:441–485.

American Psychiatric Association. 2000. *Diagnostic and Statistical Manual of Mental Disorders*. 4th ed. rev. Washington, DC: American Psychiatric Association.

American Psychiatric Association. 2013. *Diagnostic and Statistical Manual of Mental Disorders*. 5th ed. Arlington, VA: American Psychiatric Association.

Bentall, R. 2003. *Madness Explained: Psychosis and Human Nature*. London: Penguin.

Bortolotti, L. 2010. *Delusions and Other Irrational Beliefs*. Oxford: Oxford University Press.

Bradley, G. 1978. Self-serving biases in the attribution process. *Journal of Personality and Social Psychology* 36:56–71.

Brett, C. 2003. Psychotic and mystical states of being: Connections and distinctions. *Philosophy, Psychiatry, & Psychology* 9 (4): 321–341.

Clifford, W. K. 1877. The ethics of belief. *Contemporary Review (London, England)* 29:289–309.

Egan, A. 2009. Imagination, delusion and self-deception. In *Delusion and Self-Deception: Affective and Motivational Influences on Belief Formation*, ed. T. Bayne and J. Fernandez, 263–280. New York: Psychology Press.

Flanagan, O. 1991. *Varieties of Moral Personality*. Cambridge, MA: Harvard University Press.

Flanagan, O. 1992. *Consciousness Reconsidered*. Cambridge, MA: MIT Press.

Flanagan, O. 2007. *The Really Hard Problem: Meaning in the Material World*. Cambridge, MA: MIT Press.

Flanagan, O. 2009. "Can do" attitudes. *Behavioral and Brain Sciences* 32 (6): 519–520.

Flanagan, O. 2011. *The Bodhisattva's Brain*. Cambridge, MA: MIT Press.

Flanagan, O. 2015. Hallucinating Oneness. Paper delivered at Oneness Conference, City University Hong Kong, April.

Frances, A. 2013. *Saving Normal: An Insider's Revolt against Out-of-Control Psychiatric Diagnosis, DSM-5, Big Pharma, and the Medicalization of Ordinary Life*. New York: HarperCollins.

Gendler, T. 2008. Alief and belief. *Journal of Philosophy* 105:55–81.

Golin, S., F. Terrell, and B. Johnson. 1977. Depression and the illusions of control. *Journal of Abnormal Psychology* 86:440–442.

Goodman, N. 1978. *Ways of Worldmaking*. Indianapolis: Hackett.

Graham, G. 1998. Socrates and the soul of death. In *Philosophy Then and Now*, ed. S. Arnold, T. Benditt, and G. Graham, 15–34. Oxford: Blackwell.

Graham, G. 2013. *The Disordered Mind: An Introduction to Philosophy of Mind and Mental Illness*. 2nd ed. London: Routledge.

Graham, G. 2014. Being a mental disorder. In *Classifying Psychopathology: Mental Kinds and Natural Kinds*, ed. H. Kincaid and J. Sullivan, 123–143. Cambridge, MA: MIT Press.

Graham, G. 2015. *The Abraham Dilemma: A Divine Delusion*. Oxford: Oxford University Press.

Griffiths, R. R., W. A. Richards, U. McCann, and R. Jesse. 2006. Psilocybin can occasion mystical-type experiences having substantial and sustained personal meaning and spiritual significance. *Psychopharmacology* 187 (3): 268–283.

Henrich, J., S. J. Heine, and A. Norenzayan. 2010. The weirdest people in the world? *Behavioral and Brain Sciences* 33:61–135.

Jahoda, M. 1953. The meaning of psychological health. *Social Casework* 34: 349–354.

Jahoda, M. 1958. *Current Concepts of Positive Mental Health*. New York: Basic Books.

Kennedy, R., and G. Graham. 2007. Extreme self-denial. In *Cartographies of the Mind: Philosophy and Psychology in Intersection*, ed. M. Marraffa, M. De Caro, and F. Ferretti, 229–242. Dordrecht, the Netherlands: Springer.

Place, U. T. 1956/2004. Is consciousness a brain process? In *Identifying the Mind: Selected Papers of U. T. Place*, ed. G. Graham and E. Valentine, 45–52. Oxford: Oxford University Press. Reprinted from *British Journal of Psychology* (1956).

Place, U. T. 2004. From mystical experience to biological consciousness: A pilgrim's progress? In *Identifying the Mind: Selected Papers of U. T. Place*, ed. G. Graham and E. Valentine, 14–29. Oxford: Oxford University Press.

Pollan, M. 2015. The trip treatment. *The New Yorker*. February 9, 2015. http://www.newyorker.com/magazine/2015/02/09/trip-treatment.

Russell, B. 1950. *Portraits from Memory and Other Essays*. New York: Simon & Schuster. https://archive.org/stream/portraitsfrommem005918mbp/portraitsfrommem005918mbp_djvu.txt.

Sacks, O. 2015. My own life. *New York Times*. February 19, 2015. http://www.nytimes.com/2015/02/19/opinion/oliver-sacks-on-learning-he-has-terminal-cancer.html?_r=0/.

Stephens, G. L., and G. Graham. 2004. Reconceiving delusion. *International Review of Psychiatry* 16:236–241.

Stephens, G. L., and G. Graham. 2007. The delusional stance. In *Reconceiving Schizophrenia*, ed. M. Chung, K. Fulford, and G. Graham, 193–215. Oxford: Oxford University Press.

Taylor, S., and J. Brown. 1988. Illusion and well-being: A social psychological perspective on mental health. *Psychological Bulletin* 103 (2): 193–210.

Young, M. C. 2014. Do positive illusions contribute to human well-being? *Philosophical Psychology* 27 (4): 536–552.

Contributors

Richard P. Bentall, Department of Psychological Sciences, University of Liverpool

John Bickle, Department of Philosophy and Religion; Institute for Imaging and Analytical Technologies (I2AT); Mississippi State University; Department of Neurobiology and Anatomic Sciences, University of Mississippi Medical Center

Robyn Bluhm, Department of Philosophy and Lyman Briggs College, Michigan State University

Rachel Cooper, Department of Politics, Philosophy and Religion, Lancaster University

Kelso Cratsley, Department of Philosophy, University of California, San Diego

Owen Flanagan, Department of Philosophy, Duke University

Michael Frank, Department of Cognitive, Linguistic, and Psychological Sciences, Brown University

George Graham, Department of Philosophy, Georgia State University

Ginger A. Hoffman, Department of Philosophy, St. Joseph's University

Harold Kincaid, Academy of Finland Center of Excellence in the Social Sciences, University of Helsinki; School of Economics, University of Cape Town

Aaron Kostko, Center for Learning Innovation, University of Minnesota Rochester

Edouard Machery, Department of History and Philosophy of Science, University of Pittsburgh

Jeffrey Poland, Rhode Island School of Design; Science and Technology Studies, Brown University

Claire Pouncey, Psychiatrist in private practice; President, Association for the Advancement of Philosophy and Psychiatry

Şerife Tekin, Department of Philosophy and Religious Studies, Daemen College; Center for Philosophy of Science, University of Pittsburgh

Peter Zachar, Department of Psychology, Auburn University Montgomery

Index